AF572532

Microbiology and Biotechnology for Sustainable Development

Microbiology and Biotechnology for Sustainable Development

Editor

Dr. P.C. Jain

M.Sc., Ph.D., C.A.S.F. (UK)

Reader, Deptt. of Applied Microbiology & Biotechnology,
Dr. Harisingh Gour Vishwavidyalaya, Sagar, M.P. (India)

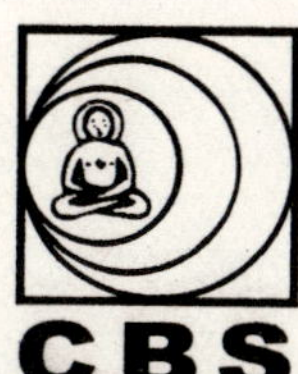

CBS PUBLISHERS & DISTRIBUTORS

NEW DELHI • BANGALORE

ISBN : 81-239-1087-8

First Edition : 2004
Reprint : 2007

Publishing Director : Vinod K. Jain

Published by :
Satish Kumar Jain for CBS Publishers & Distributors,
4596/1-A, 11 Darya Ganj, New Delhi - 110 002 (India)
E-mail : cbspubs@del3.vsnl.net.in
Website : http://www.cbspd.com

Branch Office :
Seema House, 2975, 17th Cross, K.R. Road,
Bansankari 2nd Stage, Bangalore - 560070
Fax : 080-6771680 • E-mail : cbsbng@vsnl.net

Printed at :
Asia Printograph, Delhi

Foreword

I am happy to know that Proceedings of the National Seminar on "Present Status of Microbiology and Challenges for Sustainable Development" held at Department of Applied Microbiology and Biotechnology during 5-7 March 2001 has been published in the form of a book, Microbiology and Biotechnology for Sustainable Development, highlighting the substances of the deliberations.

The microorganisms are in use as food and tools in fermentation since ancient times and as a result benefitted the man kind a great. The advent of bioprocess and recombinant DNA Technology has opened new vistas in the applicability of microorganisms in the field of energy, food and pharmaceuticals. Microbial biotechnology has been looked upon as a versatile approach for solving most difficult problems by using microbes as a tool for production of novel compounds, bioprocessing of materials and to combat problems of xenobiotics.

The implications of imposition of GATT and IPR in Indian Scenario need to be discussed at various platforms to encash the vast potential of Indian Scientific Community and to evolve strategies for our sustainable development. I am happy to see that many of important issues have been documented in the form of present proceeding.

The editor of this volume, Dr. P.C. Jain, deserves congratulations for his sustained efforts and interest in compiling this volume. I sincerely hope that this book would function as a nodal point to maintain record of our recent knowledge and to plan future strategies for our development at regional, national and global levels.

(Prof. Santosh Kumar)
Vice Chancellor
Dr. H.S. Gour V.V., Sagar

Preface

This volume contains the proceedings of National Seminar on Present Status of Microbiology and Challenges for Sustainable Development held at the Department of Applied Microbiology and Biotechnology, Dr. H.S. Gour University, Sagar from 5-7 March, 2001. It contains two sections. In Section A, there are fourteen classified reviews based on the lectures delivered during the seminar by the eminent scientists of India whose contributions are milestones in their respective fields of research while Section B of this proceeding includes 24 research papers.

Microbiology is a leading branch of applied biology and has provided a common platform to biochemists and biotechnologists for working together to ratify human sufferings and develop new technologies for poroduction of novel products to solve problems of food, agriculture and environment. However, for this we need to conserve microbial biodiversity to make use of their genetic variability for sustainable development of human society and to conserve our natures wealth. Prof. B.N. Ganguli, Prof. P.A. Alexander, Prof. S.R. Dave, Prof. S.P. Adhikari, Dr. R.K.S. Kushwaha, Dr. S.K. Deshmukh have given a comprehensive account of some aspects of microbial biodiversity in their articles and critically discussed the role of microorganisms in varied environmental conditions. Prof. Ganguli has especially raised certain issues before the microbiologists regarding microbial biodiversity highlighting the methods and enumeration strategies for culturable and unculturable microbial diversity to obtain novel bioactive molecules from them.

The book contains a number of articles from the laboratory of Prof. S.R. Dave highlighting the diversity and role of chemotrophs in solid waste bioleaching and bioremediation of heavy metals from polluted environments. Prof. Alexander highlighted the role of bacteria in leaching of low grade ores. He emphasized on the use of microorganisms for mineral exploration. The article by Dr. Adhikari gives an account of lithophytic cyanobacterial diversity while Dr. S.K. Deshmukh documented the diversity of tropical mushrooms and their secondary metabolites. In another article, Jain and Deshmukh have given valuable note on the Indian depositories and reviewed the methods of maintenance and preservation of filamentous fungi.

Sustainability in agriculture is of prime importance. Prof. B.D. Kaushik has given an elaborated account of blue-green algae based biofertilizers for improvement of rice cultivation. Dr. R.P. Thakre and his co-author have suggested new strategies for development of compost using organic waste. Degradation of our ecosystem due to sewage containing industrial effluents is an ever-increasing problem and we need to protect it by ecofreindly approaches. The above aspects have been judiciously covered by certain authors. They emphasized the use of microorganisms for bioremediation of metals from polluted water and leaching of metals using microbes as tools. Nitroaromatic compounds are produced in large amounts by chemical industries. These compounds including products of their incomplete degradation have acute toxicity while some are carcinogenic. Microbial degradation of these compounds and recalcitrants is an aspect of paramount importance. Dr. R.K. Jain and his colleagues have documented details of nitroaromatic degradation pathways in some species of bacteria.

Problems relating to human health are immense. Though the advent of antibiotics and vaccines has benefitted mankind to a great extent in controlling the bacterial and viral infections, much has to be done to develop vaccines for the killer diseases like AIDS and deadly mycotic infections in man and animals. Basu and Jain have discussed the role of microbial biotechnology in solving the problem of human health while Dr. G.P. Rai has described methodologies used in typhoid detection. Immunological aspects of fungal diseases have been discussed by Dr. Sudhir Jain and his co-authors.

Extremophiles are nature's treasure and their germplasm need to be preserved because of their adaptability to unusual environmental conditions. Article of Prof. T. Satyanarayana discusses production aspects of hyperthermostable alpha amylase while a few articles from my own laboratory have given informations about distribution of thermophilic moulds and detailed their enzymic potential. In addition other authors have presented their valuable research work in a very concise manner covering some most recent work going on in the field of Microbiology and Biotechnology.

The documentation of this nature could not have materialized but for the active cooperation of various scientists working in the field of microbiology and biotechnology and nevertheless, active research students who contributed their valuable piece of work for this book. I thankfully acknowledge suggestions and encouragement from Prof. S.C. Agrawal and wish to thank Mr. Naveen Kango, Ms. Shama J.P. Khanam and Mr. Praveen Jain for their help in reading and correcting proofs. Since the book is the outcome of the national seminar, I wish to express my deep sense of gratefulness to UGC, CSIR, DBT (New Delhi) and Dr. H.S. Gour University for their financial support to hold the seminar on Present Status of Microbiology and Challenges for Sustainable Development at Dr. H.S. Gour University.

I am thankful to CBS Publishers and Distributors for accepting the proposal for publication of this volume. The book has been compiled with utmost care but the responsibility for errors, if any, falls on me. The comments in any form will be a source of encouragement and improvement.

I am highly indebted to my family members, Mrs. Pramila Jain, Ms. Richa, Aakanchha and Vimpi and my mother Smt. R. Jain for their immeasurable support and patience observed during the compilation of this volume.

P.C. JAIN

Contents

SECTION-A

SECTION-B

Section A

Microbiology and Biotechnology for Sustainable Development (Ed. P.C. Jain),
CBS Publishers & Distributors, New Delhi (2004), pp. 3–11.

A-1

Microbial Diversity—The Challenge

Dr. B. N. Ganguli
*Emeritus Scientist of the CSIR (1994...) , General Manager and Head of Microbiology, Hoechst Centre for Basic Research, Mulund, Mumbai (1984-1994)
Distinguished Professor, Bharati Vidyapeeth Pune, (Deemed University) 2001
Agharkar Chair Professor, Agharkar Research Institute, Pune (2002...).*

Abstract

Microbial diversity is enormous and must be enumerated and exploited. Enumeration of diversity requires both classical and molecular biological approaches. Exploitation needs specific target oriented screening, a knowledge of the disease process and characterization of the microbial products. Examples of new compounds from such screens are shown. Target related screens for compounds against metabolic diseases are discussed.

Key Words: Biodiversity, Screening, Exploitation of microbes, Molecular biology, Industrial targets.

INTRODUCTION

The present status of Microbiology in the country should be a reflection of the excellence, expertise, dedication and innovative thinking of the Microbiologists of India.

A great deal of introspection is required to assess our status and to see whether we match the above statement in the context of the world wide revolution in every discipline of the sciences. Particularly the rapid advances and new discoveries in genomics and proteomics which are intrinsically and extensively related to Microbiology.

The challenge will be the ability to participate in the "state of the art" research – with its applications – as revealed by national and international publications and patents and in my personal opinion – aggressive participation in International and National Seminars such as these. Has this been happening ? Will the microbiologists of India reflect on this critically?

Inaugural Address at the National Seminar on "Present Status of Microbiology and Challenges for a Sustainable Development"; March 5-7, 2001, Dr. H. S. Gour Vishwavidyalaya, Sagar, M. P. India.

For sustainable development, it is essential to explore, exploit and conserve our Microbial Diversity. The industrial development of any country is critically dependent on the intellectual and financial investment in this area. With greater awareness of environmental protection and emphasis on "green" technologies, the use of micro-organisms and their products viz. enzymes, metabolites, nutraceuticals is increasingly important.

The intellectual and financial investment must be sufficient, adequate and over at least ten years. Such investments must come from the Government and its large number of agencies and increasingly the Industry.

The other side of the story is the ability to absorb and use both the investment and the expertise and accountability. Human resources development will play a major role.

Accountability is a key factor in the progress and success of any endeavour and must be emphasised and ensured.

At this stage I will shift the emphasis of my talk to microbial biodiversity and its exploitation.

Table 1: Strategies in the study of microbial biodiversity

1. A comprehensive and critical evaluation of the knowledge, that already exists in the country, should be made.
2. The data obtained then needs to be sorted out according to selected, known ecosystems.
3. Evaluate the accuracy and reliability of the data preferably using a common yardstick.
4. Check the data with the actuality. Are authentic libraries of micro-organisms available?
5. Choose the Biodiversity i. e. the genes, species and ecosystem that needs preservation.
6. In my personal opinion pristine ecosystems should be preserved.
7. Integrate with the world network of Microbial Resources Centres (MIRCEN)

India is basically and traditionally an agricultural nation and has both ancient practices and developed microbes that have satisfied the requirements of the poorer sections of our society for hundreds of years. Micro-organisms have been used as fertilizers, biopesticides, biodegraders and producers of selected foods. Such traditional microbes and processes need to be preserved and catalogued.

The other side is the rapid development in genetically engineered microbes – both for agriculture and for health. Integration of the traditional and the recent is a challenge.

Status of Microbial Diversity

It is well known that only 1 to 5 percent of the micro-organisms in the terrestrial, ocean and plant eco-systems have been isolated and studied. So called "uncultivable" micro-organisms exist as seen by modern DNA based techniques (Table 2 and 3). For example, the global biodiversity is estimated to be 3 to 500 million species of prokaryotes and eukaryotes in 70 phyla. Marine biodiversity alone is estimated to be 0.5 to 30 million species of macrofauna and is much greater than the terrestrial biodiversity (Bull et al., 1992; Randon, 1999; Cowan, 2000).

In the plant kingdom there are 250,000 – 750,000 species and if in each plant there are 2 to 5 endophytic fungi, as has been reported, then we are talking of millions of fungi that have not been investigated as yet (Data of Dr. Katz).

Table 2: Soil Microbial Biodiversity – Some Examples

1. The alpha, beta, gamma and delta proteobacteria are well represented.
2. Cytophagales, Actinobacteria, Low G. C. Gram positives are being detected.
3. Green non-sulphur bacteria, planctomycetes, spirochaetes known to be unusual in soil are being seen.
4. Holophaga – Acidobacterium sequences are being found, been cultured.
5. Verrumicrobia. Very few are cultured and mainly from aquatic sources. Today they appear to be rich in the soil ecosystems.
6. Novel archae: Extremophiles such as Crenarchaeota are being detected in the soils. Presumably these are mesophiles.

Table 3: Methods to Study Soil Microbial Diversity of uncultured Micro-organisms (Bull et al., 1992)

1. Isolation of bulk DNA and its analysis. Use of FISH.
2. 16 S r RNA Gene sequence analysis.
3. DNA: DNA reassociation kinetics.
4. Single Strand Conformational Polymorphisms.
5. Terminal Restriction Fragment Length Polymorphisms.
6. Electrophoretic Analysis. Denaturing – gradient gel and temperature – gradient gel electrophoresis.

Selective isolation methods yield neglected genera of actinomycetales, myxobacterial species and fungi. All of which, if exploited, can give novel skeletons. Example Ca^{2+} antagonists from fungi, antitumor compounds from actinomycetes, peptides and low molecular weight inhibitors of specific enzymes from bacteria. Neglected genera of actinomycetales such as Kibdellosporangium, Actinoplanes, Amycolatopsis, Saccharomonospora, Thermobispora have yielded new antibacterials (Ganguli, 1989).

EXAMPLES FROM MY LABORATORIES AT HOECHST

For example, from my laboratories we have isolated several new compounds, including new skeletons such as Aranorosin, Balhimycin, Mulundocandin, Mersacidin Cytorhodin, Fumifungin. All of which resulted from a specific target oriented screening (Fig. 1-5).

- Balhimycin is a new glycopeptide with a keto – amino function that is a handle for synthetic chemists (Nadkarni *et al.,* 1994).
- Mulundocandin is a lipopeptide which is today known to be active against *Pneumocystis carinii* and is active against *Candida* infection in-vio (Mukhopadhyay *et al.,* 1987a)
- Mersacidin is a new antibiotic which acts on a new target site in *Staph. aureus,* MRSA (Chattarjee *et al.,* 1992a & b).
- Aranorosin is a novel skeleton and has both anticancer and antifungal activities (Roy *et al.,* 1988).
- Cytorhodin is a new anthracycline antibiotic (Ganguli, 2002).

The metabolic potential of such cultures can be accessed in several ways. Firstly, the metagenomic approach uses the BAC (Bacterial Artificial Chromosomes) vector to clone large (> 100 kb) fragments of DNA and the resulting libraries can be expressed in *E. coli* and screened for phenotypic properties.

Entire blocks of biosynthetic genes of antibiotics can be cloned into one BAC plasmid.

Alternately, the DNA isolated from the environment can be digested and cloned into high copy number plasmid expression vectors. The resulting clones are screened for novel enzymes for example (Randon, 1999; Cowan, 2000).

Interesting Microbial Metabolites

Balhimycin
(antibacterial)

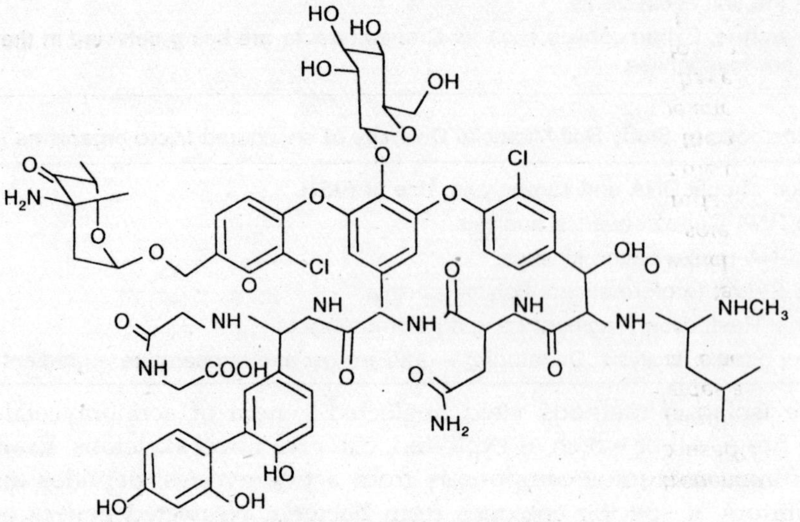

- Amycolatopsis sp
- A new glycopeptide of the vancomycin family
- MRSA active

Patents

Indian Patent No. 171883

European Patent No. 0468504 A1

CA No. 116, 150152d (1992)

Publications

J. Antibiotics, 47, 334 (1994)

J. Org. Chem., 59, 3480 (1994)

Fig. 1. Structure of Balhimycin, an antibacterial microbial metabolite

EXPLOITATION OF MICROBIAL DIVERSITY

Industries, all over the world, have made the strongest attempts to exploit the microbial diversity of this planet. Large pharmaceutical companies have been in the forefront of this, extremely aggressive, approach. There has been a proliferation of smaller but specific products oriented companies – such as Genetech, Biogen, Oncogene in the molecular biology areas and Xenova, Pharmamer, Bioleads who are in the basic microbiology area and interact with the bigger companies. Bioleads for instance offers approximately 65,000 micro-organisms from its libraries. Unfortunately the Indian Industries and the Indian academic institutes are lagging very, very far behind in these world wide efforts.

Interesting Microbial Metabolites

(A)

Cytorhodin
(anticancer)

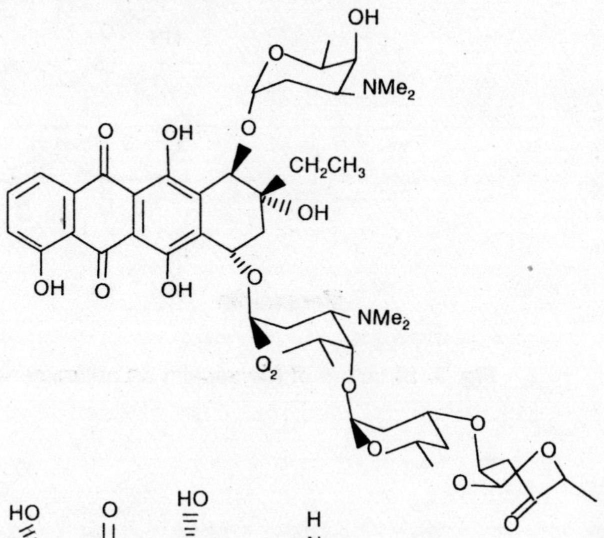

(B)

Mulundocandin
(antimycotic)

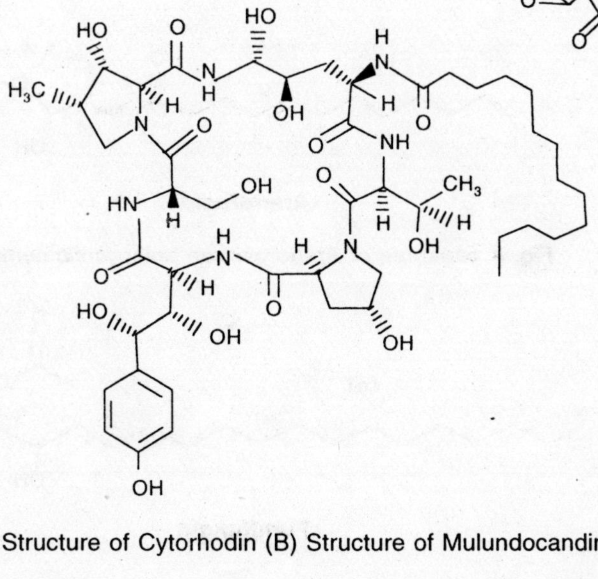

Fig. 2. (A) Structure of Cytorhodin (B) Structure of Mulundocandin

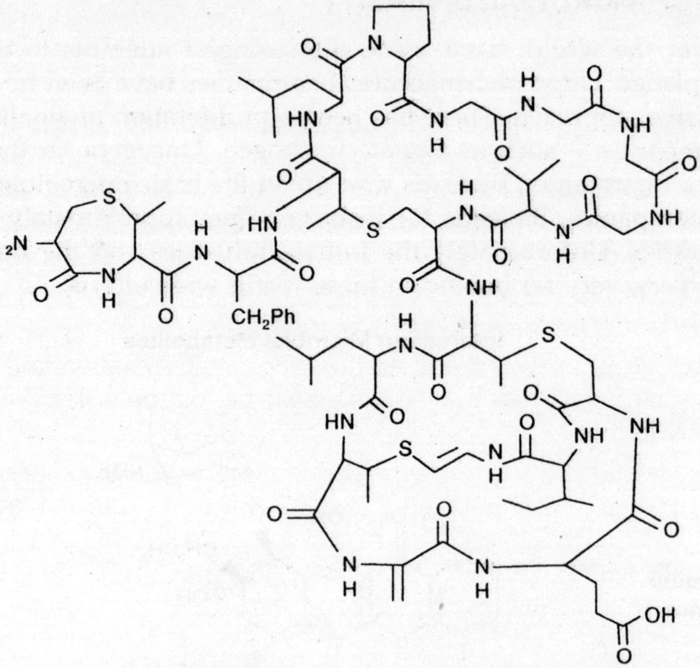

Mersacidin

Fig. 3. Structure of Mersacidin an antibacterial Compound

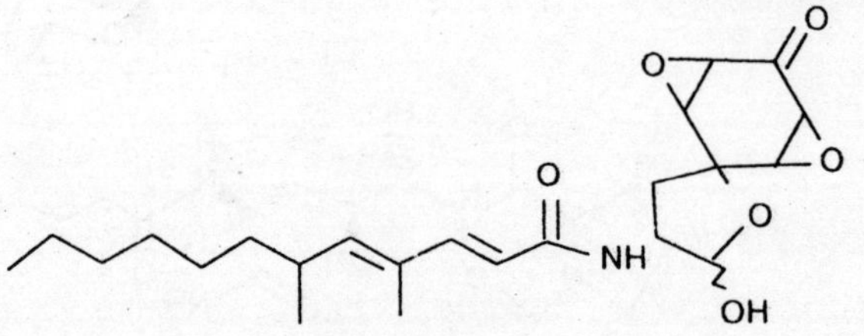

Aranorosin

Fig. 4. Structure of Aranorosin an antimycotic compound

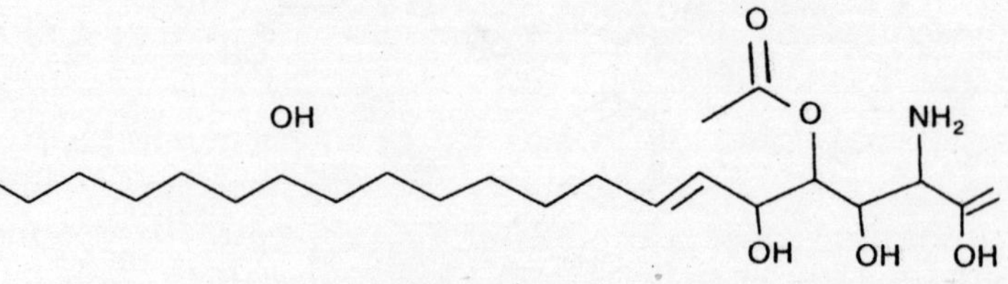

Fumifungin

Fig. 5. Structure of Fumifungin an antimycotic compound (Mukhopadhyay *et al.*, 1987b)

Selective isolation of micro-organisms has been the first step, followed by miniaturized fermentations – for example in micro-titre plates with 384 wells or even more. The broths are then put through High Thru-put Screening Assays (HTS) against a series of selected targets.

The key to New Drug Discovery Research (a multi-billion dollar sector) is to be able to find, select and produce a "novel, relevant, biological target" in the disease process – metabolic or infectious. Molecules must be found that act on that novel target. These molecules may be natural products or synthetic chemicals. This must, of course, be followed up and supported by elegant chemistry and the most sophisticated analytical hardware and software (the databases of natural products, databases of gene sequences) which is necessary to determine the structure of an identified lead molecule.

The bottle neck of the HTS is the analytics. The miniaturisation and progress in analytics has not progressed as rapidly as that of molecular biology. It is also basically highly expensive and time consuming.

I am limiting this talk to a few target areas, which some International Companies have been studying.

TARGETS USED IN INDUSTRY

Transcription Factors

Small molecules that modulate the expression of a target gene. Interactions, activations, expression, binding to DNA. Example, Nf – kappa beta is a nuclear transcription factor responsible for several metabolic diseases.

Cholestrol 7 Alpha Hydroxylase

Activation of the CYP gene to increase secretion. The CYP promoter from humans is cloned into Hep G2 cells.

Control and Function of Ice

The interleukin converting enzyme that converts Pre – IL-l b (inactive) to the active IL-l b which is responsible for septic shock, atherosclerosis and autoimmune diseases (Rheumatoid Arthritis).

Amyloid Precursor Protein

Down regulate the expression of the APP gene to prevent formation of beta amyloid deposits that cause Alzheimer's disease.

The above targets are known to be targeted by International Pharmaceutical Companies. Examples of gene expression modulating drugs exist. Aspirin inhibits IL – 1 activation of prostaglandin synthesis. Cyclosporin A and FK 506 bind to proteins which regulate the activity of select Transcription Factors. Nolvadex (Tamoxifen), Eulexin (Flutamide) regulate the expression of steroid responsive genes (Coombs, 1992).

Microbial Diversity and Examples of Products (Eligabeth, 1992; Richard, 1992)

1. From extremophiles Taq polymerase, Cellulase 103, Guar-gum liquifier, D – Hydantoinase, Heat Shock Proteins, Lipases, Proteases and Xylanases are known. A decapeptide bioadhesive is known from a marine isolate.
2. Cellulase 103 is a billion dollar product used in the textile industry and was isolated from a hyperthermophilic *Bacillus* sp. However, for industrial production it was cloned into a mesophilic Bacillus and successfully expressed.
3. From marine micro and macro-organisms, several skeletons have been isolated which have potential. Mannoalide is a phospolipase A2 inhibitor with anti-inflammatory properties. Six compounds from marine sources are under evaluation at the NCI against cancer. Bryostatin, Dolastatin, Ectinascidin, Halochondrin B, Curacin and Discodermolide Others are diterpenoids, Pseudoterosins and Methopterosin which have anti-inflammatory properties, are anti-arthritic, active against psoriasis and possibly asthma.
4. Axisonitrile is an anti-malarial.
5. A decapeptide [A1a-Lys-Pro-Ser-Tyr-Hyp-Ayp-Thre-Dopa-Lys] is a bioadhesive useful in tissue bonding and wound healing.

CONCLUSION

It is obvious that for sustainable development we must preserve our biodiversity and our established, ancient practices. On the other hand we have to integrate the enormous advances of genomics, proteomics and sophistication in chemistry and biotechnological processes into our industries and our academia. Development of human resources is a must and accountability of our scientific institutes should be ensured.

I have not touched the entire field of environmental pollution and the microbial routes that are tackling these problems. The "so called development" of our country needs to be carefully weighed against the needs and socio-economic-religious framework that exists in the rural population of India.

REFERENCES

Bull, A.T., Goodfellow, M. and Slater, I.H. (1992) Biodiversity as a Source of Innovation in biotechnology. Ann. Review. Microbial. 46 : 219-52.

Chatterjee, S., Chatterjee, S., Lad, S.J., Phansalkar, M.S., Rupp, R.H., Ganguli, B.N., Fehlhaber, H.W. and Kogler, H. (1992a) Mersacidin, a new antibiotic from *Bacillus*. Fermentation, isolation, purification and chemical characterization. J. Antibiot. 45(6): 832-838.

Chatterjee, S., Chatterjee, D.K. Jani, R.H., Blumbach, J., Ganguli, B.N., Klesel, N., Limbert, M. and Seibert, G. (1992b) Mersacidin, a new antibiotic from *Bacillus*. *In vitro* and *In vivo* antibacterial activity. J. Antibiot. 45(6): 839-845.

Coombes, J.D. (1997) New drugs from natural sources. IBC technical services publications.

Cowan, D.A. (2000) Microbial genomes – the untapped resource. Tibtech, 18: 14-16.

Elizabeth, P. (1992) In Industry: Extremophiles begin to make their mark. Science, 276: 705-707.

Ganguli, B.N. (1989) A microbial screening programme: scope and limitations. Progress in Industrial Microbiology, 27: 27-37.

Ganguli, B.N. (2002) Cytorodins, New antharocycline antitumor antibiotics IBC Tech. Services Publication, London, U.K., p. 3-20.

Mukhopadhyay, T., Ganguli, B.N., Fehlhaber, H.W., Kogler, H. and Vertesy, L. (1987a) Mulundocandin, a new lipopeptide antibiotic. II. Structure elucidation. J. Antibiotic. 40(3): 281-289.

Mukhopadhyay, T., Roy, K., Coutinho, L., Rupp, R.H., Ganguli, B.N. and Fehlhaber, H.W. (1987b) Fumifungin, a new antifungal antibiotic from *Aspergillus fumigatus* Fresenius 1863. J. Antibiot. 40(7): 1050-1052.

Nadkarni, S.R., Patel, M.V., Chatterjee, S., Vijaykumar, E.K., Desikan, K.R., Blumbach, J., Ganguli, B.N. and Limbert, M. (1994) Balhimycin, a new glycopeptide antibiotic produced by *Amycolatopsis* sp. Y-86, 21022. Taxonomy, production, isolation and biological activity. J. Antibiot. 47(3): 334-341.

Randon, M.R., Goodman, R.M. and Handelsman, I.O. (1999) The Earth's bounty – assessing and accessing soil microbial diversity. Tibtech. 17: 403.

Richard, A.K. (1992) Life goes to extremes in the deep Earth and elsewhere. Science, 276: 703-705.

Roy, K., Mukhopadhyay, T., Reddy, G.C., Desikan, K.R., Rupp, R.H. and Ganguli, B.N. (1988) Aaranorosin, a novel antibiotic from *Pseudoarachniotus roseus*. I. Taxonomy, fermentation, isolation, chemical and biological properties. J. Antibiot. 41(12): 1780-1784.

Microbiology and Biotechnology for Sustainable Development (*Ed.* P.C. Jain),
CBS Publishers & Distributors, New Delhi (2004), pp. 12–21.

A-2

Biochemical, Genetic and Molecular Analysis of Nitroaromatics Degrading Pathways in Bacteria

Gunjan Pandey*, Jim C. Spain** and R. K. Jain*
* *Institute of Microbial Technology, Sector 39-A, Chandigarh, India*
** *Air Force Laboratory/MLQ, 139 Barnes Drive, Tyndall Air Force Base, FL32403, USA*

Abstract

Nitroaromatic compounds such as nitrophenols, nitrotoluenes and nitrobenzoates are produced in large amounts by chemical industries and they are also used for large scale synthesis of explosives, dyestuff, pharmaceuticals, or precursors of aminoaromatic structures. In agriculture, some of these compounds are used as herbicides and insecticides. Nitroaromatics and products of their incomplete degradation have acute toxicity and some are carcinogenic.

At least three efficient microorganisms have been isolated and characterized viz.- Arthrobactor protophormiae, Burkholderia cepacia and Ralstonia sp. which are capable of utilizing p-nitrophenol, 4-nitrocatechol and o-nitrobenzoate as sole source of carbon and energy. The whole degradation pathway of these compounds have been thoroughly established by identifying the different intermediates using the techniques TLC, GC, GC-MS, H^1-NMR, HPLC and spectral analysis. In two of the organisms indicated above the whole degradative pathway have been found to be encoded on a large plasmid of app. 50-60 kilobase pairs and the plasmid libraries have been obtained by cloning the genes in the above case. Studies are in progress to construct the genetically-manipulated organism(s) which would not only be more efficient in their degradation abilities but also may degrade a variety of nitroaromatic compound(s).

Studies are also in progress on the molecular aspects of chemotaxis of bacteria indicated above towards nitroaromatic compounds which could prove to be very useful in enhancing the ability of motile microorganisms to locate and subsequently degrade the toxic and recalcitrant compounds present in contaminated environment.

Key Words: Degradation, Nitroaromatics, *Arthrobacter protoformiae, Burkholderia cepacia, Ralstonia sp.*

** Corresponding author.

INTRODUCTION

Environmental pollution has become a global concern due to indiscriminate use of chemicals to increase crop productivity and also due to rapid industrialization which largely results in the earth's atmosphere being contaminated with undesirable recalcitrant and xenobiotic compounds. A variety of organic pollutants released by an ever increasing number of industries are providing the direct cause of health and environmental related problems which have detrimental effects on humans an well as other living beings. Some of the widely encountered environmental pollutants include compounds ranging from halogenated aliphatics, aromatics, nitroaromatics (NACs), polycyclic aromatic hydrocarbons (PAHs), pesticides and their metabolites (Safe, 1984; Gibson and Subramanian, 1984; and Spain, 1995).

About 150 million tones of chemicals are produced annually and among these more than 5 million chemicals are known as pollutants. These chemicals enter into the environment in different forms and become pollutants by exerting an undesirable effect in the environment. India being an agricultural country, produces and consumes a huge amount of insecticides, pesticides and fertilizers, which are useful for agriculture in terms of crop productivity but pollute the waterbodies if carried there by rain or irrigation etc.

Natural organic compounds are readily biodegradable and can serve as source of carbon and energy for microorganisms that have evolved over geological time to exploit them. In contrast, xenobiotic compounds synthesized and released into the environment only recently by humans can present challenges to heterotrophic microorganisms. Presence of unusual chemical bonds or substitution with different functional groups can make a molecule resistant to microbial degradation. The vast majority of NACs detected in the environment are anthropogenic and are released into the environment because of their extensive use in the synthesis of dyes, plastics, explosives, pharmaceuticals, elastomers, insecticides and pesticides (An D, *et al.*, 1992; Munnecke, 1976; and Spain and Gibson, 1991).

Volatilization, evaporation, photooxidation, absorption and hydrolysis etc. are various physiochemical methods that are used for the decontamination of hydrocarbon contaminated sites (Hutzinger and Veerkamp, 1981). However these methods are not applicable for volatile pollutants and cannot be used to remediate sites that are contaminated with these toxic pollutants. Moreover, these methods are not very efficient and are very expensive to employ (Hebes and Schwall, 1978; and, Hutzinger and Veerkamp, 1981). Bioremediation provides an excellent alternate to this problem. Bioremediation, the degradation of toxic compounds by microbial activity, is preferred over physio-chemical methods by following reasons.

- They are friendly to the environment.
- They are cost effective.
- They lead to complete assimilation of toxic compounds.

TOXICITY OF NITROAROMATIC COMPOUNDS

The stability, persistence and toxicity that make NACs valuable to the industry render them to be hazardous when released into the environment. Some NACs are produced by incomplete combustion of fossil fuels, others are widely used as precursors of different industrially important compounds. Once released into the environment NACs undergo complex physical, chemical and biological changes. NACs are readily reduced to more reactive and, potentially more carcinogenic or mutagenic derivatives on reaching into mammalian systems. Intestinal microflora, as well as mammalian organ systems possess nonspecific reductases that catalyzes the conversion of nitro groups to more harmful nitroso and hydroxylamino groups (Venulet, and Van Etten, 1970). Epidemiological studies suggested that both amino and nitroaromatic compounds are powerful carcinogens (Anderson *et al.*, 1997). As a result, a number of NACs are listed as "Priority Pollutants" by "United States Environmental Protection Agency" (Keith and Telliard, 1976).

MICROBIAL DEGRADATION OF NACs

In recent years a number of nitroaromatic compounds has been found to be biodegradable. In most cases where biodegradation have been reported, catabolic pathways have also been elucidated (see Spain, 1995 for a review). In a few instances the gene encoding the catabolic enzyme(s) have also been cloned and sequenced. Understanding the pathway by which a pollutant is degraded is a key point in the development of an efficient bioremediation system. In light of the bacterial physiology and metabolism of degradation, systems can be designed for meeting bacterial requirements for the process of bioremediation and its control. Microbial catabolism of NACs is known to occur by one of the four mechanisms presently known.

1. An initial oxygenase reaction yielding nitrite.
2. An initial reduction yielding aromatic amines which are subjected to further catabolism.
3. A complete reduction of NACs to remove nitro group as nitrite.
4. A partial reduction of the nitro group to hydroxylamine which is further metabolized after subsequent replacements.

Isolation and characterization of *p*-nitrophenol degrading microorganisms and genetics of *p*-nitrophenol degradation.

In our laboratory, we isolated two microorganisms that are capable of utilizing *p*-nitrophenol (PNP) as the sole source of carbon and energy. They were identified as *Arthrobacter protophormiae* and *Burkholderia cepacia.* These were checked for their ability to grow on different nitroaromatic compounds. *Arthrobacter protophormiae* was able to grow on PNP, 4-nitrocatechol (NC) and *o*-nitrobenzoate (ONB) as the sole source of carbon and energy (Chauhan *et al.*, 2000). Whereas, *Burkholderia cepacia* was capable of utilizing PNP and NC (Prakash *et al.*, 1996 and Chauhan *et al.*, 2000). It is noted, many a times, that the degradation capabilities in bacteria are plasmid-encoded (Jain *et al.*, 1984; and Rani et. al., 1996). In case of *Arthrobacter protophormiae* and *Burkholderia cepacia,* Two approaches were used to establish the same: (i) by isolation of mutant strains incapable of utilizing PNP, NC and/or ONB as the sole source of carbon and energy and (ii) by determining the presence/absence of plasmids(s) in these mutant microorganisms. These two set of experiments confirmed the involvement of plasmid in the PNP, NC and ONB metabolism in *Arthrobacter protophormiae* and PNP and NC metabolism in *Burkholderia cepacia.* Plasmid cured derivatives of *Arthrobacter protophormiae* and *Burkholderia* cepacia were not able to utilize PNP, NC and ONB; and, PNP and NC respectively. Whereas transconjugants of *Burkholderia cepacia* gained PNP and NC catabolic properties. Plasmids of around 50-60 kb were found to be encoding for degradation in these strains.

BIODEGRADATION PATHWAY FOR PNP

It was found that both microorganisms indicated above released nitrite in the medium when grown on PNP as a sole source of carbon and energy, suggesting the involvement of an initial oxidative step in degradation of these compounds. Although many reports provide some information about PNP catabolic pathways, studies with *Moraxella* sp (Spain and Gibson, 1991) and *Arthrobacter* sp. (Jain *et al.*, 1994) are the only reports which give details of PNP catabolism by bacteria. In order to locate the intermediates involved in the degradation of PNP in our soil isolates, TLC and GC studies were carried out. In studies with TLC, PNP and hydroquinone (HQ) were detected in culture supernatant at different time of growth on PNP. The samples drawn after overnight growth did not show presence of PNP or any other intermediate indicating total degradation of PNP. To further confirm these samples, GC

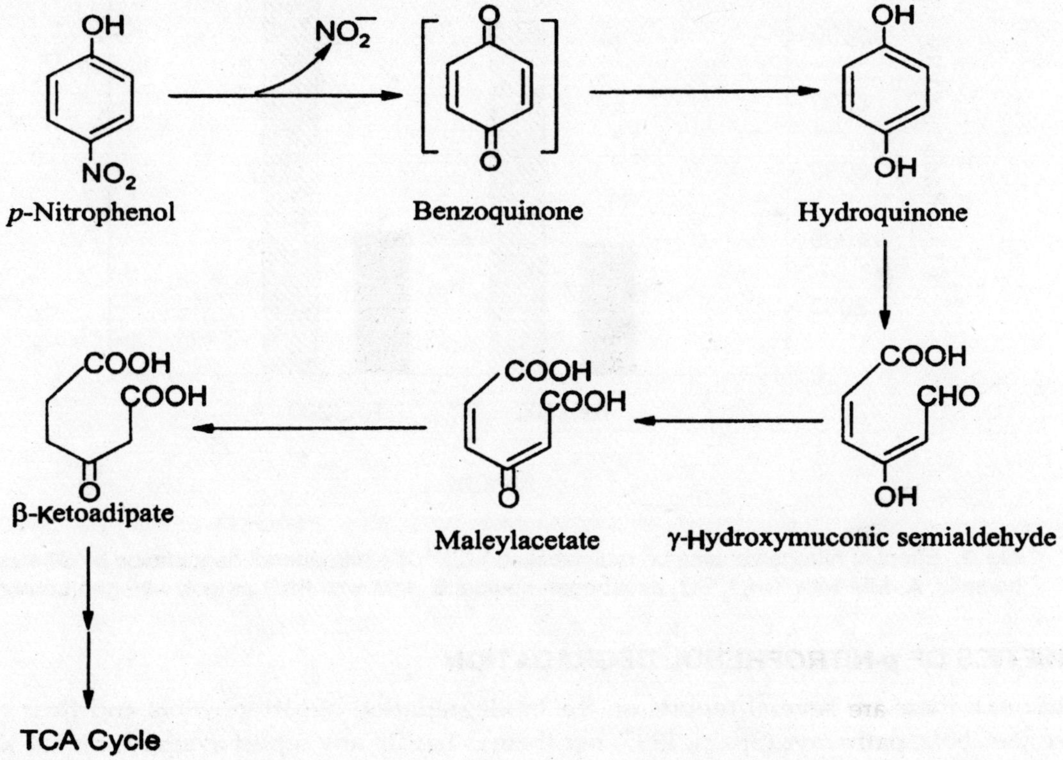

Fig. 1. Pathway of PNP degradation in *Arthrobacter protophormiae* and *Burkholderia cepacia.*

studies were carried out. The samples processed for TLC were further analyzed by GC which confirmed the results obtained by TLC. To exclude the possibility of any intracellular processing or permeability barriers of intermediates, the experiments were also carried out with crude cell extracts of *Arthrobacter protophormiae* and *Burkholderia cepacia* following growth on PNP. Following incubation of cell extracts with PNP, the intermediates were extracted and analyzed again with TLC and GC. Benzoquinone was also found to be present along with PNP and HQ (Chauhan, 2000 A and B). Presence of HQ and BQ as intermediates was further confirmed by GC-MS analysis. Rothera test (Holding and Collee, 1971) was also performed to find out whether HQ is degraded via meta or ortho cleavage pathway. Based on other studies in both these organisms it was also confirmed that β-ketoadipate was involved in the PNP catabolic pathway of both these organisms. Taken together the results obtained indicated that the degradation of PNP in both these strains occurs via BQ and HQ. Pathway is shown in (Fig. 1).

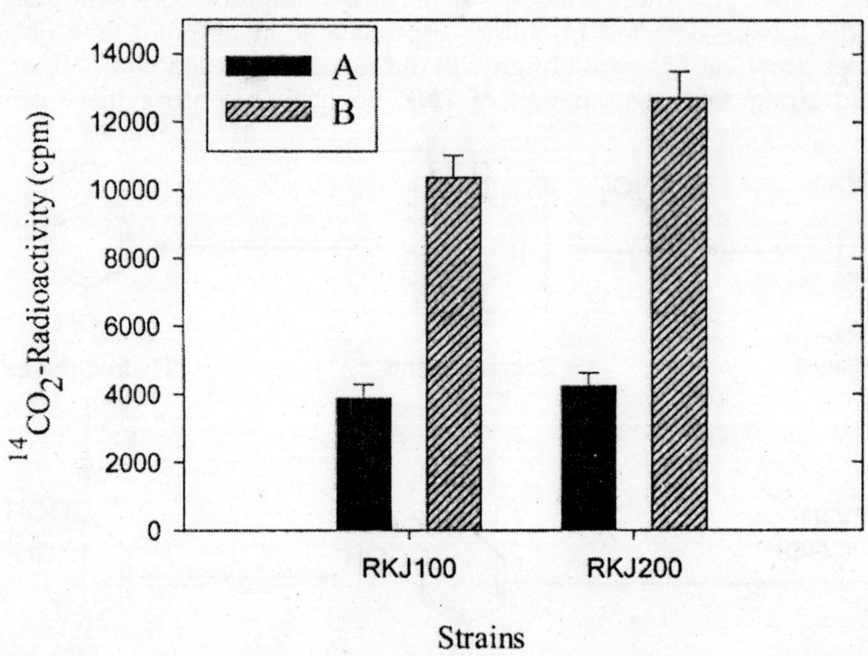

Fig. 2. Effect of nitrogen source on radiolabelled [UL-^{14}C] 4-nitrophenol degradation by different bacteria. **A**, MM with $(NH_4)_2SO_4$ as nitrogen source; **B**, MM with PNP as only nitrogen source.

KINETICS OF *p*-NITROPHENOL DEGRADATION

Although there are several reports on the biodegradation of nitrophenols and their respective metabolic pathways (Spain, 1995) but there is hardly any report available on the kinetics of PNP degradation and the effect of metabolic intermediates of PNP catabolic pathway on its degradation. *Arthrobacter protophormiae* and *Burkholderia* cepacia have been studied for their efficiency to degrade radioactive PNP in minimal medium (MM) and in nitrogen free MM. The extent of PNP degradation was estimated by measuring the evolved $^{14}CO_2$ from it as a function of microbial activity. The evolution of $^{14}CO_2$ from radioactive PNP in nitrogen free MM is about 3 fold higher as compared to MM with nitrogen sources under similar conditions (Fig. 2).

The resting cells induced with PNP were also used for studying the degradation kinetic for these two bacterial isolates. The apparent V_{max} values of PNP degradation by *Arthrobacter protophormiae* and *Burkholderia cepacia* were 0.28 and 0.23 mM, respectively, as determined by Michaelis-Menten curves (Fig. 3) drawn between PNP concentration vs rate of PNP degaration, whereas the maximum rates of PNP degradation (V_{max} values) as determined from Lineweaver-Burk plots (Fig. 4) were 7.81 and 3.38 μM PNP degraded /min/mg dry biomass respectively. To study whether the metabolite intermediate inhibits or stimulates PNP degradation, a comparative study has been done in the presence and absence of HQ and BQ, which are the intermediates of PNP degradation in these isolates. It was found that BQ and HQ inhibits the PNP degradation in Arthrobacter protophormiae noncompetitively (Fig. 5 A) and competitively (Fig. 5 B), respectively. The PNP degradation in Burkholderia cepacia was inhibited by BQ and HQ in an uncompetitive manner (Fig. 5 C, D). It was observed that β-ketoadipate did not effect PNP degradation in any case. It may be due to the reason that being the last intermediate, it enters the TCA cycle as soon as it is formed and thus does not cause a feed back effect on PNP degradation.

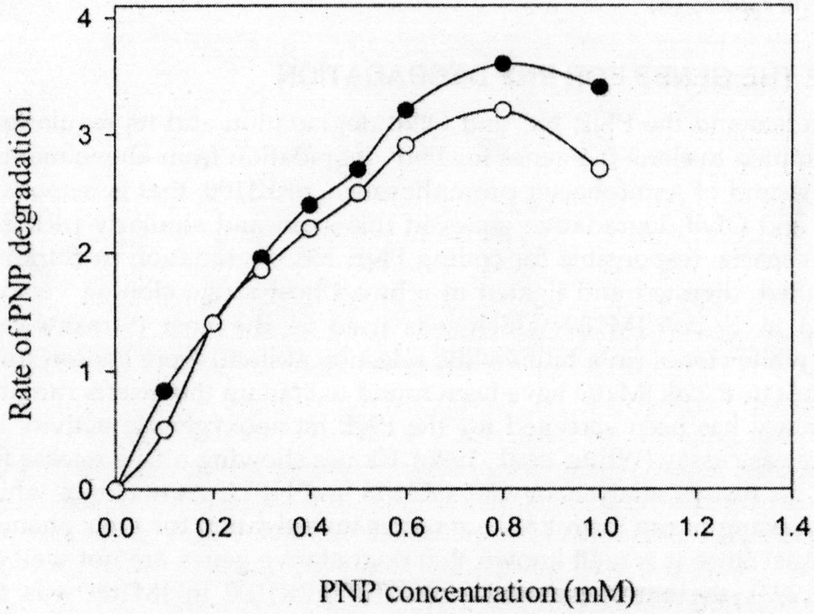

Fig. 3. Michaelis-Menten curves for PNP degradation by *Arthrobacter protophormiae* (•) and *Burkholderia cepacia* (O). Rate of PNP degradation has been measured as μmol PNP degraded $(min)^{-1}$ (mg dry biomass)$^{-1}$.

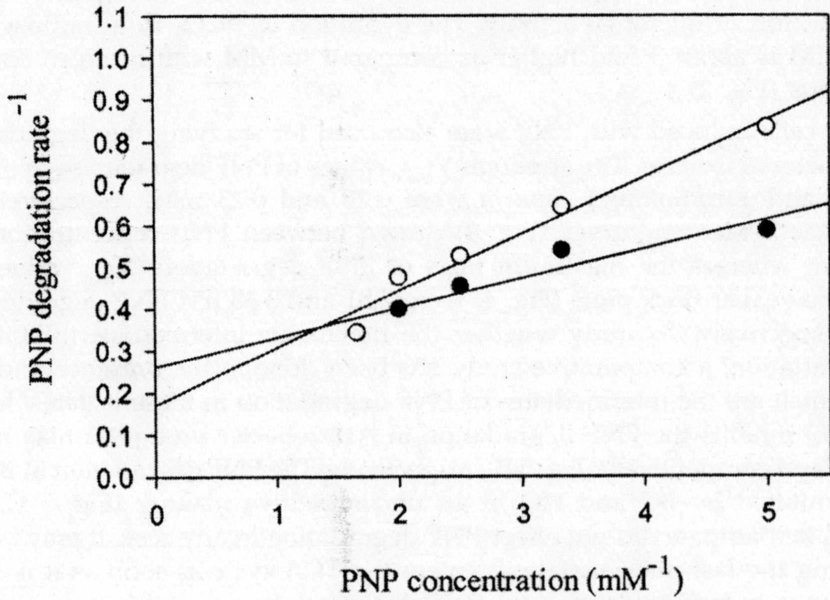

Fig. 4. Lineweaver-Burk's plots for PNP degradation by *Arthrobacter protophormiae* (O) and *Burkholderia cepacia* (●)

CLONING OF THE GENES FOR PNP DEGRADATION

In order to understand the PNP, NC and ONB degradation and its regulation in molecular detail we attempted to clone the genes for PNP degradation from above mentioned bacterial strains. The plasmid of Arthrobacter protophormiae, pRKJ100, that is responsible for coding the PNP, NC and ONB degradative genes in this srain and similarly pRKJ200, plasmid of Burkholderia cepacia, responsible for coding PNP, NC degradation in *Burkholderia cepacia* has been purified, digested and ligated in a broad host range cloning vector pLAFR3 and electroporated in *E. coli* JM109 which was used as the host (Straskwicz *et al.*, 1978). Recombinant white clones (in a blue/white selection system) were chosen for further analysis. These clones in *E. coli* JM109 have been found to contain the inserts ranging from 2 kb to 15 kb. The library has been screened for the PNP monooxygenase activity by a microtiter based nitrite release assay (White, *et al.*, 1996). Clones showing nitrite release from PNP, have been selected for further analysis by GC, GC-MS and HPLC .Few clones which were found positive for releasing nitrite form PNP are under investigation for their phenotype by HPLC and GC analysis. Since it is well known that degradative genes are not well expressed in *E. coli* (Schell, 1983), the entire plasmid library of pRKJ100 in JM109 was transformed in *Alcaligenes eutrophus* JMP222 by triparental mating and selected directly on selective plates. The recombinant clones present in *Alcaligenes eutrophus* JMP222 are currently being analyzed and characterized by physical and biochemical methods to study the molecular basis of PNP degradation in the same way as described for *E. coli* clones.

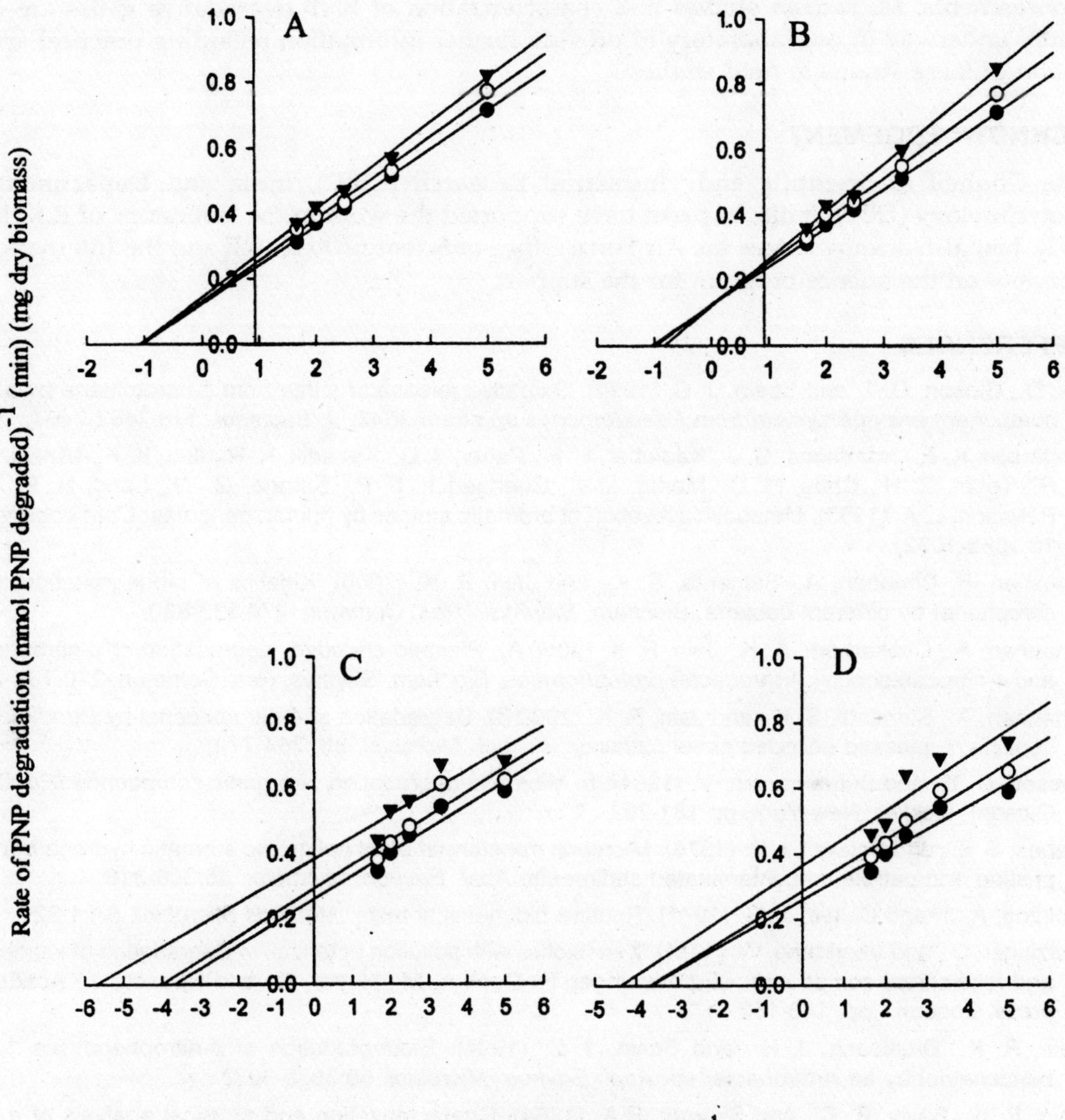

Fig. 5. Lineweaver-Burk's plots of PNP degradation. In all the figures the symbol (•) represents the case of PNP alone. *Arthrobacter protophormiae* RKJ100 (**A**: O, in the presence of 0.05 mM BQ and τ, in presence of 0.10 mM BQ; **B**: O, in the presence of 0.05 mM HQ and τ, in presence of 0.10 mM HQ); *Burkholderia cepacia* RKJ200 (**C**: O, in the presence of 0.05 mM BQ and τ, in presence of 0.10 mM BQ; **D**: O, in the presence of 0.05 mM HQ and τ, in presence of 0.10 mM HQ). (Cited from Bhushan, 2000)

Taken together these studies provides a ground for bioremediation of PNP contaminated environments. Microcosm studies and characterization of PNP degradative genes are currently underway in our laboratory to provide further information regarding practical application of these strains in field studies.

ACKNOWLEDGEMENT

The Council of Scientific and Industrial Research (CSIR), India and Department of Biotechnology (DBT), India, in parts, have supported the work in the laboratory of R.K. Jain. R. K. Jain also acknowledges the Air Force Office of Scientific Research and the International window on the science program for the support.

REFERENCES

An, D., Gibson, D. T. and Spain, J. C. (1994). Oxidative release of nitrite from 2-nitrotoluene by a two component enzyme system from *Pseudomonas* sp strain JS42. *J. Bacteriol.* 176:7462-7467.

Anderson, K. E., Hammons, G. J., Kadlubar, F. F., Potter, J. D., Kaderlik, K. R., Ilett, K. F., Minchin, R. R., Teitel, C. H., Chou, H. C., Martin, M.V., Guengerich. F. P., Barone, G. W., Lang, N. P., and Peterson, L. A. (1997). Metabolic activation of aromatic amines by human pancreas. *Carcinogenesis.* 18:1085-1092.

Bhushan, B, Chauhan, A., Samanta, S. K., and Jain, R. K. (2000). Kinetics of biodegradation of p-nitrophenol by different bacteria. *Biochem. Biophys. Res. Commun.* 274:626-630.

Chauhan, A., Chakarborti, A. K., Jain, R. K. (2000 A). Plasmid encoded degradation of *p*-nitrophenol and 4-nitrocatechol by *Arthrobacter protophormiae. Biochem. Biophys. Res. Commun.* 270:733-740.

Chauhan, A., Samanta, S. K., and Jain, R. K. (2000 B). Degradation of 4-nitrocatechol by *Burkholderia cepacia:* A plasmid encoded novel pathway. *J. Appl. Microbiol.* 88: 764-772.

Gibson, D. T., and Subramanian, V. (1984). *In* Microbial degradation of organic compounds (*Ed.* D. T. Gibson), Dekker, New York, pp 181-252.

Hebes, S. E., and Schwall, I. R. (1978). Microbial transformation of polycyclic aromatic hydrocarbons in pristine and petroleum contaminated sediments. *Appl. Environ. Microbiol.* 35:306-316.

Holding, A. J. and Collee, J. G. (1971). Routine biochemical tests. *Methods Microbiol.* 6A:1-32.

Hutzinger, O., and Veerkamp, W. (1981). Xenobiotics with pollution potential. *In* Degradation of xenobiotic and recalcitrant compounds. (*Ed.* Heisinger T., Cook A. M., Hutter, R., and Nuesch, J.) Academic press. London. pp. 146-155.

Jain, R. K., Dreisbach, J. H., and Spain, J. C. (1994). Biodegradation of *p*-nitrophenol via 1,2,4-benzenetriol by an *Arthrobacter* sp. *Appl. Environ. Microbiol.* 60:3030-3032.

Jain, R. K., Bayly, R. C., and Skurray, R.A. (1984). Characterization and physical analysis of a 3,5-xylenol degradative plasmid in *Pseudomonas putida J. Gen. Microbiol.* 130:3019-3028

Keith, L. H., and Telliard, W. A. (1976). Priority Pollutants I. A perspective view. *Environ. Sc. Technol.* 13: 416-423.

Munnecke, D. M. (1976). Enzymatic hydrolysis of organophosphate insecticide, a possible pesticide disposable method. *Appl. Environ. Microbiol.* 32:7-13.

Prakash. D., Chauhan, A., and Jain, R. K. (1996). Plasmid-encoded degradation of *p*-nitrophenol by *Pseudomonas cepacia. Biochem. Biophys. Res. Commun.* 224:375-381.

Rani., Prakash D., Sobti, R. C., and Jain, R. K. (1996). Plasmid-mediated degradation of *o*-phathalate and salicylate by an Moraxella sp. *Biochem. Biophys. Res. Commun.* 220:377-381.

Safe, S. H. (1984). *In* Microbial degradation of organic compounds (*Ed.* D. T. Gibson), Dekker, New York. pp 361-369.

Schell, M. A. (1983). Cloning and expression in *Escherichia coli* of the naphthalene degradative genes from plasmid NAH7. *J. Bacteriol.* 153:822-829.

Spain, J. C. (1995). Biodegradation of nitroaromatic compounds. *Ann. Rev. Microbiol.* 49:523-555.

Spain, J. C., and Gibson, D. T. (1991). Pathway for degradation of *p*-nitrophenol in a *Moraxella sp. Appl. Environ. Microbiol.* 57:812-819.

Straskwicz, B., Dahlbeck, D., Keen N and Napoli C (1978). Molecular characterization of cloned avirulence genes from race 0 and 1 of *Pseudomonas syringae* pv *glycinea*. J. Bacteriol. 169: 5789-5794.

Venulet, J., and Van Etten, R. L. (1970). Biochemistry and pharmacology of the nitro and nitroso groups. In The chemistry of the nitro and nitroso groups. (*Ed.* H. Fever) New York: Interscience. pp. 201-289.

White, G. F., Snape, J. R., and Nicklin, S. (1996). Biodegradation of glycerol trinitrate and pentaerythritol tetranitrate by *Agrabacterium radiobacter. Appl. Environ. Microbiol.* 62:637-642.

Microbiology and Biotechnology for Sustainable Development (Ed. P.C. Jain),
CBS Publishers & Distributors, New Delhi (2004), pp. 22–33.

A-3

Microbes in Geoenvironment

Pramod O. Alexander
Dep!t. of Applied Geology
Dr. H.S. Gour Vishwavidyalaya, *Sagar – 470003 (M.P.)*

Abstract

Microbes, including various kinds of bacteria, fungi, algae and protozoa are ubiquitous in the secondary environment. We cannot think of this planet as habitable and beautiful as it is today without them. Throughout the geological history of the earth (or for a greater part of it) the microbes have played a significant role in breaking down and shaping down the earlier rocks/minerals while forming a new and useful regime of rocks, minerals, ores and perhaps the most important of all – the fossil fuels without which our present day high tech world would have still been in the dark ages. Because of their versatility to survive at greater depth than any other organism and their capability to withstand/adjust/thrive even in toxic environment around mineral deposits of metals like As, Sb, Bi, B, Cd, Cr, Rl, Au, As, Mo, Ni, Ag including oil and gas fields, enumeration of their kind and number or even their absence in the near surface soil samples can help to detect a buried mineral deposit. It has been found so in several instances under different climatic conditions in different parts of the world. Microbial prospecting therefore needs to be developed as an additional tool for mineral exploration. It has the advantage of being easy, quick and cheaper relative to the other recognized prospecting techniques and gives a better contrast between mineralized and non-mineralized ground. Yet another application of microbes is in the field of bacterial leaching of low-grade ores, weakly mineralized rocks, solid and liquid wastes, leaching of oil sands and oil shales and desulfurization of coals. Experimental studies in these areas could be very beneficial in times to come when high grade ore deposits will be hard to find – a situation many of the nations are already facing. Selective removal of toxic metals from the aqueous system by certain microorganism is another direction in which experimental research needs to be intensified to keep our geo-hydro system clean.

Key Words: Geoenvironment, Microbes, Bio mineralization, Mineral prospecting.

INTRODUCTION

This is not a research article. It can best be described as a review cum research paper. It aims at creating awareness and interest among microbiologists to apply their knowledge and expertise for geological cum geochemical investigations while encouraging geoscientists to include microbes also among their tools for research, especially in the applied fields. The paper will be divided into three sections. The first part will be a summary of the multifarious activities of microbes in the secondary environment. The second section would be on the potential application of microbes in mineral prospecting and the third will touch upon the application of microbes in leaching low-grade ores/ rocks/ wastes as also the potential use of microbes in cleaning up our water systems. Interested readers would do well to go through the "Introduction to Geological Microbiology" (Kuznetsov *et al.*, 1963) for a better appreciation of this boundary line subject.

MULTIFARIOUS ROLE OF MICROBES IN THE SECONDARY ENVIRONMENT

Microbes, mainly bacteria make up 50% of the earth's biomass. Their arena covers parts of the lithosphere, hydrosphere, biosphere and the atmosphere. These teeny – weenie creatures are ubiquitous. Cosmo chemists are in fact looking forward to finding them even in the extraterrestrial regions of the universe. For example, the recent study on one of the twelve Martian meteorites (ALH 84001) is indicated to contain fossilized Martian bacteria (Grady *et al.*, 1994, Mckey *et al.*, 1996). Only time will tell the validity of their claim or otherwise.

If the estimates of the geological age are correct, the production of bacteria during this time should have exceeded the weight of the Earth itself. Their chemical activity including cation exchange capacity though trival individually is highly significant on a collective basis and has played a very significant role in the geological/ geochemical processes operating in the secondary environment of our planet. Their versatility makes them able to withstand even thrive in extreme environments – from Arctic cold waters to hotsprings having a temperature up to 110°C, or perhaps more; to dry desert patches to the deepest oceanic bottoms. Subsurface microbiology of recent has gone deeper and turned warmer. Bacteria that can withstand higher temperature have been recorded. Particularly remarkable is the finding of bacteria in the core samples from Triassic basin at Taylorsville Va (Ghiorse, 1999) at the depth of around 3000 meters below land surface. Studies on the microbial life of samples from even deeper horizons and hotter zones (samples taken from deep cores, mines, caves and sub sea floor) are currently in progress in many laboratories of the world with exciting results awaited.

Countless species of microorganisms are always at work like an unseen army. In the long run these microorganisms become extremely potential tool to breakdown, dissolve, destroy, metabolize, modify and build a new regime of biogeochemical order in the secondary environment. Nothing is spared from their attack once they get the favorable company of water, clays, heat, organic matter and weak chemical environment. Even the toughest artificially built material concrete, whether reinforced or not is prone to microbial attack leading to structural failure (Milde *et al.*, 1983; Sand and Bock, 1991; Zherebyateva *et al.*, 1991). The only thing is that since the microbial army is unseen by the naked eye we don't seem to realize it. The saying, 'out of sight is out of mind' cannot be more appropriate to describe the reality. Indeed our planet will suffer little chemical weathering without microbes and their metabolic end products.

Thus rocks, igneous, sedimentary or metamorphic, silicate minerals and ores (metallic and non metallic), coal, oil or gases associated with them or just plain ground water – all have had something or much to do with their formation, modification, enrichment or destruction in the past, present and will be so in future too. Some specific geological commodities via microbial activity include – limestones, marls, cherts, phosphorites, Ferruginous sandstones among sedimentary rocks and ores of Mn, Cu, Co, Pb, Zn, Ag, Au and U (among others) – mostly as sulphides or oxides and carbonates; and coal oil and sulphur among the caustobioliths. A brief review of these is given in Table 1.

Table 1: Microbes in Geoenvironement
(Bacteria, Fungi, Algae, Protozoa)

Phenomena	**Specific rock/ mineral ore** All types of Igneous, sedimentary or metamorphic rocks; Silicate, non-silicate minerals; ores, Metallic/non-metallic	**Process/ Ramark/Species**
Rock and Mineral Weathering		By metabolic products of microbes; by excretion of corrosive chemical agents that grow on rock/Mineral surface; oxidative or Reducing processes follow; lichens important weathering agents in dry environments
Sedimentary rock formation, clays, soils	Limestones, Cherts, Silccious oozes, phosphorites, Ferruginous sandstones, Ochres	A group of anaerobes, heterotrophic bacteria; algae (*Chara Corallina, Globigerina, Cyanobacteria,*), protozoa, diatoms, *Radiolaria*, phytoplanktons. *Gallionella ferrugina, Leptothrix ochracea, L. discophora* (for ochres)
Bio mineralisation	Manganese minerals. Manganese nodules	Foraminifer (saccorhiza) *Micrococcus, Hyphomicrobium, Metallogenium, Sphaerotilus, Arthrobacter, Microcystis,*
	Iron Minerals (Bog, lake, Marine)	*Hyphomicrobium, Metallogenium personatum*
		ppt ferric iron near neutrality
		Gallionella ferruginea
		Leptothrix, Crenothrix (Bog iron),
		Gallionella (Marine) *Bacterium Preciptta-tum* Algae.
	Sulphide Minerals	T. ferrooxidans
		T. thiooxidans
		various acidophilic bacteria
	Sulphur deposits	*Vibrio desulfuricans, Thiobacillus thioparus, T. thiooxidans*

(Contd.)

Phenomena	Specific rock/ mineral ore	Process/ Ramark/Species
	All types of Igneous, sedimentary or metamorphic rocks; Silicate, non-silicate minerals; ores, Metallic/non-metallic	
	Coal, oil and gas	Definite role of various kinds of bacteria in converting vegetable material to peat. Conversion of planktonic material to sapropel, the parent substance of petroleum involves active bacterial role
Isotpoe Fractionation		a kinetic process; Reaction rates for different stable isotopes in key uni-directional reactions differ sufficiently for discrimination
Microbes in Applied Geology field	Mineral Prospecting (Gold, copper, other sulphides) oil gas prospecting; Beneficiation and leaching of low grade ores, mine wastes, rocks; Beneficiation of Rock phosphate, Fertilizers from pyritiferous shales; organic fertilizer from lignite coal. Mine safety from methane gas; Desulfurization of coals; Toxic clean up of waste water.	

(Contents from various published sources)

MICROBES IN MINERAL PROSPECTING

Geomicrobial prospecting is only an extension of botanical prospecting and works on a similar principle. Right from the 1930's Soviet and American geomicrobiologists showed that the buried oil and gas fields could be detected by enumerating bacteria in the subsoil. Quite a few petroleum and gas fields were detected using this principle. Soviet scientists furnished clear proof of microorganisms, serving as signposts of buried metallic deposits later when they could detect a molybdenum ore deposit (Kuznetsov *et al.*, 1963). In spite of this geomicrobial prospecting was not in fashion for exploration work. Only during the post eighties and nineties it saw some revival in connection with gold and other base metal prospecting. It stands to logic that both the kind and number of bacteria or even its absence will reflect a particular geochemical environment. Thus bacterial count of a specific species over a known mineralized area in contrast to a non-mineralized one can be used as an indicator of economically important deposit such as toxic heavy metals, toxic non-metals or radioactive isotopes.

In practice it is feasible to study soil microorganisms by making cultures of them in various soil media. If cultures can be found that will support particular organism growth or death only in the presence of anomalous concentration of say copper or nickel, it should be possible to collect soil sample of potential area and run cultures to determine the content of particular element/s in the soil.

Soil bacteria pointing the way to deposits of gold and other metals have been one of the active research studies at the geomicrobiological laboratory of U.S.G.S., Denver, where I was also able to spend some time during the late eighties (Watterson,1983, 1985, Parduhn, *et al.*, 1986). The studies bring out two important conclusions. Firstly, like bacteria forming iron ores, they also nucleate gold nuggets. Thus many of the large gold nuggets of the world have bacteriogenic origin. A similar thing has also been reported from the University of Massachusetts (News item, Times of India, 25th July, 2001). Secondly, *Bacillus cereus,* one of the many naturally occurring bacteria in soils over buried mineralisation of gold and other heavy metals not only withstands the effects of naturally occurring penicillin that kills other bacteria in soils but uses penicillin to neutralize toxic effects of gold, copper and other heavy metals. Thus while other bacteria are killed in such mineralised grounds, *Bacillus cereus* thrives. Thus it will be a sign post for mineralisation. In some cases *Bacillus cereus* in soil showed anomalous counts even when the actual mineralisation was buried hundreds or even thousands of feet deep. Therefore, *Bacillus cereus* counts in soil and sediments in potential areas has the capability of indicating buried gold mineralisation underground. It is also true for other base metals like copper. A few of the result of these studies have been shown in a generalized way in Figs. 1-4. It was interesting to find that the same bacterial

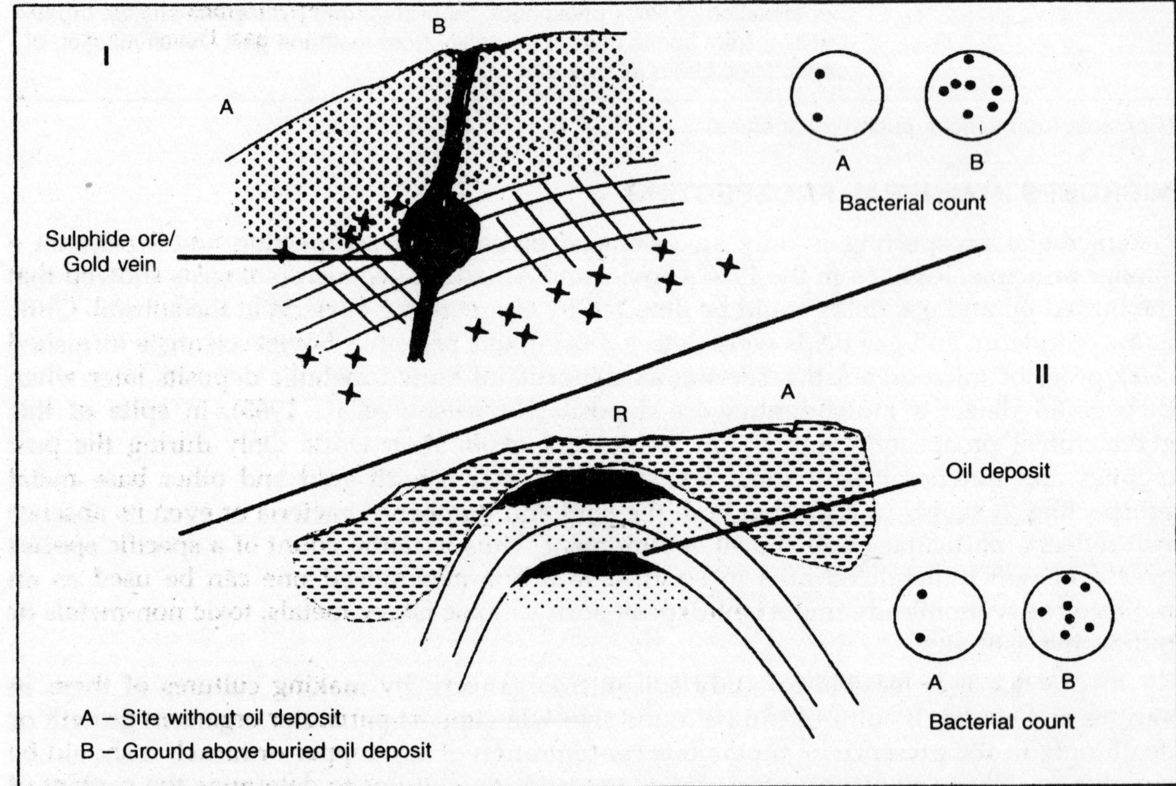

Fig. 1. Principle illustrating bacterial prospecting for metallic deposit (I) and oil deposit (II) with estimate of bacterial growth. Bacterial enumeration in soils overlying the deposit and outside it will show significant difference in kind and numbers or even absence of bacteria over the mineralised grounds relative to the non-mineralised ground will be significant.

species was also capable of distinguishing buried rock types of chemically diverse nature from one of the regions of western United States. (Alexander, 1986). It thrived in the ultrabasic rock (which incidentally is one of the primary source of diamonds) having anomalous contents of various trace elements including Cr, Ni, Co, V and U. This proves that *Bacillus cereus* is remarkably hardy and thrives in mineralized grounds under diverse climatic settings. Experimental results from the ultrabasic body within the Granitic rock are shown in Fig 3. For estimating the *Bacillus cereus* counts in soils procedure given by Watterson (1983) was adopted.

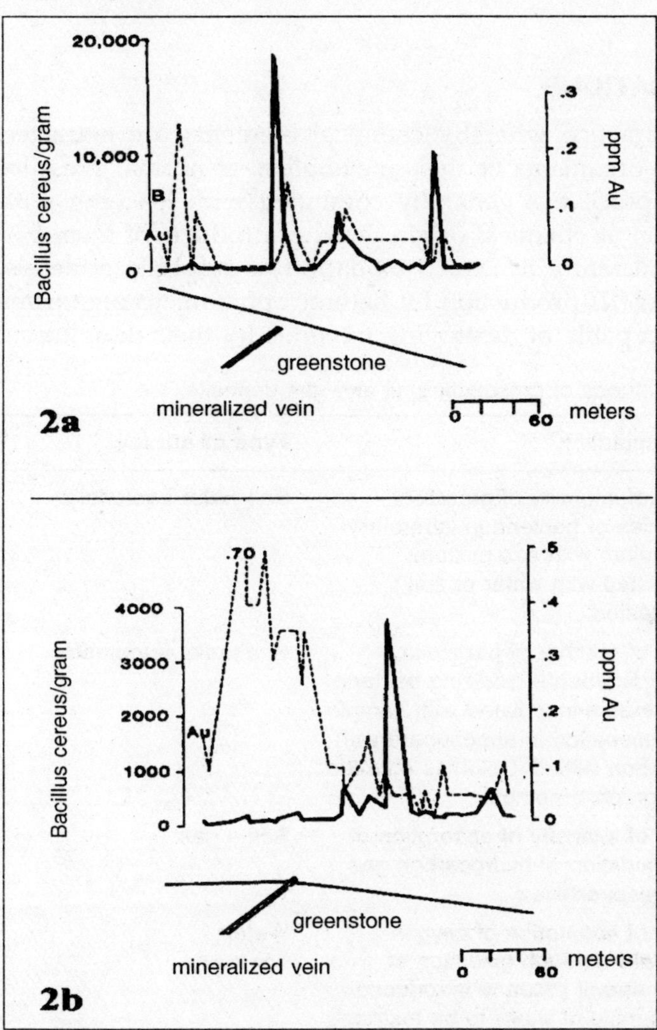

Fig. 2a. Plot of *Bacillus cereus*/gram and ppm Au in soils overlying the Evening Star gold vein, Reid Mine, Redding, California.

2b. Plot of *Bacillus cereus*/gram and ppm Au in soil overlying the Shasta gold vein, Reid Mine, Redding, California.

Microbial technique for mineral exploration has a few plus points. It is simple, quick even economic and also fairly reproducible. Another added advantage is the possibility of achieving a very strong contrast between amineralised and non mineralised ground where as the ratio of background to anomaly in geochemical soil prospecting even between 5-10 times could be called encouraging, the same may extend to 100 to 1000 times in bacterial counting technique. However, the main problem would be to achieve an explicit and aseptic working condition in the laboratory.

Microbial prospecting for oil and gas was taken up successfully even earlier than its application for metallic deposits. Scientists of the Soviet Union (Mogilevskiy, 1938, 1940) and later United States were able to detect oil and gas fields by enumerating bacteria in near surface soil which oxidize gaseous hydrocarbons as a sole source of energy. Many new discoveries were made with this technique. The basic principle involved the study of the distribution in the subsoil of bacteria, which oxidize gaseous hydrocarbons. A summary of the principle bacterial prospecting methods is given by Kuznetsov *et al.* (1963) in Table 2 while Fig. 4 gives the representative diagram of the simple bacterial procedure. In spite of fairly good results during the work of Mogilevskiy in 1953 (while sixty areas were bacterially survyed,16 structure subsequently being drilled on the basis of this study, ten out of these proved for oil and gas presence, and no oil or gas being discovered where the bacterial prospecting gave a negative result) this technique did not receive much attention later on or at the present time. The solution lies in combining bacterial prospecting with the other well recognized and currently used techniques, including geochemical, gas and seismic surveys within the scope of the overall geological and structural background. Simplicity of bacterial prospecting principle and practice should not be abandoned due to availability of other high tech techniques.

OTHER APPLIED MICROBIAL APPLICATIONS

Microbiological hydrometallurgy is a practice whereby chemical elements are extracted through the solubilizing action of micro-organisms or their metabolites at normal pressure and temperature range of 5-80°C. The process is generally combined with leaching with dilute sulphuric acid solutions of bacterial or chemical origin or other products of microbial synthesis, Two types of variations are currently in use (I) oxidation of sulphide minerals, elementary sulphur and ferrous iron and (II) production by heterotrophic micro-organisms or organic compounds, per oxides etc., capable of destroying minerals by their dissolution,

Table 2: Principal bacterial methods of prospecting oil and gas deposits

Basis of method	Method of computation	**Type of survey**
Counting of bacterial population growing in soil water or gas	1. Determination of intensity of growth of particular species of bacteria in laboratory on mineral medium with gas mixture. Medium inoculated with water or soil sample to be tested.	Soil-water-bacterial
	2. Determination of number of particular species of hydrocarbon – oxidizing bacteria. Slid mineral medium inoculated with sample to be tested; incubation in atmosphere with radioactive carbon added. Colonies counted by radio auto graphic method.	Soil radio autographic
	3. Determination of intensity of absorption of oxygen from oxidation of hydrocarbon gas in differential respirometer.	Soil – gas
	4. Determination of absorption of oxygen dissolved in water through oxidation of bubble of methane of propane introduced into isolated sample of water to be tested.	Water
Calculation of gas flow from deposit	1. Determination of intensity of development of particular species of bacteria in mineral nutrient medium within vessel placed in borehole.	Bacterial – debit

(After Kuznetsov *et al.*, 1963)

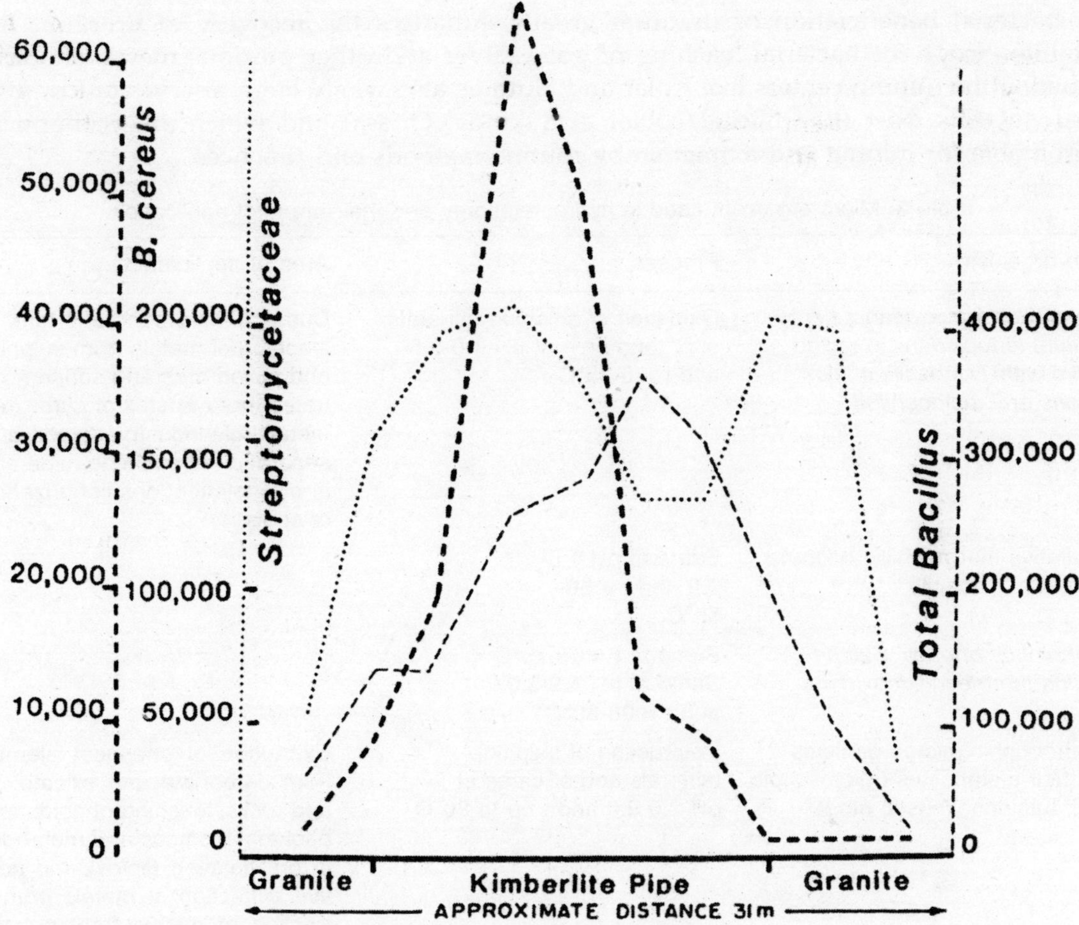

Fig. 3. Plot of streptomycetes, *Bacillus cereus* and total *Bacillus* counts for each gram of soil across Green Mountain Kimberlite pipe Colorado, USA (Alexander, 1986).

formation of complexes and oxidation of chemical elements. In Table 3 list of important microorganisms for hydrometallurgy are given, together with possible areas of application.

In short, microbes accelerate oxidation and have been successfully used in dump mining, in tank processing of metal ores, in ore flotation and extraction of metals from solutions. About 20% of US copper, these days, is extracted using bacterial leaching. In Zambia 100 tons of copper per day is extracted through bacterial leaching. For developing countries like India where there is chronic shortage of copper and other base metals and where large tonnage of old mine dumps are found bacterial extraction after proper testing and research will be a big boon for our economy especially when our known reserves are fast depleting and bacterial extraction infrastructure and methodology is relatively inexpensive and simple. There is enough scope for the technique being routinely operative at copper mining centers like

Malanjkhand and elsewhere in India. The Atomic Mineral Division, Hyderabad have found that bacterial beneficiation of uranium greatly enhances the recovery of uranium from uraninite. Scope for bacterial leaching of gold, silver and other precious metals should be studied at the mining centers like Kolar and Hutti as also where large reserves of low grade metal deposits exist (like Nickel/cobalt at Sukinda, Orissa) and which are economically unprofitable for mining and extraction by routine methods and practices.

Table 3: Micro-organism used in hydrometallurgy and their areas of application.

Micro-organism	Process	Area of application
Thiobacillus ferrooxidans, Leptospirillum ferrooxidans in mixed culture with *Thiobacillus thiooxidans* or *T. acidophilus*	Oxidation of sulphide minerals of S° and Fe^{2+} at pH 1.0-3.5 and t = 5-35°C	Dump, underground and tank leaching of metals from sulphide and mixed ores and concentrates, from wastes of pyrometallurgic industry; selective separation of sulphide minerals in ore flotation; desulphurization of coals
Facultative thermophillic bacteria similar to Thiobacilli	Same at pH 1.6-2.2 and t = 50-55°C	
Sulpholobus brierley, Sulphobacillus thermosulfidooxidans	Same at t = 45-75°C Same at pH 1.9-3.0 and t = 28-60°C	
Organotrophic microorganisms and their metabolites (microscopic fungi, bacteria, Yeasts, etc.)	Destruction of sulphide minerals and silicates at pH 2.0-9.0 and t up to 80°C	Extraction of chemical elements from carbonate and silicate ores and rocks; leaching of gold; use of bacterial biomass and metabolites in ore flotation (lipids) and selective extraction of metals from extraction of metals from solutions (Poly-saccharides and other organic compounds)

(After Karavaiko, 1982)

Within our own Bundelkhand area there are such low grade rocks/wastes which need the attention of applied microbiologists to test microbiological hydrometallurgy studies. In Sagar district itself where there is pile of volcanic rocks called basalts there are (around ten flows) some of them contain more than normal concentration of copper. In average crustal rocks the concentration of copper is around 70 ppm but in some and definitely one of the flows it is as high as 500 ppm (Alexander,1976). A large part of it is extractible by the attack of weak acids itself (Alexander, 1991) Bacterial leaching of such rocks will extract even more copper from it. At the present level of technology and need it may not be economic to extract this copper bacterially but we need to sharpen our tools and identify such material which could serve as an ore for the future. The second material is the rock-waste from diamond mining/ extraction from Panna. This material was already identified as a natural fertilizer source by the author earlier (Alexander 1985) but its abnormal concentration of several trace elements including Cr, Ni, Co, V,U will make it an ideal material for bacterial leaching for these elements. There are two plus points with it. Firstly it is a waste material – available in a couple of thousand tons annually and secondly it is available in a crushed form.

Other applied areas for bacterial treatment of geological materials include, beneficiation of rock phosphate, obtaining fertilizer from pyritiferous shales, organic fertilizer from lignite, mine safety from methane gas by converting it to oily hydrocarbons with the help of micro-organisms like species of *Aspergillus* and *Bacillus*.

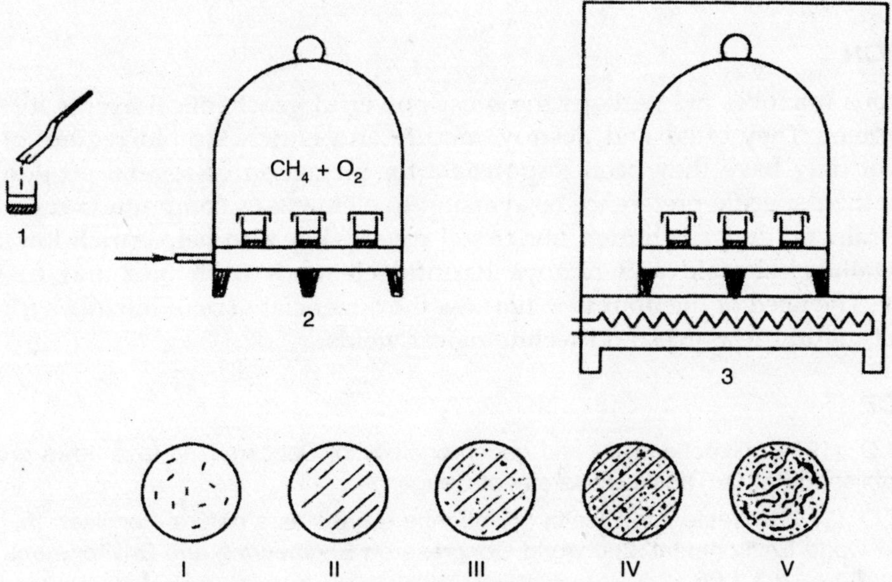

Fig. 4. Illustrating microbiological analysis of soil or water in microbiological oil and gas prospecting (after Mogilevskiy, 1953): 1, inoculation of soil or water; 2, filling of bell jar with methane and air; 3, cultivation in thermostat.

Estimate of bacterial growth:

I. Turbidity of medium bacteria discernible only Microscopically,
II. Thin transperent film,
III. Semitransparent, slightly pigmented film.
IV. Solid smooth pigmented film; V – soild, Wrinkled pigmneted film

The last two, yet very important contribution of bacteria, for increasing yield/ quality of geological resources is in the field of coal and oil. India has fairly large coal reserves, but they lack coking quality and invariably have high ash and total sulfur content. Even when they attain coking quality the high sulfur and ash content makes them unattractive for specific use. Desulfurization is the only possibility. A strain of *Thiobacillus ferrooxidans* has been found effective in removing pyritic sulfate as well as organic sulfur from such coals (Chandra and Mishra, 1988), such bacterial treatment has even improved ash content up to 50% without affecting the coking property.

Experimental / laboratory studies on the line of Chandra and Mishra (1988) need to be continued and intensified to find the most appropriate strain for desulfurization of coal specifically from coal belts of Madhya Pradesh.

Apart from the regular reserves of oil in India and the world at large, oil sands and oil shales are yet another source of oil. These have an estimated potential reserve of 14,500 – 35,000 million tons and 2,500,000 million tons respectively. However with present technology, oil extraction from these will be uneconomic. Bacterial leaching of oil sands and oil shales can make this economic and easier by making the crude oil less viscous and the total yield nearly doubled (Imhoff, 1978).

CONCLUSION

The ubiquitous microbes are perhaps the most powerful geochemical agents in the secondary environment. They build and destroy, modify and enrich the old regime of rocks and minerals. Not only have they been responsible for formation of several economic mineral deposits but their specific preference or aversion to elements/s compounds can also help us locate these mineral deposits buried under soil cover. They also help enrich low grade ores, increase metallurgical yield and remove harmful elements from ores and fuels and our hydrosphere. The need of the hour is to harness the beneficial uses of microbes for maximum utilization of natural resources and technological yields.

REFERENCE

Alexander, P.O. (1976). Geochemistry and geochronology of Deccan Trap lava flows around Sagar, M.P. Unpublished Ph. D. Thesis University of Saugar.

Alexander, P.O. (1985). Waste into Wealth : Kimberlite tailings as a natural Fertiliser. In, 'Technology for a better world Environment' 2nd world Congress on Engineering and Environment, New Delhi, Nov.85, conf. Vol. II 3.1.04

Alexander, P.O. (1986). Preliminary study of the soil bacterial population over and adjacent to three Kimberlite diatremes. 4th International Kimberlite Conf, Perth, West Aust., pp. 440-442

Alexander, P.O. (1991). Copper in Deccan basalt. *In*. Traps of Siberia and Deccan: Similarites and Differences :USSR Acad. of Sciences, Novosibirsk, pp. 108-115.

Chandra, D. (1985). Application of Microbiology in Mineral and Fuel Industries. 9th Prof.S. Ray memorial Lecture. Presidency College Calcutta.

Chandra, D. and Mishra, A.K. (1988). Desulfurization of coal by bacterial means. Resources, Conservation and Recycling. Elsevier Sci., Pub. Netherland, pp.293-308.

Ehrlich, H.L. (1998). Geomicrobiology : its significance for Geology. Earth Science Reviews, 45, pp. 45-60.

Ghiorse, W.C. (1999). 'Geomicrobiology ' *In*. Geotimes, pp. 42-43.

Grady, M.M. Wright , I.P. and Pillinger, C.T. (1997). Carbon and Nitrogen in ALH 84001 (abstract). Meteoriticam. 29, 469.

Imhoff, J.F. (1978). Bactreial extraction of Metals and Oil. Natural Resources and Development. Federal Republic of Germany, V. 8, pp. 7-12.

Karavaiko, G.I. (1982). Microbial leaching of metals. In:Commonwealth Science Council NEWS LETTER, Sep. – Oct. 1982 , pp. 6.

Kuznetsov. : K., Ivanov, M.V. and Lyalikova, N.K. (1963). Introduction to Geological Microbiology. Mc Graw Hill Book Co. New York.

Mckay, D.S., Gibson, E. K., Jr, Thomas, Keprta, K. L., Vali H, Romanek, C.S., Clementt, S.J., Chiller X. D.F., Maechling, C.M. and Zare R. N. (1996). Search for past life on Mars: possible relic biogenic activity in martian meteorite ALH 84001. Science, 273, pp. 924-930.

Milde, K., Sand W., Wolff, W., Bock E. (1983). Thiobacilli of the corroded walls of the Hamburg sewer system J. Gen. Microbiology. 129, 1327-1333.

Mogilevskiy, G.A. (1938). Microbiological Investigation in Connection with Gas Surveying : Razvedka Nedr, Nos. 8-9.

Mogilevskiy, G.A. (1940). The Bacterial Method of Prospecting for Oil and Natural Gases; Razvedka Nedr. No. 12.

Mogilevskiy, G.A. (1953). The Microbiological Method of Prosperting Gas and Oil Occurrence. Byuro Tekhn-Ekon. Tsemthefti, Gostoptekhizdat.

Parduhn, N.L., Watterson, J.R. and Silberman (1986). Distribution of *Bacillus cereus* Spores in Soil Over Subsurface Gold Deposits: A progress Report. Proc. of Denver Region Exploron. Geol. Soc. Symp "Organics and Ore Deposits" pp. 115-118.

Sand, W. and Bock E. (1991). Biodeterioration of mineral materials by microorganisms – biogenic sulfuric and nitric acid corrosion of concrete and natural stone. Geomicrobiology. J. 9, 129-138.

Watterson, J.R. (1983). The potential of microbiology in mineral Exploration, "Organic Matter, Biological Systems and Mineral Exploration" Colloquium for Mineral Explorationists and research Scientists (UCLA), 10.

Watterson, J.R. (1985). Crystalline gold in soil and the problem of supergene nugget formation: Freezing and Exclusion as Genetic mechanisms. Precambrian Research, 30, pp. 321-335.

Zherebytaeva, T.M.; Lebedeva, E.V. and Karavaiko., G.I. (1991). Microbiological corrosion of concrete structures of hydraulic facilities Geomicrobiology. J. 9, pp.119-127.

Ehrlich, H.L. (1998). Geomicrobiology; its significance for Geology. Earth Science Reviews, 45, pp. 45-60.

Umbreit, W.W. (Ed). (1964). Advances in Applied Microbiology. Academic Press, New York.

Watterson, J.R. (1884). A procedure for estimating *Bacillus cereus* in soil and stream sediments. U.S. geological Survey Open File report. 84-482:11 p.

Microbiology and Biotechnology for Sustainable Development (Ed. P.C. Jain),
CBS Publishers & Distributors, New Delhi (2004), pp. 34–41.

A-4

Solid Waste Bioleaching for Environmental Clean-up and Sustainable Development

S.R. Dave
*Department of Microbiology, School of Sciences, Gujarat University,
Ahmedabad 380 009. Email : shaileshrdave@hotmail.com*

Abstract

Intensive mining and increased industrial activities have generated huge tonnes of low-grade ores, tailing and industrial solid materials. These waste materials are piled up at the mining site or used as landfill inspite of the presence of toxic metals. Under natural environmental conditions, metals from these wastes are solubilized and create a potential environmental hazard. The basic problem of metal removal from such solid waste is that "the metal content is too low to be worth mining but sufficiently high to be of environmental concern." Chemical methods used to remove toxic metals are unattractive due to high cost, operational difficulties and large acid or lime requirements. The industrial wastes such as tailing, slag, galvanic sludge, filter dust, fly ash etc. serve as solid substrate for microbial processes and can be considered for remediation and recovery of toxic and valuable metals respectively. Metal contaminated wastes have been microbiologically treated using variety of lithotrophic and organotrophic microorganisms. Metals from waste are extracted mostly by the formation of acid, redox reactions and/or complexing agents produced by the concerned organisms. The bioleaching efficiencies mainly depend on the concentration of reduced sulphur compounds, content of organic carbon, buffering capacity, presence of bioleaching organisms, temperature and other environmental factors prevailing during the process.

The problems of bioremediation of toxic metals from the waste are quite different from those of bioremediation of organic pollutants. As metals are non biodegradable they can only be transformed to less toxic state, solubilized or precipitated out from the waste. Bioleaching technology must be seen in the context of a future in which industrial technologies have to be more in harmony with global material cycle within the biosphere. There are numerous advantages of bioleaching process compared to chemical and pyrometallurgical leaching techniques. Bioleaching represents a "clean technology" process with a low cost and energy input as compared to conventional thermal solid waste treatment techniques. The process is friendly to human and the environment. Thus, application of biohydrometallurgy to solid waste opens an important field of research to support sustainable development. The overview of metal bioremediation will be discussed.

Keywords: Bioleaching, solid waste, bioremediation, biohydrometallurgy.

INTRODUCTION

Advances in science and technology since the industrial revolution have increasingly enabled humans to exploit natural resources. However, this has created unprecedented disturbances in global elemental cycles and resulted in the generation of huge tonnes of low grade ores, tailings and industrial solid waste to problematic or even harmful levels (Liu and Suflita, 1993).

Sewage treatment plants also usually generate millions of tonnes of residual sludge world-wide every year (Hayes *et al.*, 1980). The treatment and final disposition of such solid waste often constitutes the most expensive stage in the treatment of waste. In strictly economic terms, disposal options have always seemed more attractive than investment in waste-treatment technology (Hamer, 1993). Thus until very recently, the practice of oceanic dumping, landfilling and incineration appears to be widely accepted solid waste management methods (Davis, 1987; Bruce and Davis, 1989; Blais *et al.*, 1992). However, the presence of potentially toxic concentration of metals and pathogens represent major constraint in implementation of above practices (Bruce and Davis, 1989).

The disposal methods of heavy metal containing solid waste should be prevented because under natural environmental conditions, metals from these wastes are spontaneously solubilised due to natural weathering processes and uncontrolled microbial activities (Horvath and Gruiz, 1996; Moore and Luoma, 1990).

The potential health hazard associated with the land disposal of such waste is the metal uptake by plants and the subsequent accumulation of metals in the food chain via plants and animals. Plant grazing animals tend to accumulate Cd, Cu, Fe, Mn, Ni, Se and Zn (Lester *et al.*, 1983; Scheltinga, 1987) metals which are leached from the polluted soils may be mobilised into surface and ground waters.

The basic problem of metal removal from such solid waste is that, the metal content is too low to be worth mining but sufficiently high to be of environmental concern (Bosecker, 1999). Chemical methods such as chlorination, ion exchange, acid hydrolysis, use of chelating agents etc. used to remove toxic metals are found to be unattractive due to high cost, operational difficulties and large acid or lime consumption (Blais *et al.*, 1992; Tyagi and Couillard, 1987).

Biohydrometallurgical technologies are already successfully applied in the mining industry to leach out valuable metals from low grade ores and concentrates (Dave, 1980; Torma, 1988; Rossi, 1990; Menon, 1995; Menon and Dave, 1995; Agate, 1996; Brombachar *et al.*, 1997; Tipre *et al.*, 1998; Tipre, 1999). In last two decades, attempts to extract toxic metals from industrial and municipal solid waste by the generation of organic and inorganic acids have been done (Dave, 1991; Tyagi, 1992; Dave, 1995a; Bosecker, 1997; Donati *et al.*, 1997).

When the process is employed for the metals that are more valuable than toxic, it is called 'Biorecovery', but when it is used for metals that are toxic but not intrinsically valuable, the process is referred to as 'Bioremediation'. In the light of the expected shortage of non-renewable resources and accumulation of huge quantity of metal containing solid waste, increased efforts are absolutely necessary to find out new sources of raw materials and eco-friendly processes with the aid of new or improved technologies. A possible solution for these is the use of microbiological leaching processes (Dave, 1995b).

Genesis of solid waste

Intensive mining and ore processing are responsible for the production of billions of tonnes of low grade ores and tailings all over the world. These wastes are normally piled up surrounding the mining sites or ore processing plants. Other mineral industrial activities are responsible for the generation of waster products such as fly ash, slag, incineration cinders, filter dust (Horvath and Gruiz, 1996; Brombachar *et al.*, 1999). During any waste water treatment, the volume of the sludge generated amounts to approximately 1% of the volume of waste water treated, with solids content of 1 to 7% (Lester *et al.*, 1983; Davis, 1986). The amount of sludge produced has recently increased due to higher levels of sludge treatments and use of chemical precipitation for phosphorus removal. This precipitation also removes a large proportion of many of the toxic metals, which then become concentrated in the sludge. The United States generates municipal solid wastes at an average rate of 176 Kg per person per year resulting in about 40 million tonnes of waste per year (Christy *et al.*, 1999). The production of sludge in Europe in 1990 was about 10 million tonnes (Scheltinga, 1987). The production of sewage sludge in Canada is about 1 million tonnes per year (Webber, 1988). The produced sludge is mainly classified as primary, primary digested anaerobically, aerobically digested, anaerobically digested, secondary activated, etc. (Blais *et al.*, 1992). Even relative short life times of electrical and electronic equipments are responsible for an increased amount of waste production. In Switzerland and Germany alone, approximately 0.1 and 1.5 million tonnes of electrical appliances have to be disposed yearly. The disposal process results in about 4% dust residues. These residues contain metals like Al, Cu, Zn, Sn, Pb and Ni in concentrations of 24, 8, 3, 2, 2 and 2 %(w/w) respectively. In addition to these, precious metals like Ag and Au are also present in small amounts (Brandl *et al.*, 1999).

Sediments from rivers and docks also contain high amounts of toxic metals. When all these solid wastes are exposed to air and water, the toxic metals from them get mobilised.

Microorganisms involved

The most widely used microorganisms are *Thiobacillus ferrooxidans* and *Thiobacillus thiooxidans* (Colmer and Hinkle, 1947; Colmer *et al.*, 1950). These organisms tend to live in acidic environments, such as sulphide deposits, acid mine drainage, hot-springs and volcanic fissures. They attack several forms of sulphur and oxidize them to sulphate ion. Although *Thiobacillus ferrooxidans* and *Thiobacillus thiooxidans* are very essential to the bacterial leaching of metals, they are by no means the only organisms with an important role in the process. Acidophilic bacteria such as *Leptospirillum ferrooxidans, Thiobacillus organoparus,*

Thiobacillus acidophilus, Acidiphillum cryptum and thermoacidophilic bacterium *Sulfolobus acidocaldarius* are reported to be important for metal extraction from tailing, low grade ores, sludge and other metal containing industrial waste (Leroux *et al.*, 1978; Norris, 1983). The optimum pH for the activity of these organisms range between pH 2 to 3.5, they are known as acidophilic iron and/or sulphur oxidisers. Several moderate acidophilic thiobacilli have also been reported for sulphur oxidation with higher and wider pH range for their activity. They reduced the pH of the synthetic medium from pH as high as 7.5 to as low as 2.2. These organisms decrease the pH of the medium with the rate of 0.3 to o.4 units per day.

Apart from autotrophic bacteria, the mixture of chemoorganotrophic *Bacillus* spp., *Clostridium* spp. were reported to solubilize heavy metals from industrial waste. Solubilization of metals by metabolites of *Aspergillus niger, Penicillium simplicissium, Candida lipolytica, Rhizopus arrhizus* etc. is documented in the literature (Dave and Natarajan, 1981; Burgstaller and Schinner, 1993; Strasser *et al.*, 1994).

Mechanism of metal extraction

A variety of autotrophic and heterotrophic bacteria, fungi and archaea are known to catalyse metal extraction from ores, solid waste, mine tailings, industrial and sewage sludge. The ability of microorganisms to leach and mobilize metals from solid materials comprises three main principles, namely (1) redox reactions (2) formation of organic or inorganic acids and (3) the excretion of complexing agents.

Redox reaction and inorganic acid production

The important aerobic autotrophic organisms associated with the metal extraction process are *Thiobacillus ferrooxidans* and *Thiobacillus thiooxidans.* Their carbon requirements are fulfilled by CO_2 from the atmosphere and the energy required for the CO_2 fixation is derived from the oxidation of ferrous, sulphur and reduced sulphur compounds to ferric or sulphate by the direct (equation 1) or by the indirect (equation 2 and 3) process (Lundgren and Silver,1980; Sand *et al.*, 1999; Tributsch, 1999).

$$MS + 2O_2 \xrightarrow[\textit{Thiobacillus thiooxidans}]{\textit{Thiobacillus ferrooxidans}} M^{+2} + SO_4^{-2} \qquad (1)$$

$$4FeSO_4 + O_2 + 2H_2SO_4 \longrightarrow 2Fe_2(SO_4)_3 + H_2O \qquad (2)$$

$$4Fe_2(SO_4)_3 + 2MS + 4H_2O + 2O_2 \longrightarrow 2M^{+2} + 2SO_4^{-2} + 8FeSO_4 + 4H_2SO_4 \qquad (3)$$

Reaction 1 and 2 take place enzymatically under the active participation of both the species of *Thiobacillus,* whereas reaction 3 takes place chemically without the role of microorganisms. A cyclic process between reaction 2 and 3 results in more and more solubilization of the metals. Moreover, the excess H_2SO_4 generated during this process further enhances the metal extraction. Bacterial leaching of heavy metals from anaerobically digested sludge has been well investigated by Wong and Henry (1984) and Jain and Tyagi (1992) and more than 60% solubilization of Cd, Zn, Ni and Cu was reported in 12 to 14 days of time (Tyagi, 1992; Jain and Tyagi, 1992; Wong and Henry, 1984).

Organic acid production

Heterotrophic microorganisms are known to contribute to the release of heavy metals from rocks, minerals and solid waste. The heterotrophic microorganisms require organic carbon for their growth and energy supply. Heterotrophic metal extraction is mainly due to the production of organic acids and other metabolic compounds (Burgstaller and Schinner, 1993; Strasser *et al.*, 1994, Sayer *et al.*, 1995).

$$\text{Carbohydrate} \xrightarrow[\textit{Aspergillus}\text{ sp.}, \; \textit{Penicillium}\text{ sp.}]{\textit{Actinomucor}\text{ sp.}} \text{Oxalate/malate, gluconate, citrate etc.} \quad (4)$$

$$\text{Organic acids + Insoluble metal} \longrightarrow \text{Soluble metals} \quad (5)$$

When *Pseudomonas putida* was exposed to fly ash in glucose containing medium, the pH decreased from 8 to 4 and the organism produced citric acid which acted as leaching agent for the extraction of Cd, Ni, Zn and Cu (Krebs *et al.*, 1997).

Applications and patents

Mine and solid waste materials viz. tailing, fly ash, filter dust, galvanic sludge, sewage sludge and slag often represent significant amount of toxic and valuable metal containing materials. For such waste, microbial processing can be economically effective and is thought to be a useful process to recover or recycle the metal. As can be seen from the Table 1, recent patents on the bioleaching process show the application of *Thiobacillus, Aspergillus, Penicillium, Pseudomonas,* and *Bacillus* etc. for the recovery of metals from various industrial wastes.

Table 1: Patent applications since 1990 for the biohydrometallurgical processing of coal fly ash, soil and industrial waste.

Treated Material	Microorganisms	Recovered metals
Integrated circuits	Mixture of Gram-positive cocci and Gram-negative rods with *Sulfolobus*	Ga, Ge
Municipal sludge	*Thiobacillus thiooxidans* *Thiobacillus thioparus*	Cd, Cr, Cu, Mn, Ni, Pb, Zn
Coal fly ash	*Thiobacillus thiooxidans*	Al, Ti, Co
Soil	Endogenous microorganisms, *Thiobacillus thiooxidans, Thiobacillus ferrooxidans*	Ba, Cd, Co, Cu, Hg, Ni, Pb, Zn etc.
Iron oxide-metal coprecipitates	*Clostridium* sp.	Cd, Cr, Ni, Pb, Zn
Industrial waste	Chemoorganotrophic bacteria	Cu, U
Industrial sludge	Activated sludge	Heavy metals

Only a few patents have been published concerning biohydrometallurgical process. Most of the patents covering biological leaching process deal with the leaching of low grade ore. In last one decade, nine patents have been published for metal extraction from fly ash, industrial waste, municipal sludge and contaminated soil (Brombachar *et al.*, 1997). The removal of toxic metals from the solid waste and soil can drastically reduce disposal costs, and furthermore precious metals could be recovered.

Perspective for solid waste bioleaching

Bioleaching opens an important field of research to support sustainable development. According to the Agenda 21 established at the Earth Summit in Rio de Taneiro '92, it is must to do progress towards a more environmentally friendly technology for winning of mineral resources (Keating, 1993; Krebs, 1997). The application of bioleaching process for solid waste treatment is a step in this direction. Solids from waste incineration such as slag and ash, dust residues from shredding of electronic waste etc. are considered "artificial ores" or secondary metal resources.

It could be possible to recycle the leached and recovered metals so that the metal manufacturing industry can reuse them as raw materials. In addition, the costs of disposing such sludges are reduced by such biological treatment, because the residues can be deposited at lower cost in landfills or can be used for construction purpose (Krebs, 1997; Brandl *et al.*, 1999).

Bioleaching represents a 'clean technology' process with a low cost and energy, as compared with conventional thermal solid waste treatment process. Of course, the technology is still in its infancy. Industry views this as a very promising technology for sustainable development.

REFERENCES

Agate, A.D. (1996). Recent advances in microbial mining. *World J. Microbiol. Biotechnol.* 12 : 487–495.

Blais, J.F., Tyagi, R.D., Auclair, J.C. and Lavoie, M.C. (1992). Indicator bacteria : Reduction in sewage sludge by a metal bioleaching process. *Water Res.* 26 : 487-495.

Bosecker, K. (1997). Microbial recycling of mineral waste products. *Acta. Biotechnol.* **7** : 487-497.

Bosecker, K. (1999). Microbial leaching in environmental clean-up programmes. In *Biohydrometallurgy and the environment towards the mining of the 21st century. Proc. Intl. Biohydrometallurgy Symp.* (*Ed.* Amils, R. and Ballester, A.), Elsevier, Spain, pp 533-536.

Brandl, H. Bosshard, R. and Wegmann, M. (1999). Computer-munching microbes: Metal leaching from electronic scrap by bacteria and fungi. In *Biohydrometallurgy and the environment towards the mining of the 21st century. Proc. Intl. Biohydrometallurgy Symp.* (*Ed.* Amils, R. and Ballester, A.), Elsevier, Spain, pp 569-576.

Brombachar, C., Bachofen, R. and Brandi, H. (1997). Biohydrometallurgical processing of solids : A patent review. *Appl. Environ. Biotechnol.* 48 : 577-587.

Brombachar, C., Bachofen, R. and Brandi, H. (1999). Microbial metal recovery from industrial waste. *Proc. 4th World Cong. With Company Displays.* Geneva, Switzerland.

Bruce, A.M. and Davis, R.D.C. (1989). Sewage sludge disposal : current and further options. *Water Sci. Technol.* 21 : 1113-1128.

Burgstaller, W. and Schinner, F. (1993). Leaching of metals with fungi. *J. Biotechnol.* 27 : 91-116.

Christy, A.D., Myers, M.J., Gagliano, W.R.B. and Tuovinen, O.H. (1999). Solid state bioreactor design for laboratory scale landfill studies. In *Phytoremediation and innovative strategies for specialized remedial actions* (*Ed.* Leeson, A. and Alleman, B.C.), Battelle Press, Columbus, Ohio, pp 181-186.

Colmer, A.R. and Hinkle, M.E. (1947). The role of microorganisms in acid mine drainage. *Science.* 106 : 253-256.

Colmer, A.R., Temple, K.L. and Hinkle, M.E. (1950). An iron-oxidizing bacterium from the acid drainage of some bituminous coal mines. *J. Bacteriol.* 59 : 317-328.

Dave, S.R. (1980). Microbiological and bioleaching studies on metallurgical bacteria cultured from Indian sulphidic mine water. Ph.D. Thesis, The University of Mysore, Mysore, India.

Dave, S.R. (1991). Bioremoval of metal from waste. *Proc. National Symp. Application of Geomicrobiology in India.* 48-53.

Dave, S.R. (1995a). Biooxidation of metals from sludge by mix bacterial culture. *Proc. Acad. Environ. Biol.*, 4 : 39-42.

Dave, S.R. (1995b). Bioremediation of metals-An attractive potential microbial technology. *Proc. 3rd Int. Conf. Appropriate Waste Mgmt. Technologies for Developing Countries.* 773-779.

Dave, S.R. and Natarajan, K.A. (1981). Leaching of copper and zinc from oxidised ores by fungi. *Hydrometallurgy.* **7** : 235-242.

Davis, R.D. (1986). Cadmium in sludges used as fertilizer. *Experientia Supplementum.* 50 : 55.

Davis, R.D. (1987). Use of sewage sludge on land in the United Kingdom. *Water Sci. Technol.* 19 : 1-8.

Donati, E., Pogliani, C. and Boiardi, J.L. (1997). Aerobic leaching of covellite by *Thiobacillus ferrooxidans. Appl. Environ. Biotechnol.* 47 : 636-639.

Hamer, G. (1993). Bioremediation : a response to gross environmental abuse. *TIBTECH.*, 11 : 317-319.

Hayes, T.D., Jewell, W.J. and Kabrick, R.M. (1980). Heavy metals removal from sludge using combined biological/chemical treatment. *Proc. 34th Ind. Waste Conf.*, pp 529-543. Purdue University, West Lafayette.

Horvath, B. and Gruiz, K. (1996). Impact of metalliferous ore mining activity on the environment in Gyongyosoroszi, Hungary. *Sci. Total Environ.* 184 : 215-227.

Jain, D.K. and Tyagi, R.D. (1992). Leaching of heavy metals from anaerobic sewage sludge by sulfur-oxidzing bacteria. *Enzyme Mircob. Technol.* 14 : 376-383.

Keating, M. (1993). Erdgipfel 1992-Agenda fur eine nachhaltinge Entwicklung. Centre for our Common Future, Geneva.

Krebs, W., Brombachar, C. Bosshard, P.P., Bachofen, R. and Brandl, H. (1997). Microbial recovery of metals form solids. *FEMS Microbiol. Rev.* 20 : 605-617.

Leroux, N.W., Wakerley, D.S. and Perry, V.P. (1978). Leaching of minerals using bacteria other than *Thiobacillus.* In *Metallurgical applications of bacterial leaching and related microbiological phenomena.* (*Ed.* Murr, L.E., Torma, A.E. and Brierley, J.A.)., Academic Press, New York, pp 167.

Lester, J.N., Strerrit, R.M. and Kirk, P.W.W. (1983). Significance and behaviour of heavy metals in waste water treatment process : II. Sludge treatment and disposal. *Sci. Total. Environ.* 30 : 45-83.

Liu, S. and Suflita, J.M. (1993). Ecology and evolution of microbial populations for bioremediation. *TIBTECH.* 11 : 344-352.

Lundgren, D.G. and Silver, M. (1980). Ore leaching by bacteria. *Ann. Rev. Microbiol.* 34 : 263-283.

Menon, A.G. (1995). Biotechnology of complex sulphide ore processing. Ph.D. Thesis, Gujarat University, Ahmedabad, India.

Menon, A.G. and Dave, S.R. (1995). Observation on heavy metal extraction from the tailings of Zawar mines. *Proc. Acad. Environ. Biol.* 4 : 43-48.

Moore, J.N. and Luoma, S.N. (1990). Hazardous waste from large-scale metal extraction. *Environ. Sci. Technol.* 24 : 1278-1285.

Norris, P.R. (1983). Iron and mineral oxidation with *Leptospirillum* like bacteria. In *Recent Progress in Biohydrometallurgy* (*Ed.* Torma, A.E. and Rossi, G.)., Associazione Mineraria Sarda, Cagliari, Italy, pp 83.

Rossi, G. (1990). Biohydrometallurgy. McGraw-Hill Book Company, New York.

Sand, W., Gehrke, T., Jozsa, P.G. and Schippers, A. (1999). Direct versus indirect bioleaching. In *Biohydrometallurgy and the environment towards the mining of the 21st century. Proc. Intl. Biohydrometallurgy Symp* (*Ed.* Amils, R. and Ballester, A.), Elsevier, Spain, pp 27-49.

Sayer, J.A., Raggett, S.L. and Gadd, G.M. (1995). Solubilization of insoluble metal compounds by soil fungi : development of a screening method for solubilizing ability and metal tolerance. *Mycol. Res.* 99 : 987-993.

Scheltinga, H.M.J. (1987). Sludge in agriculture : the European approach. *Water Sci. Technol.* 19 : 9-18.

Strasser, H., Burgstaller, W. and Schinner, F. (1994). High yield production of oxalic acid for metal leaching processes by *Aspergillus niger. FEMS Microbiol. Lett.* 119 : 365-370.

Tipre, D.R. (1999). Scale-up of bioextraction process for the polymetallic concentrate. Ph.D. Thesis, Gujarat University, Ahmedabad, India.

Tipre, D.R., Vora, S.B. and Dave, S.R. (1998). Improved metal extraction by selected *Thiobacillus ferrooxidans* consortium from polymetallic concentrate. *J. Sci. Indus. Res.* 57 : 805-808.

Torma, A.E. (1988). Leaching of metals. In *Biotechnology* (*Ed.* Rehm, H.J. and Reed, G.) VCH Verlag, Weinheim, pp 367-400.

Tributsch, H. (1999). Direct versus indirect bioleaching. In *Biohydrometallurgy and the environment towards the mining of the 21st century. Proc. Intl. Biohydrometallurgy Symp* (Eds. Amils, R. and Ballester, A.), Elsevier, Spain, pp 51-60.

Tyagi, R.D. (1992). Microbial leaching of metals from municipal sludge : Effects of sludge solids concentration. *Proc. Biochem.* 27 : 89-96.

Tyagi, R.D. and Couillard, D. (1987). Bacterial leaching of metals from digested sewage sludge. *Proc. Biochem.* 114-117.

Webber, M.D. (1988). Controle de la concentration de metaux lourds dans les sols apres epandage de boues degout municipales : l' approche canadienne. *Sci. Tech. Eau.* 21(1) : 45-51.

Wong, L. and Henry, J.G. (1984). Decontaminating biology sludge for agricultural use. *Water Sci. Technol.* 17 : 575-586.

Microbiology and Biotechnology for Sustainable Development (Ed. P.C. Jain),
CBS Publishers & Distributors, New Delhi (2004), pp. 42–58.

A-5

Potential of Microorganisms for the Management of *Lantana camara* in India: Possibilities and Prospects

A. K. Pandey, Archana Pandey, G.M. Shrivastava and R.C. Rajak
Department of Biological Science, R.D. University
Jabalpur-482 001 (M.P.) India

Abstract

Lantana camara *L., native of tropical America popularly known as Sadabahar was probably introduced in India at the beginning of 20th Century as an ornamental and hedge plant. It is now creating serious hazards in India and very difficult to control through conventional methods of weed control. Ever since this weed became a menace, several control methods are being recommended. Role of microorganism in sustainable management of weed has now been recognized as one of the most important way to control such weeds. Therefore, the possibilities of exploitation of microbes are briefly discussed in this article.*

Key Words: *Lantana camara,* herbicides, microorganisms, fungi.

INTRODUCTION

Lantana camara L., native of tropical America is a globally important weed, which was introduced in India at the beginning of 20th Century as an ornamental and hedge plant. It is one of the top ten most noxious weeds of the world. It imposes serious allelopathic effects to most of the forest and other native vegetations besides, responsible for serious illness to human and animals. Many control methods viz. Physical, Chemical or even Biological control through insect have been tried. However, these methods of its control have failed due to or the other reason. Herbicidal potential of the microorganism especially Fungi have attracted a large group of scientist world over. *Lantana* is also attacked by several organisms, therefore the present article aimed to highlight the possibilities of the exploiting of microorganism as herbicides for the management of *Lantana camara*.

A. The weed, *Lantana camara* L.

Lantana camara (Angiospermae, Dicotyledones, lignosae, verbenales, verbinaceae) is a native of the tropical America viz., Mexico, Central America, South America, South and North Argentina (Swarbrick, 1986). It has several popular names such as White saga, Kayakit, Cariaqito, Big saga (English), Wild saga, Mavisou, Mille fleurs, Sauge, Verveine, Malbisou, Pinyin etc. in various countries of the world (Duke and Ayensu, 1985). Taxonomy of weed has been extensively reviewed in several publications (Louw, 1948; Smith and Smith, 1982; Spies and Du Piessis, 1987; Bansal, 1988; Neser and Cilliers, 1989). It was introduced as an ornamental and hedge plant to other areas of the world in late 1700's, 1800's and in early 1900's (Denton *et al.*, 1991). Now it is widely distributed in tropical, subtropical and temperate regions of the world and has been reported as a weed from 47 countries (Holm *et al.*, 1977).

Holm and Herberger (1969) listed it as one of the ten world's worst weeds. According to Holm et al (1977) it has infested millions of hectares of natural grazing lands in Asia and Africa and some areas of India its invasion of cultivated land has led to the shifting of entire village. It can withstand to a wide range of climatic and edaphic conditions ranging from a rainfall of 200 to 30 inches / annum and found to be highly drought resistant. It grows well on nutrient rich and poor soils, in low lying as well as on high hill slopes up to a height of 4500 ft. above sea level. Vigorous growth of *Lantana* can be seen even in hot and dry climate with a bare depth of soil between two rocks. It is a poor competitor under dense shade conditions and grows profusely in acidic soil. It cannot withstand frequent tillage. This is the reason that our cultivated areas under crops and orchards have so far been free from this weed (Bansal, 1988; Pandey and Pandey, 2001).

It was probably introduced in India during 1809 as an ornamental and hedge plant and It is also popularly known as Chadurangi, Ghaneri (Mar.), Pulikhumpa (Tel.), Unnichedi (Tam.), Ghanidalia (Guj.), Rai Muniya, Panbidia (M.P.), Arippu (Mal.), Natahugida, Hesika (Kan.), Phulnu, Punch Phool, Baraphulun, Bunch berry, red phulanoo, kukri (pahari Hindi) etc. in India (Ambasta, 1986). In India, the plant is most abundant in the scrub-type forests of the Deccan Plateau, parts of the Vindhyas, Chhota Nagpur and Assam, while it is sparsely distributed in delta regions, particularly those on the eastern coast (Gujral and Vasudevan, 1983; Gupta and Pawar, 1984). Although the plant is now spread to almost all the states but the density is more in certain parts of Aandhra Pradesh, Bihar, Madhya Pradesh, Rajasthan, Himanchal Pradesh, Kerela, Orrisa, Punjab, Tamilnadu, Kashmir, Delhi, Karnataka and Assam (Singh *et al.*, 1988). In Madhya Pradesh and Chatisgarh, it is considered as one of the major threat for resurgence of forest trees (Pandey, 2000).

In recent years it has covered almost all the uncultivated land whether forests, pastures, railway lines, road sides, grazing lands or hilly tracts. Initially *Lantana* was confined to marshy foothills but due to its capability to withstand the adverse climatic conditions, it has now present upto 2000 m and can be seen almost every where. The weed normally spread though the fruit (seeds) being edible and largely devoured by birds, which pass the seeds perhaps far away where fruit was gathered. Sometimes the weed is also spread through the cuttings and trasnporting of shrubs for fuel and animal bedding purposes (Kanwar and Kharwara, 1988; Pandey and Pandey, 2001).

The weed is known to impose serious allelopathic effects on the nearby vegetations due to the release of toxins by seeds, leaves, twigs, roots, inflourescence and their residues. (Acchireddy and Singh, 1984; Mersle and Singh, 1987; Wadhwani and Bhardwaja, 1981; Sahid and Sugau, 1993). The allelochemicals were found to be polar and slightly acidic and might be phenolic in nature (Achhireddy *et al.*, 1985). *Lantana* has also been reported to be a "Symptom less carrier" of spike disease of Sandal (Nayar and Srimathi, 1968). Its thickets are also said to be breeding sites for feral pigs and insect vectors of diseases (CIBC, 1982). *Lantana* is also known to be highly hazardous to human and animal health. Several poisoning cases have been reported from different parts of the world (Gopinath and Ford, 1969; Sharma *et al.*, 1988).

In India, cases of *Lantana* toxicity have been frequently observed in the field, which lead to high morbidity and mortality (Sharma *et al.* 1981; Singh *et al.* 1988; Sharma, 1988). Sharma *et al.* (1981) reported the presence of lantadene (Lantanin) as high as 6-7 mg/gm dry weights. The course of illness and severity of symptoms depends upon the quantity of foliage eaten. The survival rate varies from one location to another. In India the survival of affected animals has been very rare and the symptomatic treatments used are not very effective. Furthermore, if the affected animals survive they subsequently exhibit illness and their rearing is not possible (Sharma *et al.*, 1981). Besides these, the weed is also known to directly affect humans. *Lantana* leaves are very rough, causing skin irritation on contact and give off an offensive smell causing headache and giddiness thereby making it irksome to harvest any other products in the vicinity of *Lantana* bushes (Sharma *et al.*, 1988). In additions, green fruits are toxic to children (Wolfson and Solomons, 1964). However, ripe fruits are very commonly eaten by children without any overt adverse effect. The nature and chemical structure of toxic principles have extensively been discussed in several publications (Louw, 1948; Barton and De Mayo, 1954; Barton *et al.*, 1956; Hart *et al.*, 1996 a,b; Beeby 1978).

B. Management Strategies

a. Physical and Cultural: Utilization of manual energy, animal power, or fuel to eradicate the weed, uprooting and burning of the plants and subsequent fodder tree plantation have been recommended to control this weed (Sharma *et al.*, 1983; Sharma, 1988). It has also been recommended that the bulk of *Lantana* should be burned or bulldozed and then the pasture sown with a shade tolerant grass and a climbing legume (Hannan- Jones, 1998). However, wide spread burning is not possible in conservation area or in many inaccessible areas. It is also ineffective as there is usually inadequate fuel to maintain a fire and their root may not be killed.

b. Chemical herbicides: The large-scale foliar application of herbicides is usually restricted to hand or powered spot application to infestations in plantations or along the edges of natural vegetation and pasture. However aerial applications with helicopter as used in some countries is possible in some more open locations. However, indiscriminate use of pesticides for the past few decades or so has done great harm to humans, animals, vegetation and the environment as a whole (Pandey *et al.*, 1996 a, b). As the public's and resource manager's demand for safer herbicides increases and legislative constraints continue to reduce the amount of herbicides used in developing countries, there is increased pressure to develop and improve environmentally friendly weed control strategies.

c. Microbial Management: *(i) Microbial herbicides:* Biological control of *Lantana* through insect have seriously attempted by many workers which has been excellently reviewed by Denton *et al.* (1991) and Pandey and Pandey (2001). Some phaenroganic parasites have also tried against this weed (Rajak *et al.*1985; Pandir, 1985). However, shorter life cycle, difficulty in mass production, storage, transportation and application and lace of consistency in the effectiveness are the major constraints in their application as bio-control agents.

Biological control by exploiting different categories of microorganism has attracted the attention of a large group of workers worldwide. It has reached to a point where four distinct strategies have been clearly defined. These are Classical, Bioherbicidal (= mycoherbicidal), Phytotoxic biorationals and Integrated Weed Management Programme. Biological, technological and economical perspectives of these strategies have been excellently reviewed in many publications (Freeman, 1987; Charudattan, 1991; Templeton and Heiny, 1989; Templeton *et al.*, 1986; Templeton, 1992; Auld, 1990; Hasija *et al.* 1994; Auld and Morin, 1995; Prasad, 1999; Pandey *et al.*, 1996, a b, 97; Pandey, 1999, 2001; Hoagland, 1990,1999, 2001). *L. camara* is also known to attack by a variety of organisms, which are briefly discussed herewith.

The weed, *Lantana* is also attacked by a variety of pathogens. They include fungi, bacteria, viruses, mycoplasma etc. that exhibits levels of parasitism ranging form obligate parasitism to saprophytism. Amongst these, fungal pathogens are ranked first as for their suitability as biocontrol agent is concerned which is also evidenced by the patenting and commercialization of many of them as mycoherbicides (Pandey, 1999).

A thorough and extensive survey of literature on the pathogens of *L. camara* showed that the weed is attacked by more than 130 fungal species / strains in different parts of the world including India (Table 1). Amongst these more then 90% of fungal strains have been reported from India. However, unfortunately no systemic and serious evaluation of these has been attempted in this country. More than 25 fungi have been observed to attack living leaves and two pathogen viz, *Sclerotium rolfsii, Diplodia lantanicola* and *Corynespora cassicola* incites severe collar, stem or twig blights. According to Barreto *et al.* (1995) *Ceratiobasidium lantanae-camarae, Mycovellosiella lantanae var. lantanae, Prospodium tuberculatum, Micropustulomyces muscilagenosus and Puccinia lantanae* etc. have significant pathogenic potential and could be developed as mycopherbicides for the management of noxious weed *Lantana.*

Table 1: Fungi Associated with *Lantana camara L.*

Name of the pathogen	PPI	References
Acanthostigma (= Nematostoma) lantanae (Henn.) Thesis	NM	Stevenson (1975)
Aecidium lantanae Ramchandra Rao	DS, LL	Rao (1965), Tilak and Rao (1966); Hiratsuka and Commins, 1963; Commins, 1940

(Contd.)

Name of the pathogen	PPI	References
Aleurodiscus sp.	NM	Barreto *et al.* (1995)
Alternaria sp.	NM	Barreto *et al.* (1995)
A. alternata (Fr.) Keissler	LL	Pandey (2000)
Anhellia lantanae (Viegas)Arx	NM	Evans (1987)
Anthostomella spirilla Panwar and Kaur	DS	Panwar and Kaur (1976)
Aphanostigme lantanae Srin. and Sathe	DS	Srinivasulu and Sathe (1970)
Bagnisiella australis Speg.	DS	Rangaswami *et al.* (1970), Patil and Thite, (1977), Anahosur (1969)
B. mangiferae Tilak and Ramachandra Rao	DT	Vaidya (1975)
Calospheria lantanae Tilak and Nagre	DT	Tilak and Nagre (1964), Rizwi (1977)
Calospora lantanae Anahosur	DT	Anahosur (1969)
Capnodium sp.	DT	Patil and Thite (1977), Johnston (1960), Rangaswami *et al.* (1970)
Ceratobasidium lantanae-camarae Evans *et al.*	LL	Barreto *et al.* (1995)
Cercospora sp.	NM	Orieux and Felix (1968)
Cercospora canescens Ellis and Martin	NM	Orieux and Felix (1968)
Cercospora lantanicola Chupp	LL	Chupp (1954)
Cercospora lantanae-aculeatae Yen	NM	Rajak and Rajak (1981)
Cercospora lantanae-camarae Yen and Gilles	LL	Rajak and Rajak (1981)
C. lantanae-camarae Rajak and Rajak	LL	Rajak and Rajak (1981)
C. lantanae indicae Munjal, Lal and Chona	LL	Patil (1975), Patil and Thite (1978)
Ceratosphaeria bicellula Panwar and Kaur	DS	Panwar and Kaur (1976)
Cercospora lantanae Tilak and Kale	DS	Tilak and Kale (1967)
Cladosporium oxysporum Berk. and Curtis	NM	Barreto *et al.* (1995)
Cochiloboluslunatus (Walk) Boed	LL	Pandey (2000)
Colletotrichum capsici (Syd.) Butler and Bisby	NM	Sarbhoy *et al.* (1986)
C. dematium (Pers. exFr.) Grove	LL	Pandey (2000)
Comatricha lurida Lister.	DT	Singh and Puspawathy (1966)
Corynespora cassiicola (Berk. and Curtis) Wei	LT	Agarwal and Sarbhoy (1984), Pandey, (2000)
Comatrich lurida Lister	DT	Singh and Puspawathy (1966)
Dendryphiella aspera Barreto and David	LL	Barreto *et al.* (1995)
Diatrype cryptostegiae Tilak	DT	Rao (1966c), Rizwi (1977)
D. chloroscarca Berk. L Br.	DT	Evans (1987)
D. pavattae Patil	DT	Patil and Thite (1978)
D. lantanae Earle.	DT	Gaikwad (1973), Patil (1975), Ahmed (1967)
Diatrypella citriocola Ellis and Evans	DT	Rizwi (1977)
Didymosphaeria donacina (Niessl.) Sacc.	DL	Anahosur (1971)

(Contd.)

Name of the pathogen	PPI	References
D. futilis (Berk. and Br.) Rehm.	DT	Reddy (1973)
Diplodia lantanicola Ahmad	DL	Ahmad (1967)
Diplodia lantanicola Ahmad	LT, LS	Rao (1966c), Ahmad, (1967)
Epiphyma (=Botryosphaeria) *nervisequens* (Chardon) Mill and Burton	NM	Barreto *et al.* (1995)
Eutypa aspera (Nitschke) Fuckel	NM	Barreto *et al.* (1995)
Eutypa lantanae Patil	Dead branches	Patil (1983)
Eutypella russodes (Berk. and Br.) Berl	Dead twigs	Jadhav *et al.* (1978)
Fusarium oxysporum Schl. ExFr.	Seedlings	Pandey, (2000)
Gloeosporium sp.	NM	Norse (1974)
Godronia lantanae (Cash) Seaver	NM	Farr *et al.* (1989)
Haplosporella lantanae Kachroo	Dead twigs	Kachroo (1966), Agarwal and Sarbhoy (1983), Pandey, (1990)
Helicosporium Hohnel.	Decaying twing	Chouhan and Panwar (1980)
Helminthosporium mauritianum Cooke.	Dead twigs	Saikia and Sarbhoy (1980)
Hendersonia sp.		
H. velutinum Link.	Dead twigs	Saikia and Sarbhoy (1980)
Hypoxylon notatum Berk. and Curt.	Twigs	Pande (1972, 1974)
Hysterium lantanae Tilak and Ramchandra	Dried stem	Tilak and Rao (1966)
Leptosphaeria conithyrium (Fuckel.) Sacc.	Twigs	Panwar and Gehlot (1973)
L. haemitites (Rob.) Niessl	Twigs	Evans, (1987)
L. isocellula Panwar and Kaur	Dead twigs	Panwar and Kaur (1977)
L. rajasthanensis Panwar and Kaur	Dead twigs	Panwar and Kaur (1977)
Macrovalsaria megalospora (Mont.) Sivanesan	Dead twigs	Panwar and Kaur (1977)
Massarina mucosa Panwar and Kaur	Dead twigs	Panwar and Kaur (1976)
M. tricellula Panwar and Kaur	Dried stem	Panwar and Kaur (1975)
Meliola sp.	NM	Barreto *et al.* (1995)
Meliola ambigua Pat. and Gaillard	NM	Barreto *et al.* (1995).Piening (1962), Stevenson (1975), Baker and Dalee (1951), Farr *et al.* (1989)
Meliola cookeana Speg.	NM	Farr *et al.* (1989)
Meliola durantae Gaillard	NM	Barreto *et al.* (1995)
Memnoniella echinata (Riv.) Gall.	Twigs	Agarwal and Sarbhoy (1979)
Merulius corium (Pers.) Fr.	Dead twigs	Bakshi and Singh (1988)
Metasphaeria abuensis Panwar and Kaur	Dead twigs	Panwar and Kaur (1976)
Microdiplodia minuta (Ellis and Tracy)	Dead twigs	Evans (1987)

(Contd.)

Name of the pathogen	PPI	References
Micropustulomyces mucilaginosus Barreto	Dead twigs	Barreto *et al.* (1995)
Mycovellosiella lantanae (Chupp) Deighton var. *Lantane cercospora lantanae* chupp = *Cladosporium trichophilum* Petrak and Giferri = *Chactotrichum lantanae* petrak)	LL	Norse (1974), Waterson (1947), Chupp (1954), Stevenson (1975), Farr *et al.* (1989), Deighton, (1974), Barreto *et al.* (1995).
Mycovellosiella lantanae (Chupp) Deighton var. *Cubensis* Deighton	LL	Deighton (1974)
Myrothecium roridum Tode ex Fr.	LL	Johnston (1960), Tripathi and Udit Narain (1985)
Mysterographium multiseptum Panwar and Kaur	DT	Panwar and Kaur (1977)
Nectria wegeliniana (Rehm) Rehm ex Strasser *N. polyporina* Petch.	NM	Barreto *et al.* (1995) Patil and Thite, (1977)
Oidium sp.	NM	Butler and Bisby (1960)
Oidium erysiphoides Fr.	NM	Viegas (1961)
Oospora spp.	LL	Barreto *et al.* (1995)
Ophiobolus lantanae Ramchandra Rao	LL	Rao (1966d)
Ostropa indica Kale and Tilak	Twigs	Patil and Thite (1977)
Patellaria lantanae Rao	DT	Rao (1967)
Periconia cookei Mason and Ellis	LL	Gupta *et al.* (1983)
Perisporiopsis lantanae (Stevens) Barreto (*Perisporina lantanae* Stevens)	LS	Barreto *et al.* (1995), Evans (1987)
Peroneutypell echidna (Cook, Deighton) B	DS stem	Barreto *et al.* (1995)
Pestalotiopsis guepinii stey (Desm)	LL	Pandey (2000)
Phoma lantanae Verwood and Duplossis	LL	Singh and Agarwal (1974), Gorter (1981)
Phoma sp.	NM	Barreto *et al.* (1995)
P. multirostrata (Mathur *et al.*) Doren and Boevan.	LL	Pandey (2000)
Phomopsis lantanae (Costa and Camara) Sutton (= *Phomopsioides lantanae* Costa and Camara)	LL	Sutton (1980)
Phyllosticta lantanae - verae Trotter (as *P. lantanicola*)	NM	Stevenson (1975)
Phyllosticta lantanae Pass.	NM	Norse (1974)
Phyllosticta lantanicola Stevenson	LL	Stevenson (1975)
Phyllosticta sp.	NM	Barreto *et al.* (1995)
Physalospora abdita (Berk. and Curtis) Voorhees	NM	Farr *et al.* (1989)
Pithomyces ellisii Rao and Chary	DS	Rao and Chary (1972)
Pleospora herbarum	DS	Rao (1966a)
P. lantanae Jadhav, Somani and Wangikar	DT	Jadhav *et al.* (1978)
P. wehmeyerii Pande	DT	Pai (1968)

(Contd.)

Name of the pathogen	PPI	References
Prospodium tuberculatum (Speg.) Arthur (= Uredo tuberculata speg. = *Puccinia tuberculata* speg.)	LL	Barreto *et al.* (1995), Evans (1987), Stevenson (1975), Dale (1955)
Protostroma indica Mhaskar and Rao	DS	Mhaskar and Rao (1972)
Pseudocercospora formosana (Yamam.) Deighton (= *Cercospora formosana* Ysamam.)	NM	Peregrine and Ahmed (1982), Leather and Hor (1969), Yamamoto (1934), Yen and Lim (1980), Deighton (1976)
Pseudocercospora guianensis (Stevens and Solheim) Deighton (= *Cercospora guianensis*	LL	Chupp (1954), Hino and Tokeshi (1978)
Puccinia lantanae Farl. (= *Micropuccinia lantanae* (Farl.) Arthur and Jackson)	LL	Evans (1987), Norse (1974), Dade (1940), Baker and Dale (1951), Rios (1982), Stevenson (1975), Farr *et al.* (1989)
P. natalensis Dietel and Syd.	LL	Piening (1962), Evans (1987)
Ramularia sp.	Leaves	Evans (1987)
Rhizoctonia sp.	NM	Orillo and Valdez (1959), Farr *et al.* (1989)
Rhizoctonia solani Kuhn	NM	Farr *et al.* (1989)
Rosencheldia paraguaya Speg.	NM	Viegas (1961)
Sarcinella palwanensis (Syd.) Sahni	LL	Patil and Thite (1977)
Sclerotium rolfsii Sacc.	Leaves, stem	Pandey (2000)
Scolecobasidium sp.	NM	Barreto *et al.* (1995)
Scolecopeltidium lantanae Bat. and Lima	NM	Barreto *et al.* (1995)
Septoria lantanae Garman	Leaves	Garman (1915), Barreto *et al.* (1995)
Septoria lantanifolii Bat. and Bezerra	Leaves	Barreto *et al.*(1995)
Spegazzinia sundra Subram.	Stem	Desai and Patwardhan (1974), Rao and Anahosur (1971)
Sphaerulina sp.	NM	Barreto *et al.* (1995)
Stictis lantanae Tilak and Nanir	Dried stems	Tilak and Nanir (1975)
Stictis radiata (L.) Pers.	NM	Barreto *et al.*(1995)
Subramania poonensis Pande	Dead stems	Pande (1973), Desai and Patwardhan (1974)
Teichospora lantanae Ramchandra Rao	Dried stems and branches	Rao (1966b)
Teichosporella lantanae Tilak	Stems	Tilak (1966)
Torula harbarum f. sp. quaternalla Sacc.	Fallen culms	Agarwal and Sarbhoy (1979)
Tryblidaria maharashtrensis Anahosur	Twigs	Anahosur (1969)
T. pongamiae Ramachandra Rao	Dead stems	Tiwari *et al.* (1981)
Tryblidiella rufula (Spegg.) Sacc.	Leaves	Muthappa (1967)
Tubeufia helicomyces Hohnel	Dead Twigs	Chauhan and Panwar, 1980
Tympanopsis lantanae Ramchandra Rao	Dead stems	Rao (1965), Tilak and Rao (1966)

DT = Dead Twigs DS = Dead Stem LL = Living Leaves
NM = Not mentioned LS = Living stem LT = Living Twigs

Realizing the need and importance of its management, a microbial control programme has been undertaken which yielded several potentially pathogenic fungi (Table-2). Five isolates viz; *Lantana camara* LC#20, *Cochilobolus lunatus* LC#35, *Corynespora cassicola* LC#61, *Fusarium oxysporum* LC#34, and *Sclerotium rolfsii* LC# 58 were incited severe infection and responsible for complete death of the plant. (Pandey, 2000; Pandey and Pandey, 2001a). Similarly many other pathogen viz; *Alternaria* sp. LC# 17, *Colletotrichum dematium* LC#52, *Pestalotiopsis guepinii,* and *Phoma multirostratata* were also responsible for significant damage to weed. On the basis of overall performance *A. alternata* LC#20, which incited severe leaf blight and also colonized on growing tips and twigs of the weed was finally selected for development as mycoherbicide. The pathogen caused more than 83.30% ± 4.71 and 73.33% leaf area damage and mortality of seedlings respectively. Richard's broth medium was a most suitable growth medium supported maximum growth and sporelation when supported with other 25° ± 1°C, 4.2 pH, Potassium nitrate (N), sucrose (C), 1.75: 1 C/N ratios. Conidial germination and infectivity were also very high in such environment. For maximum mortality it requires slightly higher humidity supported by moderate temperature and longer dew duration (18-20 hrs.). Glyphosate (Chemical herbicide) and two other pathogen i.e. *Corynospora cassicola* LC#61 and *Cochilobolus lunatus* LC#35 were highly compatible with the pathogen and failed to infect economically important trees and crop plants. (Pandey, 2000; Pandey and Pandey, 2000; 2001).

Table 2: Origin and Pathogenecity Of Fungi From *Lantana* In M.P.

Name of Pathogens	Acces. No.	Origin of Isolates	Lesion Type	Detached
Alternaria sp.	LC-4	Bb, BC	LDB	3
	LC-5	Bb	LLB	3
	LC-17	PB	LDB	4
	LC-20	BC	LDB	5
Colletortichum dematium	LC-52	SP	A	3
Colletotrichum gloeosporioides	LC-16	BC	SB	2
Curvularia sp.	LC-35	BC	LLB	5
	LC-40	BH	SB	2
	LC-44	Ab	LLB	2
	LC-46	Ma	LDB	3
Fusarium sp.	LC-7	Bb	W	1
	LC-13	PB	SB	3
	LC-34	BC	W	5
	LC-45	Ma	W	2
Helminthosporium sp.	LC-9	Bb	SB	2
Pestalotia sp.	LC-2	Bb	LLB	2

(Contd.)

Name of Pathogens	Acces. No.	Origin of Isolates	Lesion Type b leaf assayc	Detached
Phoma sp.	LC-32	BC	LT	5
	LC-37	R	LDB	3
	LC-39	BH	SB	1
Phomopsis sp.	LC-3	SP	SB	1
Unidentified	LC-38	R	SLB	2
	LC-18	K	SB	1
	LC-19	PG	LLB	1
	LC-24	KG	LDB	1
	LC-25	UC	LDB	4-5
	LC-28	D	SB	2
	LC-29	D	SB	1
	LC-41	TG	SC	1
	LC-42	R	LDB	2
	LC-50	PB	SB	1

Source: Pandey and Pandey (2001).

A. Abbreviations for origins : AB = Abhanpur; Bb = Bhad - bhadha; BC = Bio-Science Campus; BH = Bergi Hills; D = Dindori; KG = Kashtal ghati; Ma = Maiher; PB = Pat Baba Hills; Pg = pathar Gaon; R=Rampur; SP = Sita Pahari; T=Tilwara Ghat.

B. Abbreviations for the types of lesions associated with the fungus in the field; A=Anthracnose; LLB=Large, light brown lesions; LDB=Large, dark brown lesions; LT=large ten lesions surrounded by a magenta discoloration; SB=Small brown lesions: Sc=Small circular lesions similar to type LT;W=Wilt.

C. Detached leaf rating: 0=No effect; 1=Up to 20% leaf area necrotic; 2=Up to 40% leaf area necrotic; 3=Up to 60% leaf area necrotic; 4=Up to 80 % leaf area necrotic; 5=Up to 100 % leaf area necrotic. The range of reactions for three leaf pieces is shown.

(ii) Phytotoxic metabolites: Microbial Biodiversity is considered as an invisible and vast source of large number of secondary metabolites / biochemicals. Microbes are referred as the "Biochemical factories" as they produce diverse biologically active compounds (secondary metabolites) under natural / extremeophilic conditions due to their metabolic plasticity. Highly destructive role of several such compounds as evidenced by plant diseases has attracted the attention of weed scientists world over for their exploitation in the management of weeds (Hoagland, 1990, 1999, 2001, Saxena and Pandey, 2001, Pandey, 2001). Despite of several reports of pathogenic and nonpathogenic fungal isolates, phytotoxicity of secondary metabolites of none of them has been evaluated. Recently Saxena and Pandey (2001) evaluated herbicidal potential of cell free culture filtrates of more then 20 fungi and observed very high herbicidal activity against *Lantana* in CFCF of *Alternaria alternata* LC#18. Acute chlorosis followed by death of plant parts sprayed was observed (Saxena *et al.,* 2001). Saxena (2000) reported maximum phytotoxic metabolites production in Richards broth fermentation medium at 30° ± 1°C, 4.0 pH, 21 days incubation containing sucrose (Carbon), Potassium nitrate

(nitrogen) and 4C: 2N ratio. Similarly Pandey *et al.* (2001) reported very high herbicidal activity of secondary metabolites obtained from eight fungi and CFCF from *Phoma herbarum* FGCC#03 was the most effective. Benzene fractions of CFCF of this isolate have maximum toxicity. Chandla (1999) have also reported significant phytoxicity of CFCF of two strains of streptomyces (GF#01 and GF#02). Crude culture filtrates of strains of *Streptomyces sp.* (GF_1 and GF_0) were also produces severe chlorosis followed by hyponasty and defoliations in the weed, *Lantana* (Chandla, 1999).

CONCLUSION

The advent and early success of the comical herbicides has stimulated the idea of crop and forestry production in a weed free environment, and up until recently, the clean crop-forestry productions have been the ultimate aim of weed control. Resulting environmental contaminations, difficulties in controlling specific weed species and increasing consumer pressure against all pesticide use have contributed to a re-examination of weed control strategies. This resulted into the extensive evaluation of several microorganisms and finally commercialization of few of them as microbial herbicides (Pandey, 1999). Preceeding discussions clearly indicate that the weed, *Lantana camara* is associated with a large number of potential pathogenic and non-pathogenic fungi and actinomycetes. Amongst pathogenic forms, *Alternareia spp. Phoma sp., Corynespora cassicola, Coehliobolus lunatus, Fusarium oxysporum etc.* have very high herbicidal potential. Secondary metabolites of several nonpathogenic forms both fungi and actinomycetes associated with the weed, may also have significant herbicidal activity against this weed or may lead to the discovery of new eco-friendly safer herbicides sometimes saprophytic organisms also act as secondary invaders and caused significant damage to the concerned plants. This may be the other way to utilize saprophytic organisms. Therefore, a development of effective organism as either microbial herbicide or characterization and exploitation of their secondary metabolites for herbicide activities are urgently needed. These may offer more environmental friendly alternatives to chemical herbicides. They could also be used where weeds have developed resistance to conventional herbicides.

ACKNOWLEDGEMENTS

Authors are highly grateful to Dr. G. P. Agarwal and Dr. S. K. Hasija, Emeritus Professors for their valuable suggestions for the preparation of the manuscript. Financial assistance provided by Indian Council of Forestry Research and Education (ICFRE), DehraDun and DOEn, NewDelhi are also thankfully acknowledged.

REFERENCES

Acchireddy N.R. and Singh M. (1984). Allelopathic effects of *Lantana* (*Lantana camara*) on milkweed vine (*Morrenia odorata*). *Weed Sci.* 32, 757-761.

Acchireddy N.R., Singh M., Acchireddy L.L., Nigg H.N. and Naggy S. (1985). Isolation and Partial Characterization of Phytotoxic compounds from *Lantana* (*Lantana camara*). *Chem. Ecol.* 11, 979-988.

Agrawal D.K. and Sarbhoy A.K. (1984). New host records for dematiaceous hyphomycetes. *Indian Phytopath.* 37: 586.

Agrawal D.K. and Sarabhoy A.K. (1979). Studies on dematiaceous hyphomycetes of India-V. *Indian Phytopath.* 32, 637-639.

Agrawal D.K. and Sarbhoy A.K. (1983).Additions to fungi of India. *Indian Phytopath.* 36, 748-751.

Ahmad S. (1967). Contribution to the fungi of west Pakistan-VI. *Biologia* 13,15-42.

Ambasta S.P. (1986). The useful plant of India. *Council of Scientific and Industrial Research* (CSIR), New Delhi. 918.

Anahosur K.H. (1969).Some noteworthy Ascomycetes from Maharastra India. *Sydowia* 23, 63-68.

Auld B. A. (1990). Mycoherbicides: One alternative to chemical control of weeds. *In*: (*Ed.* C. Basset, L J. Whitehouse and J.A.Zabkiewicz), *Alternatives to the chemical control of weeds. Proc Int Conf Roturcia*, New Zealand Ministry of Forestry No. 155. 71-73.

Auld B.A.and Morin L (1995). Constraints in the development of Bioherbicides. *Weed Technol.* 9(3), 638-652.

Baker RE.D and Dale W.T. (1951). Fungi of Trinidad and Tobago. *Mycological Papers* 33, 1-123.

Bakshi B.K. and Singh B. (1988). The Indian species of *Merulius. Indian Phytopath.* 41, 70-75.

Bansal G. L(1988). Weed biology of *Lantana* and *Ageratum* sp. *Proc Sem on control of Lantana and Ageratum,* H P K V V Palampur. 10-13.

Barreto R.W., Evans H.C.and Ellison C.A. (1995). The mycobiota of the weed *Lantana camara* in Brazil, with particular reference to biological control. *Mycol Res.* 99(7), 767-782.

Barton D.H.R., De Mayo P. and Orr J.C. (1956). Terpenoids Part XXIII. Nature of lantadene A. *J. Chem. Soc.,* 4160-4162.

Barton D.H.R. and De Mayo P. (1954). Terpenoids Part XVI. The constitution of rehmannic acid. *J Chem Soc,* 900-903.

Beeby P.J. (1978). Chemical modification of triterpenes from *Lantana camara.* 22 - β-ester analogues of lantadene A. *Aust. J. Chem.* 31, 1313-1322.

Butler E.J.and Bisby G.R.(1960). The fungi of India. *The Indian Council of Agricultural Research,* New Delhi.

Chandla Poonam (1999) Screeing and evaluation of phytotxic metabolitcs of some indigenous microbes for the management of *Lantana camera. M.Sc. Microbiology Dissertation* R.D. Univercty, Jabalpur-1 (M.P.)

Charudattan R (1991). The mycoherbicides approach with plant pathogens. *In:* (*Ed.* D O Te Beest), *Microbial control of weeds*, Chapman and Hall Inc., USA. 25-57.

Chouhan J.S. and Panwar K.S. (1980). Hyphomycetes of Mt. Abu. *Indian Phytopath.* 33, 285.

Chupp C.(1954). A monograph of the fungus genus *Cercospora. Ithaca* New York USA..

CIBC (1982). Biological control of *Lantana camara. Commonwealth institute of Biological control.* Status paper 3, 1-4

Commins G.B. (1940). The genus *Prospodium* (Uredinales). *Lloydia.* 3: 1-78.

Dade H.A. (1940). A revised list of Gold cost fungi and plant diseases. *Kew Bulletin.* 6, 205-247.

Dale W.T.(1955). A preliminary list of Jamaican Uredinales. *Mycol. Pap.* 60, 1-21.

Deighton F.C.(1974). Studies on *Cercospora* and allied genera. 5. *Mycovellosiella* Rangel and new species of *Ramulariopsis. Mycol. Pap.* 137, 1-75.

Denton G.R.W., Muniappan R.and Marutani M.(1991). Status and natural enemies of the weed *Lantana camara* in Micronestia. *Trop. Pest. Manage.* 37(4), 338-44.

Desai S.H.and Patwardhan P.G.(1974). Addition to Hyphomycetes of Maharashtra. *J. Univ. Poona* 46, 127-133.

Duke J.A.and Ayensu E.S. (1985). Medicinal plants of China. Vol. 2, *Reference Publications Inc.* Michigan 705.

Evans H.C. (1987).Fungal pathogens of some subtropical and tropical weeds and the possibilities for biological control. *Biocontrol News Information* 8(1), 7-30.

Farr D.F. Bills G.F, Chamuris G.P.and Rossman A.Y.(1989). *Fungi of plants and plant products in the United States.* APS Press. St. Paul. MN U. S. A.

Freeman T.E. (1987). Microbial herbicides. *In:* (eds) N.S.Subbarao, *Advances in Agricultural Microbiology.* 419-428 Oxford and IBH Publishing Ltd.

Gaikwad Y.B. (1973). The genus *Didymosphaeria* Fuck. in India. *Maharashtra Vigyan Mandir Patrika* 8, 16-20.

Garman P. (1915). Some Porto Rican Parasitic fungi. *Mycologia* 7,333-340.

Gopinath C and Ford E.J.H. (1969). The effect of *Lantana camara* on the liver of sheep. *J. Path.* 99, 75-85.

Gorter G.J.M.A. (1981). Index of plant pathogens and diseases they cause in wild growing plants in South Africa. *Sci. Bull. Dept. Agr. Fish., Republic of South Africa* 398, 1-84.

Gupta Durga, Chowdhry P.N. and Padhi B. (1983). Some phytopathogenic fungi of ornamental plants from India. *Indian Phytopath.* 36, 244-246.

Gupta M. and Pawar A.D.(1984). Role of *Teleonemia scrupulosa* Stal in controlling *Lantana camara. Indian J. Weed Sci.* 16(4), 221-226.

Hannan M.A. and Jones (1998). The seasonal response of *Lantana camara* to selected herbicides. *Weed Research* 38, 413-423.

Hino and Tokeshi (1978). Some pathogens *Cercosporiosis* collected in Brazil. *Japan Technical Bulletin.* 11: 1-61.

Hiratuska Y. and Cummins G.B. (1963). Morphology of spermogonia of the rust fungi. *Mycologia* 55: 487-507.

Hoagland R.E. (1990). Microbes and Microbial products as herbicides. *Amer. Chem. Soc. Symp. Ser. No. 439.* Washington DC 389.

Hoagland R.E. (1999). Plant pathogens and microbial products as agents for Biological weed control. *In:* (*Ed.* J.P. Tiwari, J.N. Lakhanpal, Jagjit Singh, Rajni Gupta and D.P. Chambola) *Microbial Biotechnology.* APH Publishing Corporation, New Delhi-110002, India.

Hoagland R.E. (2001). The genus streptomyces: a rich source of novel phytotoxins. *In:* (*Ed.* Ishwar Prakash) *Ecology of Desert environment*, Scientific publishers, Jodhpur, India. 139-169.

Holm L.G., Plucknett Pancho J.V. and J.P. Herbergur (1977). *The worlds worst weeds.* East West Center Book, University Press of Hawaii, Honolulu 609.

Jadhav A.N., Somani R.B. and Wangikar P.D. (1978). Some interesting fungi around Akola-11. *Indian Phytopath.* 31: 47-51.

Johnston A. (1960). A supplement to a host list of plant diseases in Malaya. *Mycological Papers* 77: 1-30.

Kachroo J.V. (1966). Three new species of *Haplosporella* Speg. *Mycopath. et Mycol. Appl.* 28: 49-53.

Kanwar B.S. and Kharwara P.C. (1988). Infestation of *Lantana* and *Ageratum* in Kangra Valley in Himachal Pradesh. *Proc. Seminar on control of Lantana and Ageratum* HPKV, Palampur, 4-10.

Leather R.J. and Hor M.N. (1969). A preliminary list of plant diseases in Hongkong. Department of Agriculture and Fisheries Hongkong. *Agriculutral Bulletin.* 2:1-64.

Louw, P.G.J. (1948). Lantadene A., the active principle of *Lantana camara* L. part II. Isolation and Lantadene B and the oxygen functions of lantadene A and lantadene B. Onderstepoort. *J. Vet. Sci. Anim. Ind.* 18: 197-202.

Mersle W. and Singh M. (1987). Allelopathic effect of *Lantana* of some agronomic crops and weeds. *Plant Soil.* 98: 25-30.

Mhasker D.N. and Rao V.G. (1972). *Protostroma indica* sp. nov. from India *Curr. Sci.* 41: 111-112.

Muthappa B.N. (1967). *Ryblidiella rufula* (Spreng) Secc on diverse substrate and its systemic position. *Nova Hedwigia* 14: 395-401.

Nayar R. and Srimathi R.A. (1968). A symptomless carrier of sandal spike disease. *Curr. Sci.* 37: 567-568.

Neser S. and Cilliers C.J. (1989). Work towards biological control of *Lantana camara* perspectives. *In: (Ed.* E.S. Delfcsse) *Proc. VII Int. Sym. Biol. Contr. Weeds 1st Sper. Patol. Veg.* (MAF) 363-369.

Norse D. (1974). Plant diseases in Barbados. *Phytopathol. Pap.* 18: 1-38.

Orieux L. and Felix S. 1968. List of plant diseases in Mauritius. *Phytopathol. Pap.* 7:1-48.

Orillo F.T. and Valdez R.B. (1959). Four disease of Coffeo hitharto undescribed in the Philippines. *Philippine Agriculture* 42: 292-302.

Pai H.S. (1968). Two species of *Phyllosticta* and a common ascigerous stage on *Sapinadus* L. *Mycopath et Mycol. Appl.* 35: 121-128.

Pande A. (1972). Contribution to the Xylariaceae of Western India. *VI. J. Univ. Poona* 42: 85-86.

Pande A. (1973). *Subramania poonensis* sp. Nov. from Maharashtra *Curr. Sci.* Poona 42: 651.

Pande A. (1974). Contribution to the Xylariaceae of Western India. *VI. J. Univ. Bombay* pi. 63: 164-167.

Pandey A.K. (1990). The Genus *Haplosporella:* a Review. *In: Perspectives in Mycological Research-I (Ed.* K S Bilgrami and S K Hasija) Today and Tomorrow's Printers and Publishers, New Delhi-5.

Pandey A.K. (1999). Herbicidal potential of microorganism: present status and future prospects. *In: (Ed.* R. C. Rajak), *Microbial Biotechnology for Sustainable Development and Productivity.* Scientific Publications. Jodhpur, Rajasthan. 87-105.

Pandey A.K., Gaythri S., Rajak R.C. and Hasija S.K. (1996a). Possibilities and prospects of microbial management of *Parthenium hysterophorus* L. in India. *In: Perspectives in Biological Science. (Ed.* V Rai, M L Naik and C Manoharachary), School of Life Science, Pt. R. S. Shukla University Raipur. 253-269.

Pandey A K, Mishra J, Rajak R.C. and Hasija S.K. (1996b). Potential of indigenous strains of *Sclerotium rolfsii* Sacc. for the management of *Parthenium hysterophorus* L. a serious threat to biodiversity in India. *In: Herbal Medicines Biodiversity and Conservation Strategies, (Ed.* R. C. Rajak and M K Rai), International Book distributors, Dehradun. 104-138.

Pandey A.K., Rajak R.C. and Hasija S.K. (1997). Potential of indigenous *Colletotrichum* species for the management of weeds in India. *In: Achievements and Prospects in Mycology and Plant Pathology. (Ed.* S S Chahal, I B Parashar, H S Randhawa and S Arya), International book distributors. 9/3 Raipur Road Dehra Dun-India.

Pandey A.K. (2000). Microorganisms associated with weeds: Opportunities and challenges for their exploitation as herbicides. *Nt. J. Mendel* 17 (1-2), 59-62

Pandey A.K. and Pandey Archana (2001). *Lantana camara* L: Taxonomy, Biology and status of its Biological management, *In: Contemporary trend in Entomology, Environmental Biology, Physiology and Microbiology. (Ed.* S.M. Singh and C.T. Gujar), Japson printers and publication, Jabalpur. (M.P.)

Pandey A.K., Chandla Poonam and Rajak R.C. (2001). Herbicidal potential of secondary metabolites of some fungi against *Lantana camara* L. *J. myco. Pl. pathol.*31 *(in press)*

Pandey A.K., Rajak R.C. and Hasija S.K. (2001) Biotechnological development of ecofriendly mycoherbicides. *In: Innovative Approach in Microbiology.* (*Ed.* Maheshwari D.K., and R.C. Dube). Bishen Singh Mahendrapal Singh, Dehradun India. 1–21.

Pandey S. Jr. (2000). Mycoherbicidal potential of some fungal pathogens for the management of *Lantana camara* L. *Ph. D. Thesis,* R. D. University, Jabalpur-1 (M.P.).

Pandey, Santosh and Pandey A.K. (2000). Mycoherbicidal potential of some fungi against *Lantana camara* L.: a preliminary observation. *J. Trop. Forestry* 16: 28-32.

Pandir Y P S (1985). *Acta Botenica. Mica.* 13(2): 298-300.

Panwar, K.S. and Gehlot, C.S. (1973). Two species of *Leptosphaeria* new to India. *Curr. Sci.* 42: 734.

Panwar, K.S. and Kaur, S.J. (1975). A new species of *Massarina* Sacc. *Curr. Sci.* 44: 523-524.

Panwar, K.S. and Kaur, S.J. (1976). Ascomycetes of Mt Abu Rajasthan. *Kavaka* 4:77-80.

Panwar, K.S. and Kaur, S.J. (1977). Ascomycetes of Mt. Abu, Rajasthan III. *Kavaka* 5: 41-48.

Patil, M.S. (1975). Some *Ceroospora* species from Kolhapur-II. *Botanique.* 6: 219-226.

Patil, M.S. and Thite, A.N. (1977). Some Deuteromycetes fungi from Maharashtra I. *Maharashtra Vigyan Mandir Patrika.* 12: 28-35.

Patil, M.S. and Thite, A.N. (1978). Fungal flora of Amboli (Ratnagiri). *J. Shivaji Univ. (Sci.).* 18: 219-224.

Patil, M.S. (!983). Studies in pyrenomycetes of Maharastra-111. *Indian Phytopath.*

Peregrine, W.T.H. and Ahmad K.B.(1982). Brunei: a first annotated list of plant diseases and associated organisms. *Phytopathol. Pap.* 27: 1-87.

Piening, L.J. (1962). A check list of fungi from Ghana. *Ghana Ministry of Agriculture Bulletin.* 2: 1-130.

Prasad Raj (1999). Role of Microbial Bioherbicides in Biological control of weeds in forestry. *In: Microbial Biotechnology for Sustainable Development and Productivity,* (*Ed.* R C Rajak), Scientific Publisher, Jodhpur 88-93.

Rajak, R.C. and Rajak, R.N. (1981). A new species of *Cercospora* from India. *Indian Phytopath.* 35: 282-284.

Rajak, R.C., Rai, M.K. and Pandey, A.K. (1985). New host records of *Cuscuta reflexa. J. Trop. Forestry* 1 (11).

Rangaswami, G, Seshadre, V.S. and Lucy Channamma, K. A. (1970). Fungi of South India. *University of Agricultural Sciences*, Banglore. 193.

Rao, V.J. and Anahosur, K.H. (1971). Some interesting fungi imperfectai from India. *Sydowia* 25; 51-53.

Rao Ramchandra (1965). A new species of *Tympanopsis* from India. *Mycopath et Mycol Appl.* 27: 238-240.

Rao Ramchandra (1966a). Some additions to fungi of India-1. *Mycopath et Mycol Appl.* 28: 45-48.

Rao Ramchandra (1966c). Fungi on *Lantana camara* L. *Mycopath. et Mycol Appl.* 28: 133-136.

Rao Ramchandra (1966d). Some new noteworthy fungi from India II. *Mycopath et Mycol Appl.* 29: 187-188.

Rao Ramchandra (1967). Two new species of *Patellaria* from India. *Mycopath et Mycol. Appl.* 31: 29-32.

Rao, V.J. and Chary, S. J. (1972). A new *Pithomyces* from India. *Curr Sci.* 41:822-823.

Reddy, S.M. (1973). Some additions to Indian species of *Didymosphaeria Indian Phytopath.* 26: 642-45.

Rios, E.A.E. (1982). Catalogo do Enfermeda des de ias plantas on la, publica de panama. Published by the auther; Maxico city Maxico.

Rizwi, M.A. (1977). Ascomycetes of Bihar-1. *Proc Bihar Acad. Agric. Sci.* 25:102-105.

Sahid, I.B. and Sugav, J.B. (1993). Allelopathic effect of *Lantana camara* and siam weed (*Chromolaena odorara*) on selected crop. *Weed Sci.* 41: 303-308.

Saikia, U.N. and Sarbhoy, A.K. (1980). Hyphomycetes of North East India. *Indian Phytopath.* 33: 637-640.

Sanders, D.A. (1946). *Lantana* poisioning in Cattle. *J. Ama. Vet. Med. Assoc.* 119: (833) 139-141.

Sarabhoy, A.K., Agrawal D.K. and Varshney J.L. (1986); Fungi of India (1977-1981). Associated publishing company; New Delhi India 271 pp.

Saxena, S. and Pandey, A.K. (2001). Microbial metabolites as ecofriendly agrochemicals for the next millennium. *Appl. Microbiol. Biotechnol.* 55: 395-403

Saxena Sanjai (2000). Efficacy of microbial metabolites on some fungi to enhance their mycoherbicidal potential for the management of *Lantana camara* L. *Ph. D. Thesis,* R. D. University, Jabalpur M.P.

Saxena, Sanjai and Pandey, A.K. (2000). Preliminary evaluation of fungal metabolites as natural herbicides for the management of *Lantana camara. Indian Phytopath.* 53 (4): 490-49.

Seawright, A.A. (1963). Studies on experimental intoxication of sheep with *Lantana camara.* Aust. Vet. J. 39: 340-344.

Seawright, A.A. (1964). Studies on the pathology of experimental *Lantana* (*Lantana camara*) poisioning of sheep. *Pathol. Vet.* 1: 504-599.

Sharma, O.P. (1988). The noxious plant *Lantana camara*-overview of the toxicity of *Lantana* in animals. *Clinicals Toxicology* 18: 1077-1094.

Sharma, O.P., Makkar, H.P.S. and Dawra, R.K. (1988). A review of noxious plant *Lantana camara. Toxicon* 26: 975-987.

Sharma, O.P., Makkar, H.P.S. Dawra, R.K. and Negi, S.S. (1981). A review of the toxicity of *Lantana camara* L. in animals. *Clinical Toxicology* 18: 1077-1094.

Singh, C.M., Angiros, N.N. and Gautam, S. K. (1988). Profiles of *Lantana*-A review. *Proc. Seminar Control Lantana and Ageratum.* HPKV, Palampur 58-65.

Singh, Hardev and Pushpawathy, K.K. (1966). The slime moulds of Delhi-II *Mycopath. et Mycol. Appl.* 28: 265-272

Singh, S.M. and Agrawal, G.P. (1974): Some Spheropsidales new to India. *Indian phytopath.* 27:244-246.

Smith, L.S. and Smith, D.A. (1982). The naturalised *Lantana camara complex in estern Australia.* Old Bot Bull no. 1. 1982. Old Dept. Prim Ind. Brisbane, 26.

Spies, J.J. and Du Plessis, H. (1987). Sterile *Lantana camara.* Fact or theory S. Afr *J. Plant. Soil.* 4(4): 171-4.

Srinivasulu, B.V. and Sathe, P.G. (1970). Genus *Aphanostigme* from India. *Sydowia* 24:75-78.

Stevenson F L (1917). Porto Rican fungi old and new. *Transaction of the Illinois Academic of Science* 10: 162-218.

Stevenson, J.A. (1975). Fungi of Puerto Rico and the amercian virgin Island. Contribution of read herbarium 23:1-747.

Sutton Brianc (1980). The coelomycetes fungi imperfecti with pycnidia acervuli and stromata. commonwealth Mycological institute kew survey England.

Swarbrick, J.T. (1986). History of the *Lantanas* in Australia and origins of the weedy biotypes. *Plant Prot. Quart.* 1(3): 115-21.

Templeton, G.E. (1990). Weed control with pathogens: Future needs and directions. *In: Microbes and microbial products as herbicides.* (*Ed.* R C Hoagland) ACS Symposium series 439, American Chemical Society. Washington DC 320-329.

Templeton G.E. (1992). Regulatory encouragement of Biological control with plant pathogens. *In:* Regulations and guidelines: *critical issues in Biological control* (*Ed.* R. Charudattan and H.W. Browning) *Proc.* USDA CSRS Nat. Work Institute Food Agr. Sci. Univ. Florida, Gainesville. 61-63.

Templeton, G.E. and Heiny D.K. (1989). Improvement of fungi to enhance mycoherbicidal potential. *In: Biotechnology of fungi for improving plant growth.* (*Ed.* J.M. Whipps and R.D. Lumsden) Cambridge University Press, Cambridge U K. 127-151.

Templeton, G. E., Weideman G L and Smith R J Jr (1986). Biological weed control. *In*: *Research methods in weed science IIIrd edition* (*Ed.* N.D. Campered), Southern weed Science Society 309 West Clark Stree, Champaign, 1L 61820. 100-109.

Tilak, S.T. (1966). Contribution to our knowledge of Ascomycetes of India-VIII. *Mycopat et Mycol. Appl.* 29: 125-127.

Tilak, S.T. and Kale, S.B. (1967). Contribution to our knowledge of Ascomycetes of India-XVI. *Sydowia.* 21: 295-301.

Tilak, S.T. and Nagre, R.S. (1964). A new species of *Calosphaeria* from India. *Mycopath et Mycol Appl.* 22: 291-292.

Tilak, S.T. and Nanir, S.P. (1975). The genus Stictis Pers from India. *Revue De Mycologie Tom.* 39: 119-123.

Tilak, S.T. and Rao, R. (1966). The Genus *Hysterium* in India. *Mycopath et Mycol. Appl.* 30: 155-160.

Tiwari, D.P., Rajak, R.C. and Nikhara, M. (1981). A new species of *Phomopsis* causing leaf spat disease of *Tectona grandis* L. *Curr Sci.* 50: 1002.

Tripathi, R.C. and Udit Narain (1985). Some new host records of *Myrothecium roridum* from India. *Indian Phytopath.* 38: 394.

Vaidya, J.G. (1975). Contribution to Ascomycetes of Maharastra, India. Some new host records. *J. Ind. Bios. Assoc.* Nagpur 1: 33.

Viegas, A.P. (1961). Indice de fungos da America do suk instituto Agronomico de Campinas: Sao Paulo, Brazil.

Wadhwani, C. and Bharadwaj, T.N. (1981). Effect of *Lantana camara.* extract on fern spore germination. *Experientia* 37: 245-246.

Waterson, J.M. (1947): The fungi of Bermuda. Department of Agriculture, Bermuda, Bulletin 23: 1-305.

Wolfson, S.L. and Solomons, T.W.G. (1964). Poisoning by fruit of *Lantana camara* L. An acute syndrome observed in children following ingestion of green fruit. *Ann. J. Dis. Child.* 107: 1073.

Yamamoto, W. (1934). *Cercospora* Arten aus Taiwan (formosa) II. *J. Soc. Trop. Agr.* Taiwan 6: 599-608.

Yen, J. and Lim, C. (1980). Cercospora and alied genera of Singapore and Malay peninsula. Garden Bulletin, Singapore 33: 151-263.

Microbiology and Biotechnology for Sustainable Development (Ed. P.C. Jain),
CBS Publishers & Distributors, New Delhi (2004), pp. 59–70.

A-6

Diversity of Keratinophilic Fungi in Soil and on Birds

R.K.S. Kushwaha and Madhu Gupta
Department of Botany, Christ Church College, Kanpur 208 001 India
Email: rks_kushwaha@yahoo.co.in

Abstract

Keratinophilic and allied fungi were isolated from soil of four different habitats by using hair bait technique and from dropped off feathers by incubating them directly in moist chambers. 37 isolates, belonging to different species of six genera ie. Acremonium, Myceliophthora, Chrysosporium, Malbranchea, Microsporum and Trichophyton were isolated from soil samples of crop fields, gardens, forests and zoo. While, 30 isolates belonging to 4 genera ie. Chrysosporium, Myceliophthora, Microsporum and Trichophyton representing 11 species and two sterile mycelial forms were obtained from 33 feather samples. Distribution of these fungi in soils and on birds is discussed in present paper.

Keywords: Keratinophilic fungi, birds, zoo, forest, soil garden, crop field.

INTRODUCTION

The ability of keratinophilic fungi and dermatophytes to decompose and parasitize keratinous substrates is closely associated with and depends upon the utilization of keratin. Fungi capable of colonizing keratinous substrates such as human hair, skin, nails, feathers, hooves, horns and nails are widely spread in nature. Among the multitude of fungal species known to colonize keratin some are able to parasitize human and animals causing disease. These keratinophilic fungi include genera *Chrysosporium, Trichophyton, Epidermophyton, Microsporum, Myceliophthora, Malbranchea* and their related forms.

Soil is recognized as the basic substrate for keratinophilic fungi. The studies from several countries reported their occurrence in soil [Table 1]. Sufficient data has accumulated in the past few years on the ecology and distribution of such fungi from several parts of the world [Ajello and Alpert, 1972; Kushwaha and Agrawal, 1976; Sur and Ghosh, 1980 a,b; Guarro *et al.*, 1981; Abdel-Fattah *et al.* 1982, Nigam and Kushwaha, 1986, 1989a, b, 1990; Kushwaha, 2000]. The frequency of occurrence of geophilic dermatophytes and related keratinophilic fungi in a particular habitat depends on the frequency of animals visiting it. [Pugh and Mathison, 1962; Garg, 1966, Randhawa and Sandhu, 1965; Sur and Ghosh, 1980; Deshmukh and Agrawal, 1983]. Keratinophilic fungi and dermatophytes have been commonly isolated from soil by hair baiting method.The first report of distribution of keratinophilic fungi in Indian soil can be traced back to 1955 when Dey and Kakoti reported the occurrence of *Microsporum gypseum* from Assam. Reports on the isolation of these fungi of identical nature were also composited from other states of India [Randhawa and Sandhu, 1965; Kushwaha and Agrawal, 1976; Shrivastava and Kushwaha, 1983; Jain *et al.,* 1985; Nigam and Kushwaha, 1989 a, 1990; Dixit and Kushwaha, 1990; Awasthi and Gotewal, 1990].

The distribution of keratinophilic and allied fungi on birds was studied by several workers in India and abroad [Emmons, 1995; Pugh, 1972; Rees, 1967; Pugh and Evans, 1970; Sheridan, 1971; Hubalek, 1974, 2000; Sur and Ghosh, 1980; Dixit and Kushwaha, 1991]. Pugh [1966 a,b] investigated keratinophilic fungi on feathers removed from living birds and in nest materials. He also studied cellulolytic and keratinophilic fungi associated with certain Indian birds and reported variation in mycoflora of the birds of two countries. It has long been suspected that numerous fungi are carried by birds and their feeding habits and flights are good sources of fungal transport. The distribution of numerous fungal species on birds, however, has long being question. Indian reports of keratinophilic fungi on birds are confined to few surveys.

Keratinophilic and allied fungal species were isolated from soil by using hair baiting technique and from dropped off feathers by incubating directly in moist chambers. Isolated fungi were cultured and maintained on suitable media, in water cultures, as lyophilized cultures and dry cultures. Sub cultures were deposited in international culture collections.

Table 1: Percentage prevalence of keratinophilic fungi in India and different countries.

Fungus	Country	Percent Prevalence
Acetheca purpurea	India	1.14
Acremonium obelvatum	India	1
Acrodontium album	India	–
Ajellomyces dermatitides	India	1.14
Ameruroascus oblatus	Spain	–
Anixiopsis flavescens	India	1.09
Aphanoascus flavescens	France	8
Aphanoascus terreus	India	7.3
Aphanoasus sp.	India	2.5-19.5
Arthroderma benhamjae	India	3.29
A.biplanata	Nepal	–

(Contd.)

Fungus	Country	Percent Prevalence
A.ciferri	India	2.19
A.cuniculi	India, Jordan	1.09-32.0
A.gerteleri	India	7.3
A.glorie	Italy	–
A.insigulari	Japan	–
A.quadrifidum	India, Japan, Poland	–
A.flavescens	India	6.21
A.simii	India	–
A.tuberculatum	India	3.4
A.uncinatum	Japan	13.5
Arthroderma sp.	Egypt, Jordan	–
Arthrographis kalari	India	–
Auxarothron conjugatum	India	1.14
A.reticulatum	India	1.14
Botryotrichum keratinophilum	India	–
Chrysosporium asparatum	Angers district, India	1.8-7.1
C.carmichaeli	Kuwait	1.1-1.0
C.crassitunicatum	India	–
C.dermatidis	–	–
C.evolceauni	Germany, India Jordan, Poland Spain, Italy	0.41-2.19
C.europae	Spain	–
C.farinicola	India	100
C.geophilum	India	–
C.georgi	–	–
C.indicum	India, Italy, Kuwait, Poland	1.1-48.25
C.inops	–	–
C.keratinophilum	Angers district, Egypt, Jordan, India, Japan, Kuwait, Magnesia, Nigesia, Poland	1.09-88.3
C.lobatum	Neetherland	
C.lucknowense	India	0.82-11.0
C.luteum	–	–
C.mephiticum	India	–

Occurrence of keratinophilic and related fungi from different habitats

Six genera namely *Acremonium* [4 species], *Chrysosporium* [14 species], *Myceliophthora, Malbranchea, Microsporum* and *Trichophyton,* one species each were isolated during a study while using three types of keratinous substrates i.e. human hair, buffalo hair and chicken feathers from four habitats. The per cent distribution and relative density of each fungus in different habitats are given in Tables 2 and 3.

Table 2: Percent distribution of keratinophilic and allied fungal genera in different habitats.

Per cent occurrence	Cropfield 75	Garden 100	Forest 83.3	Zoo 87.5	Distribution Per cent
Fungus isolated					
Acremonium sp.	0	20.0 [2]	16.6 [2]	0	10.5
Chrysosporium sp.	12.5 [1]	20.0 [2]	8.3 [1]	12.5 [1]	13.2
C.indicum	12.5 [1]	20.0 [2]	0	12.5 [1]	2.6
C.evolceanui	0	10.0 [1]	0	0	10.5
C.keratinophilum	0	8.3	12.5 [1]	5.3	
C.pannicola	12.5 [1]	0	0	12.5 [1]	5.3
C.queenslandicum	12.5 [1]	0	0	12.5 [1]	5.3
C.tropicum	25.0 [2]	30.0 [3]	16.6 [2]	25.0 [2]	23.7
Chrysosporium anamorph of *Arthroderma tuberculatum*	0	10.0 [1]	0	0	2.6
Chrysosporium anamorph of *Gymnoascus demonbreunii*	0	10.0 [1]	0	0	2.6
Myceliophthora vellera	0	0	0	12.5 [1]	2.6
Malbranchea sp.	0	0	8.3 [1]	0	2.6
Microsporum gypseum	0	10.0 [1]	16.6 [2]	0	7.9
Trichophyton flavescens	0	0	8.3 [1]	0	2.7
Total isolates	6	14	10	7	
Average number of fungi/habitat	0.75	1.4	0.83	0.88	

Figures in parentheses represent the number of isolates.

Table 3: Relative density of keratinophilic and allied genera in different habitats

Fungal genera	Habitat				
	Crop field	Garden	Forest	Zoo	Per cent RD
Chrysosporium	100 [6]	78.6 [11]	40.0 [4]	85.7 [6]	73
Myceliophthora	0	0	0	14.2 [1]	2.1
Malbranchea	0	0	10.0 [1]	0	2.1
Microsporum	0	7.1 [1]	20.0 [2]	0	8.1
Trichophyton	0	0	10.0 [1]	0	2.7
Acremonium	0	114.3 [2]	20.0 [2]	0	10.8

Acremonium species were isolated from garden and forest soil. *Chrysosporium evolceanui* was isolated from garden soil and exhibited 10.5 per cent distribution. *C. indicum* was isolated from all the habitats studied except forest. The distribution of this fungus was maximum in garden soil. *C. keratinophilum* was isolated from the soil of forest and zoo while *C. pannicola* was recovered from crop field and garden soil. *C. queenslandicum* could be isolated from crop field and zoo. *C. tropicum* was most prevalent and frequently trapped from all the habitats studied. The maximum distribution of this fungus was observed in garden soil and minimum was in forest soil. *Chrysosporium* anamorph of *Arthroderma tuberculatum* and *Chrysosporium* anamorph of *Gymnoascus demonbreunii* were isolated from garden soil exhibiting 10.0 per cent distribution in each habitat. *M. vellera and Malbranchea* sp. were restricted to zoo and forest soil. *M. gypseum* was isolated from soil of garden and forest. *T. flavescence* could be isolated from forest soil respectively. The relative density of *Acremonium* sp. varied from 14 to 20 per cent in garden and forest soil while that of *Chrysosporium* varied from 100 to 40 per cent.

The perusal of data provide an information on the nature of distribution of various *Chrysoporium* sp. and allied fungi in different habitats. *C. tropicum* was found most frequent among various isolates of *Chrysosporium* studied. This fungus was trapped from all the four habitats. This widespread occurrence of *C. tropicum* is in correlation with earlier reports. Randhawa and Sandhu [1965] reported it from cattle field in Punjab, while Garg [1966] reported its isolation from garden, cultivated field and riversand. Cattle field soils have been earlier described as suitable habitat for the occurrence of *C. tropicum* [Deshmukh and Agrawal, 1993 a; Singh and Agrawal, 1983]. Other reports have confirmed its isolation from poultry farm, crop field and forest soil. Nigam and Kushwaha [1986] isolated *C. tropicum* from house dust, nutritionally very poor habitat. These reports indicated the wide distribution of *C. tropicum* in Indian soils of different climatic conditions.

C. idicum was found very common in its occurrence and was isolated from the soils of crop field, garden and zoo. Saksena [1993] isolated this fungus from forest soil also along with the habitats mentioned above. Earlier reports indicated the presence of this fungus both in soils of plains and hills of India. However, soils of plains confirmed the greater preponderance of *C. indicum* in usual habitats than on the hills. It is observed that the men and animal dwelling areas and soil rich in organic and keratin substances favoured the distribution of *C. indicum*. Isolation of this fungus is in accordance with previous reports from India. *C. evoleauni* was found associated with garden soil in the present attempt. Its isolation from garden soil has already been reported [Garg, 1966]. This author also reported it from soil of farm, water course bank and hills of India. Other reports showed the existence of this fungus in soil of various states of India.This fungus have been also isolated from house dust [Nigam and Kushwaha, 1986], poultry farm and petrol residue [Singh, 1992]. *C. keratinophilum* was isolated from forest and zoo. Its isolation from India has been reported by several workers [Garg, 1966; Jain, 1983; Deshmukh and Agrawal, 1985; Jain et al 1985; Nigam and Kushwaha, 1986]. The infection potential of C. keratinophilum and C. tropicum in white mouse was established by Hubalek and Hornick [1977]. *C. pannicola* was found to be associated with soil of crop field and garden. It was reported for the first time from house dust in India [Nigam and Kushwaha, 1986]. *C. queenslandicum* was recorded from crop field and zoo

Chrysosporim anamorph of *A. tuberculatum* and *Chrysosporrim* anamorph of *G. demonbreunii* was very much restricted in its distribution, being isolated from garden soil only. Nigam [1987] and Dixit [1991] isolated *Chrysosporium* anamorph of *A. tuberculatum* from soil of college campus. The restricted distribution of Chrysosporium anamorph of *G. demonbreunii* and *C. queenslandicum* indicated their presence from soil with low nutritional levels.

In the present study two unidentified species of *Chrysosporium* were reported from garden and one each from crop field, forest and zoo. The high per cent of distribution of various species of *Chrysoporium* in different habitats may be due to the fact that soil of these habitats was rich in organic, inorganic and keratin substrates. The ability to digest these substrates easily by the species of *Chrysosporium* has been confirmed [English, 1965]. Nigam [1987] while studying the ecology of *Chrysosporium* elaborated its competitive survivability with other fungi present in the environment. She has also found *Chrysosporium* to be widely distributed. The genus *Acremonium* was isolated in the present study from forest and garden. It was earlier isolated from house dust and zoo [Nigam and Kushwaha, 1989 a; Saksena, 1993]. *M. vellera* was reported from zoo. Previous report of isolation of *Myceliophthora* is from college campus soil [Nigam and Kushwaha, 1990], from hospital waste [Dixit, 1991] and from forest soil [Saksena, 1992]. *Malbranchea* species was recorded from forest soil. This fungus appears to be common in distribution in India [Kushwaha and Agrawal, 1976; Jain and Agrawal, 1979; Jain 1983; Dixit, 1991].

Isolation of *M. gypseum* was made in the present study from garden and forest soil. This dermatophyte was first isolated from Assam soil later reported in swimming pool, baren yard, chicken house and dairy farm where the soil was presumably intermixed with keratin substrates. Jain [1983] also reported colonization of peacock feathers buried in soil of poultry farm and cattle field. Nigam and Kushwaha [1986] found it in house dust and Dixit [1991] isolated this fungus from all the habitats he studied. There are evidences for the saprophytic existence of this fungus which disclose the wide spread occurrence of *M. gypseum* in garden and soil. Another dermatophyte *T. flavescens* was isolated from forest soil in the present study. This fungus was also reported from cattle field, garden, playground and hospital waste.

Recovery of soil inhabiting keratinophilic and allied fungi from different keratinous baits

Black human hair, buffalo hair and chicken feathers were used as keratinous substrates during isolation of keratinophilic fungi and related dermatophytes from soil [Table 4]. Thirty fungi were isolated from these keratinic substrates. All the isolated fungal species appeared on human hair except *Chrysosporium* anamorph of *Arthtroderma tuberculatum*.This fungus was recovered from chicken feathers. *C. tropicum* was recorded most frequently on all the baits while *C. indicum* was also isolated from all the baits but with low frequency. Feathers were unable to show any growth of *Myceliophthora, Malbranchea, Microsporum* and *Trichophyton*. However, animal hair showed the appearance of *M. gypseum*. This fungus was also trapped from human hair during this study.

Occurrence of keratinophilic and allied related fungi on birds feather

The keratinophilic fungi, which occurred on five Indian birds are listed in Tables 4, 5 and 6. A total of 30 keratinophilic fungal isolates belonging to 4 different genera representing 11 species and 2 sterile mycelium were isolated from 33 feather samples. Chicken feathers yielded the maximum number of fungi. The average number of isolate per bird was maximum on chicken and minimum on house, crow. The isolated genera with their respective relative density were *Chrysosporium* [76.6], *Myceliophthora* [10.0], *Microsporum* [3.3] and sterile mycelium [6.6].

Table 4: Keratinophilic and allied fungal genera isolated from dropped off feathers of Indian birds.

Fungus	Accession number	Birds feather
Chrysosporium sp.	GPCK 278	Chicken
Chrysosporium sp.	GPCK 288	Pigeon
Chrysosporium sp.	GPCK 293	Chicken
Chrysosporim indicum	GPCK 281	Pigeon
Chrysosporim indicum	GPCK 285	Chicken
Chrysosporim indicum	GPCK 286	House sparrow
Chrysosporim indicum	GPCK 287	Chicken
Chrysosporim indicum	GPCK 294	Chicken
Chrysosporim indicum	GPCK 298	Pigeon
Chrysosporium keratinophilum	GPCK 292	Pigeon
Chrysosporium keratinophilum	GPCK 324	Chicken
Chrysosporium pannicola	GPCK 280	Chicken
Chrysosporium pannicola	GPCK 282	House sparrow
Chrysosporium queenslandicum	GPCK 275	Chicken
Chrysosporium queenslandicum	GPCK 277	House sparrow
Chrysosporium queenslandicum	GPCK 284	Chicken
Chrysosporium queenslandicum	GPCK 295	Pigeon
Chrysosporium queenslandicum	GPCK 297	Parrot
Chrysosporium queenslandicum	GPCK 302	House sparrow
Chrysosporium tropicum	GPCK 276	Chicken
Chrysosporium tropicum	GPCK 279	Chicken
Chrysosporium tropicum	GPCK 283	Pigeon
Chrysosporium tropicum	GPCK 296	Chicken
Myceliophthora sp.	GPCK 290	Chicken
Myceliophthorra anamorph of Ctenomyces serratus	GPCK 291	Chicken
Myceliophthora vellera	GPCK 299	Pigeon
Microsporum gypseum	GPCK 268	Pigeon
Trichophyton mentagrophytes	GPCK 334	Pigeon
Sterile mycelium		Crow
Sterile mycelium		Parrot

Chrysosporium sp. were dominant on dropped feathers of all the birds studied except the feathers of crow. Total of 6 species of *Chrysosporium* were isolated. Among these *C. indicum* and *C. queenslandicum* were found associated with feathers of domestic chicken, pigeon and house sparrow. The later fungus was also associated with parrot. *C. keratinophilum* and *C. tropicum* were also isolated from chicken and pigeon. *C. pannicola* was reported from chicken and house sparrow. *M. gypseum* and *T.mentagrophytes* were also found to be restricted with the feathers of chicken in this study. *M. vellera* was reported from feather of pigeon while *Myceliophthora* species and *Myceliophthora* anamorph of *Ctenomyces serratus* was trapped from feather of chicken. The least frequency of occurrence was seen in the feathers of crow as it could yield only sterile mycelium. Another isolate of sterile mycelium was obtained from the feather of parrot.

Table 5: Occurrence of keratinophilic and allied genera on some Indian birds.

	Chicken	Pigeon	House sparrow	Crow	Parrot	Total	Isolation rate [%]
Percent occurrence	75.0	71.4	60	25	50	63.5	
Fungus isolated							
Chrysosporium sp.	10.0 [2]	7.4 [1]	0	0	0	3	5.8
C.indicum	10.0 [2]	21.4 [3]	20.0 [1]	0	0	6	11.5
C.keratinophilum	5.1 [1]	7.1 [1]	0	0	0	2	3.8
C.pannicola	5.1 [1]	0	20.0 [1]	0	0	2	3.8
C. queenslandicum	10.0 [2]	14.3 [2]	20.0 [1]	0	25.0 [1]	6	11.5
C.tropicum	15.0 [3]	7.1 [1] 0	0	0	0	4	7.7
Myceliophthora sp.	20.0 [1]	0	0	0	0	1	1.9
Myceliophthora anamorph of *Ctenomyces serratus*	20.0 [1]	0	0	0	0	1	1.9
Myceliophthora vellera	0	7.1 [1]	0	0	0	1	1.9
Micosporum gypseum	5.1 [1]	0	0	0	0	1	1.9
Trichophyton mentagrophytes	5.1 [1]	1	1.9				
Sterile mycelium	0	0	0	25.0 [1]	25.0 [1]	2	3.8
Total isolates	15	9	3	1	2	30	

Figures in parentheses represent the number of isolates.

During the present study four genera including 11 fungal species with 2 sterile mycelia were isolated. Among *Chrysosporium* isolates, *C. indicum* and *C. queenslandicum* were the most common fungal species associated with five Indian birds. *C. indicum* was isolated by Sur and Ghosh [1980]. Dixit and Kushwaha [1991] isolated it from feathers of chicken. In the present study this fungus was isolated from the feathers of pigeon and house sparrow along with chicken feathers. The isolation of this fungus from chickens confirmed its association with this bird. *C. tropicum* was also found to be wide spread with its isolattion rate of 7.7 per cent. Among the 72 feather samples *C. tropicum* was more than 33 per cent. Dixit and Kushwaha [1991] found that *C. lucknowense* and *C. tropicum* were the most common fungal species associated with birds in Kanpur. This fungus has also been isolated from black headed gulls. *C. pannicola* was isolated from the feathers of chicken and house sparrow. *C. keratinophilum* was found associated with chicken and feathers of pigeon.

Table 6: Relative density of keratinophilic and allied fungal genera associated with bird's feathers.

Fungal	Birds					
	Chicken	Pigeon	House sparrow	Crow	Parrot	%RD
Chrysosporium	84.6 [11]	88.8 [8]	100 [3]	0	50 [1]	76.6
Myceliophthora	0	11.1 [1]	0	0	0 [0]	10.0
Microsporum	7.7 [1]	0	0	0	0 [0]	3.3
Trichophyton	7.7 [1]	0	0	0	0 [0]	3.3
Sterile mycelium	0	0	0	50.0 [1]	50 [1]	6.6

Figures in parenthese represent the number of isolates.

Among dermatophytes, *M. gypseum* and *T. mentagrophytes* were recorded from chickens. Earlier reports on the occurrence of these fungi revealed that *Microsporum* species were found on birds of other countries also. Padhye *et al.* [1967] found *M. gypseum* as second common most species, next to *C. tropicum,* from the feathers of partriges and quails. Dermatophytes have from time to time being recorded on birds. However, their pathogenecity has not been certain. *T. mentagrophytes* was isolated from the feathers of chicken during the present study without ascertaining its pathogenecity. This fungus have also been isolated from chickens and pigeons.

Three isolates of *Myceliophthora* namely *Myceliophthora* anamorph of *C. serratus, M. vellera* and *Myceliophthora* sp. were recorded. Padhye *et al.,* [1967] reported conidial stage of *Ctenomyces serratus* from the feathers of an unidentified bird. In the present attempt the feathers used for the isolation could not be recognised but the site of collection was college campus. Nigam and Kushwaha [1990] reported this fungus from the soil collected from the same site. This may be due to the fact that keratinophilic mycoflora on feathers are considerably influenced by the occurrence of these fungi in soil of areas frequently visited by particular bird species. To a certain extent, the colonization of bird feathers by keratinophilic fungi is a reflection of qualitative and quantitative representation of microfungi in soil of biotype inhabited or frequented by birds, although it can not rely on the close ecological association with soil substrates, such as in the case of small terrestrials [Dixit, 1991].

This dependence was also indicated in the presented study, which demonstrated a rich flora of keratinophilic fungi on chicken, pigeon and house sparrow with the average number of fungi per bird. These birds are very similar in their, terrestrial ground feeding habits, thus the birds come in close contact with soil as these take dust baths. Thus geophilic fungal species are removed with a greater frequency from them. The influence of active contact with soil and the influence of cavity nesting upon the higher frequency of keratinophilic fungi were also proved by Hubalek [1974].

The average number of fungi per bird were 0.6 in the present study while Dixit and Kushwaha [1993] recorded it as 0.4. This value is very low in comparision to the birds surveyed in Britain. Pugh [1965] recorded 2.3 fungi per bird. Variation in occurrence of keratinophilic fungi on India and foregin birds might be due to the differences in their habits and habitats. The variation in mycoflora may also due to possible differences in the microenvironment of the feather where the fungi are logged. Pugh and Evans [1970] pointed out that feather fats determined the distribution both qualitatively and quantitatively of keratinophilic fungi on birds. This is also suggestive for some selective relationships of kerratinophilic fungi and Indian birds [Dixit and Kushwaha, 1991]. Isolates obtained from the feather after surface sterilization indicate their ability to penetrate the feather while it was still on the birds and thus provide indirect evidence for the growth of keratinophilic fungi on birds [Pugh and Evans, 1970]. The change in the mycoflora of various environments which the birds visit directly affects the mycoflora of the bird as well. The data revealed that maximum number of keratinophilic fungi are recorded on feather of chicken. The results are correspondent to Dixit and Kushwaha [1991]. It was suggested that the distribution of fungi on birds depend upon body temperature of bird, feather fat and climatic conditions including topography.

ACKNOWLEDGEMENTS

This work was financially supported by University Grants Commission, New Delhi.

REFERENCES

Abdel-Fattah, H.M., Moubasher, A.H. and Maghazy, S.M. (1982). Keratinophilic fungi in Egyptian soil. Mycopathologia 79:49-53.

Ajello, L. and Alpert, E.M. (1972). Survey of Easter Islands soils for for keratinophilic fungi. Mycologia. 64:161-166.

Awasthi, P.B. and Gotewal, S. (1990). Prevalence of keratinophilic fungi in certain soils of Rohilkhand division in relation to edaphic factors. Proc. Natl. Acad. Sci. 76:37.

Deshmukh, S.K. and Agrawal, S.C. (1983a). Prevalence of dermatophytes and other keratinophilic fungi in soils of Madhya Pradesh [India]. Mykosen 26:574-577.

Deshmukh, S.K. and Agrawal, S.C. (1983b). Isolation of keratinophilic fungi from coastal habitats of Goa [India]. Kavaka 11:53-54.

Deshmukh, S.K. and Agrawal, S.C. (1985). Degradation of human hair by some dermatophytes and other keratinophilic fungi. Mykosen 28:463-466.

Dey, N.C. and Kakoti, L.M. (1955). *Microsporum gypseum* in India. J.Indian Med. Assoc. 25: 160-164.

Dixit, A.K. (1991). Occurrence and antagonistic studies of keratinophilic fungi with special reference to Microsporum species. Ph.D.Thesis, Kanpur University, Kanpur.

Dixit, A.K. and Kushwaha, R.K.S. (1990). Keratinophilic fungi of Andaman Islands, India. Indian J. Microbiol. 30:349-350.

Dixit, A.K. and Kushwaha, R.K.S. (1991). Occurrence of keratinophilic fungi on Indian birds. Folia Microbiologia 36:383-386.

Emmons, E.W. (1955). Saprohytic sources of Cryptococcus neoformans associated with pigeon [Columba livia]. Amer. J.Hyg. 62-227-235.

English, M.P. (1965). The saprophytic growth of non-keratinphilic fungi on keratinized substrates and a comparision with keratinophilic fungi. Trans. Brit. Mycol. Soc. 48:219-235.

Garg, A.K. (1966). Isolation of derrmatophytes and other keratinophilic fungi from soil in India. Sabouraudia 4:259-264.

Guarro, J., Punzola, L. and Calvo, M.A. (1981). Keratinophilic fungi from soil of Tarragona, Cataluyna. Mycopathologia 76;69-71.

Hubalek, Z. (1974). Fungi associated with free living birds in Czechoslovakia and Yugoslavia. Acta. Sci. Ne. Brno. 8:1-62.

Hubalek, Z. (2000). Keratinophilic fungi associated with free-living mammals and birds. In: Biology of dermatophytes and other keratinophilic fungi (*Ed.* Kushwaha, R.K.S. and Guarro, J). Revista Iberoamericana de Micologia, Bilbao, Spain 93-103.

Hubalek, Z. and Hornic, M. (1977). Experimental infection of white mouse with Chrysosporium and Paecilomces. Mycopathologia 62:173-178.

Jain, P.C. (1983). Prevalence of keratinophilic fungi in soil of Madhya Pradesh and Uttar Pradesh. India. Geobios New Reports 2:10-13.

Jain, P.C. and Agrawal, S.C. (1979). Some additions to Indian Malbranchea. Kavaka 7.69-72.

Jain, Madhu, Shukla P.K. and Shrivastava, O.P. (1985). Keratinophilic fungi and dermatophytes in Lucknow soil and their global distribution. Mykosen 28:98-101.

Kushwaha, R.K.S. (2000). The genus *Chrysosporium*, its physiology and biotechnological potential. In: (Ed. Kushwaha, R.K.S. and Guarro, J.) Biology of dermatophytes and other keratinophilic fungi. Revista Iberoamericana de Micologia, Bilbao, Spain 66-76.

Kushwaha, R.K.S. and Agrawal, S.C. (1976). Some keratinophilic fungi and related dermatophytes from soil. Proc. Indian. Natl. Sci. Acad. 42:102-110.

Nigam, Neeta (1987). Studies on Chrysosporium and allied fungi from soil.Ph.D.Thesis, Kanpur University, Kanpur.

Nigam, Neeta and Kushwaha, R.K.S. (1986). Keratinophilic fungi in house dust of Kanpur. Proc. Natl. Acad. Sci.India 56:39-37.

Nigam, Neeta and Kushwaha, R.K.S. (1989a). Some new reports on keratinophilic fungi. Curr.Sci. 58:1374.

Nigam, Neeta and Kushwaha, R.K.S. (1989b). Occurrence of non-keratinophilic fungi on keratin. Trans.Mycol. Soc. Japan 30:1-8.

Nigam, Neeta and Kushwaha, R.K.S. (1989c). Decomposition of feathers and hairs by keratinophilic fungi. Indian J. Microbiol. 29:241-244.

Nigam, Neeta and Kushwaha, R.K.S. (1990). Occurrence of keratinophilic fungi with special reference to *Chrysosporium* species in India. Sydowia 42:200-208.

Padhye, A.A., Pawar, V.H. Sukapure, R.S. and Thirumalachar, M.J. (1967). Keratinophilic fungi from marine soils of Bombay, India. Part I Hindustan Antibiot. Bull. 10:138-141.

Pugh, G.J.F. (1965). Celluloytic and keratinolytic fungi recorded on birds. Sabouraudia 4:85-91.

Pugh, G.J.F. (1966a). Fungi on birds in India. J. Indian Bot. Soc.45:296-303.

Pugh, G.J.F. (1966b).Association between birds nest, their pH and keratinophilic fungi. Sabouraudia 5:49-63.

Pugh, G.J.F. (1972). The contamination of birds feather by fungi. Sabouraudia 114:172-177.

Pugh, G.J.F. and Mathison, G.E. (1962). Studies on fungi in coastal soils. III. An ecological survey of keratinophilic fungi. Trans.Brit.Mycol.Soc.45:567-572.

Pugh, G.J.F. and Evans, M.D. (1970). Keratinophilic fungi associated with birds. I. Fungi isolated from feathers, nests and soil. Trans.Brit.Mycol.Soc.54:233-240.

Randhawa, H.S. and Sandhu, R.S. (1965). A survey of soil inhabiting dermatophytes and related keratinophilic fungi of India. Sabouraudia 4:71-79.

Rees, R.G.(1967). Keratinophilic fungi from feathers of domestic fowl. Sabouraudia 6:19-28.

Saksena, V. (1993). Studies on anamorph and teleomorphs of Arthtroderma and related fungi. Ph.D.Thesis. Kanpur University, Kanpur.

Sheridan, J.E. (1971). The kerosene fungus *Amorphotheca resinae* as a natural component of air spora and bird feathers Newzealand J. Sci.14:1094-1096.

Shrivastava, J.N. and Kushwaha, R.K.S. (1983). Dermatophytes from Indian soils. III Internatl.. Myco. Cong. 638.

Singh, K. V. and Agrawal, S.C. (1983). Keratinophilic fungi from some substrates on central India. Geobios 10:165-171.

Sur, B. and Ghosh, G.R. (1980a). Keratinophilic fungi from Orissa, India I isolation from soil. Sabouraudia 18:269-264.

Sur, B. and Ghosh, G.R. (1980b). Keratinophiiic fungi from Orissa, India II Isolation from feathers of wild birds and domestic fowls. Sabouraudia 18:275-280.

Microbiology and Biotechnology for Sustainable Development (Ed. P.C. Jain),
CBS Publishers & Distributors, New Delhi (2004), pp. 71–83.

A-7

The Maintenance and Preservation of Filamentous Fungi

P.C. Jain and S. K. Deshmukh*
Department of Applied Microbiology and Biotechnology
Dr. H.S. Gour Vishwavidyalaya, *Sagar 470 003, India*

Abstract

The various methods of the maintenance and preservation of filamentous fungi viz. maintenance by subculturing, storage in sterile distilled water, under mineral oil, drying on silica gel, soil storage, freeze-drying, cryo-preservation and preservation using liquid nitrogen are described here. Control of mite infestation and use of black light to induce sporulation in fungal cultures is highlighted.

The need to have culture collections with ultra modern techniques for varied groups of microorganisms is emphasized at regional and national level. The need of a national collection for reference strains including a gene bank with identification services, where cultures can be deposited for patent purposes with a data base connected to the regional culture collections is also emphasized.

Key Words: Fungi, Preservation, Freeze-Drying, Cryo-preservation, Liquid Nitrogen.

INTRODUCTION

Fungi are widely used in different sectors of society and are known to produce a large number of secondary metabolites (Turner, 1971; Turner and Aldridge,1983). They are used for the production of drugs, pesticides, enzymes, vitamins and acids. They are also part of food processes i.e. cheese, bread, wine, beer and yoghurt. Fungi also form an important group that cause diseases in human beings and animals. It is frequently stated that biodiversity generally is greater in tropical climates than in temperate climates. Hawksworth (1991) estimated that some 1.5 million species of fungi were likely to exist, compared to the 69,000 or so recorded; out of these only 11,500 (17 %) are represented in all the collections. Evidence

* Dept. of Natural Products, Quest Institute of Life Sciences, Nicholas Piramal India Limited, Post Box No. 17753, L. B. S. Marg, Mulund (W), Mumbai 400 080. India

for the richness of the fungal biota of tropical region is also quoted in the same article. This is why many culture collections are coming up in developing countries.

Many reviews are available on preservation techniques of microorganisms (Smith, 1988; Stockdale *et al.*, 1989; Smith and Onions, 1994; Singh, 1995 and Smith, 1997). Liquid nitrogen and lyophilization (freeze-drying) are the best methods available and are essential for the preservation of irreplaceable isolates and for the maintenance of genetic stability: both prove to be excellent long-term storage techniques. However, for the successful use of any of the methods, it is essential that the culture should remain in good condition. Optimum growth and sporulation will lead to better survival after preservation; poor cultures are rarely improved by preservation.

This article gives a comprehensive list of the methods of maintenance of fungal cultures. It is recommended that each isolate should be maintained by at least two of the methods. The choice of the method will depend largely on the extent to which equipment and facilities are available in the laboratory.

PRESERVATION AND MAINTENANCE BY SUBCULTURING

Many fungi can be kept in good condition for several years by routine subculturing on agar medium slopes in screw capped bottles or plugged tubes and this was the only method available in early collections. However, the fungi must be transferred to fresh agar at intervals as nutrients become exhausted and the built-up waste products may become inhibitory. A mass spore transfer is by far the best method and mycelium transfer should only be used where no spores are available (Onions,1971). Dehydration may also occur. The maximum period between subculturing varies widely according to the isolate and the laboratory conditions (temperature, humidity), from as little as 2 weeks to 6 weeks or longer. Transfer once a month is suitable for most pathogenic fungi maintained at an average ambient temperature of 20°C.

The transfer is a selective process and should be carried out by a person who knows the fungi. Subculturing of the collection should not be assigned to an untrained person. Long-handled needles with the tip of the needle bent at a right angle are most suitable for handling fungi. When fungi are grown in artificial conditions they may undergo genetic changes to produce atypical strains more suitable to the condition provided. Many fungi tend to degenerate and lose the ability to sporulate.

This method is still used for working collections holding a small number of cultures that are in constant use. However, this is a very time consuming and labor-intensive exercise, especially when a large number of organisms are kept.

If well-grown cultures are transferred to the cold-room or refrigerator, it should be ensured that bottle caps are not screwed down tightly as metabolism may continue at a reduced rate and oxygen starvation may occur. Transfer to the fresh medium should be carried out at intervals of 1 month to 1 year depending on the species. As a general rule, under refrigeration the storage period for non-cold sensitive strains is doubled. This will reduce the interval between the transfer of the culture to a fresh medium as the metabolic rate of the fungus is lowered, drying out by evaporation occurs more slowly and movements of mites is reduced. Some fungi are sensitive to storage at low temperature and suffer chill injury that may cause permanent damage and eventually death.

CONTROL OF MITE INFESTATION

Fungal cultures are susceptible to infestation with mites. These small animals, commonly of the genera *Tryoglyphus* and *Tarsonemus,* occur naturally in soil and on almost any organic material. The first sign of mites is usually bald non-sporing patches on the colony or lines of small bacterial or fungal colonies where the mites have walked. These can be seen by the naked eye as tiny white dots. They are detected more easily by examination under a low power - binocular microscope, particularly around the apex of the agar slope. The damage caused by these mites is tremendous; on one hand they eat the culture and heavy infestation can completely strip a culture and on the other hand they carry fungal spores and bacteria on and in their body from one culture to another culture and contaminate the other cultures.

Some of the methods used for controlling infestation by mites in laboratories are as follows:

1) Destroy all cultures contaminated with mites.
2) Isolate the cultures that have been in contact with contaminated cultures and examine frequently for mites.
3) Wash all benches, incubators and culture cabinets with an acaricide such as 0.2% v/v Acetelic (ICI) or a strong phenolic disinfectant such as Hycolin (William Pearson Ltd.).
4) Place a culture of importance that is mite-infested in a deep freezer at - 20°C for 3 days before subculturing. Cultures of non-sporulating fungi which will not survive the short term cold storage may be covered with a layer of mineral oil and sub-cultured after 24 hours. Eggs of mites are more resistant to such treatment than adults and the procedure may have to be repeated two or three times (Stockdale *et al.*, 1989).
5) Snyder and Hansen (1946) recommended that sealed bottles below the screw caps or above the cotton wool plugs (well pushed down) with sterile cigarette papers using copper sulfate glue (Gelatin 20g; Copper sulfate 2.0g and water 100 ml). The pores of the papers allow respiration but prevent movement of mites, thus protecting clean cultures and isolating the infected ones. Care is taken to ensure that the seal is effective.
6) Smith (1971) recommended the use of disposable plastic bottles with plastic caps which when screwed down still allow respiration but exclude mites.
7) Smith (1978) described a method using screwed lids with a hole sealed with metricel that is said to give complete protection.

STORAGE IN STERILE DISTILLED WATER

Dispense 1-2 ml of distilled water into small screw-capped bottles and sterilize by autoclaving. Remove aerial mycelium from the surface of a mature (preferably sporulating) culture, using a mounted needle or inoculating wire and taking care not to remove any of the agar medium, and transfer it to the water. The vials are stored at room temperature or in a cooling cabinet at 4°C in the dark.

This is a simple, inexpensive, and effective way to store fungi and is equally good for sporulating and non-sporulating cultures. In this case the caps of the vials are closed and the cultures are safe from contamination and from mites. Contamination may occur on removal of the mycelia, therefore a stock culture should be kept in reserve. A point to note is that some tubes may have poor seals and the collection should be checked every 6 months for signs of evaporation and water loss.

The revival of the culture stored in sterile distilled water is achieved by removing the aerial mycelia aseptically and placing on a suitable medium. Castellani (1939) introduced this method for preservation of some pathogenic fungi. Many types of dermatophytes have been kept in sterile water with little or no deterioration for over 10 years. Some morphological changes have been noted in a number of tubes and it is thought that accidental transfer of the agar medium to the tube enables growth and mutation to take place during storage. This method was reported for the preservation of fungi (Boeswinkel, 1976; Hartung de Caprieles *et al.*, 1989). Castellani (1967) reported that the water storage method can be used for the preservation of human pathogenic fungi. Other fungi including phytopathogenic fungi (Figueiredo and Pimentel, 1975: Boeswinkel, 1976), oomycetes (Clark and Dick, 1974) entomophthorales, pyrenomycetes, gesteromycetes, hyphomycetes (Ellis, 1979) and ectomycorrhizal fungi (Marx and Danial, 1976) have all survived using this technique. This technique is a very valuable labour saving technique for the maintenance of ectomycorrhizal fungi (Heinonen-Tanski, 1989; Heinonen-Tanski and Holopainen, 1994).

PRESERVATION AND MAINTENANCE UNDER MINERAL OIL

Well grown cultures on Potato dextrose agar (PDA) slants are covered to a depth of 1 cm above the top of the slant with twice autoclaved (121°C for 15 minutes) liquid paraffin (medicinal paraffin, specific gravity 0.830- 0.890). Care should be taken in this regard since any exposed mycelium bits can act as wicks to dry out the culture. If the slants are made short, less oil is required. The oil is prepared and added separately to individual tubes, because dry spores on the surface of the culture may be dislodged at the time of addition and infect the oil applicator if it is used for multiple additions. This reduces the chances of contamination. McCartney bottles with rubber liners removed from the caps (the oil used in this method reacts with the rubber liners in metal caps of culture bottles) are useful for this purpose as they stand on their own, but test tubes are quite suitable. It is important to use good healthy cultures, preferably well sporulated. This method of preservation is particularly useful in tropical climates as it prevents drying out of the cultures, does not allow penetration of mites, requires no expensive apparatus and is easy to use.It also slows down metabolic activity.

The revival of a culture maintained in mineral oil is achieved by removing a small amount of the fungal colony on a mounted needle and draining away as much as possible on the neck of the culture bottle. The inoculum is then streaked onto a suitable agar medium (PDA). More than one subculture may be necessary after revival as the growth rate can very often remain slow because of adhering oil. Better results may be obtained by inoculating midway down an agar slope and allowing oil to drain and the fungus to grow up the slope away from the oil.

Survival is generally good but morphological changes have been reported in several dermatophytes. There are chances of naturally occurring mutants becoming dominant over the wild type. The occurrence of sectoring as an expression of mutants is increased after storage under a layer of mineral oil. Constant supervision is required by a fungal expert to ensure that the original strain rather than the variant or mutant is transferred. This method is very simple and has been used from very early days (Buell and Weston, 1947; Little and Gordon, 1967; Smith and Onions, 1983).

DRYING ON SILICA GEL

McCartney bottles are filled with medium-grain plain 6-22 mesh non indicating silica gel and sterilized in dry heat (180 °C for 3 hours). The bottles are kept in a tray of water to a depth above the level of the silica gel. The water is frozen by placing the tray in a deepfreezer (-7°C to -24°C). As silica gel liberates heat when moistened with water, the technique depends upon keeping the cultures at a temperature cool enough not to damage the spores during preparation. Spore suspensions are prepared in sterile 5% (w/v) skimmed milk and added to the silica gel crystals in the tray of frozen water using a Pasteur pipette and are wetted three quarters to avoid over-saturation. The gel bottles are left in the ice bath for about 20 minutes till the ice around them has melted a little. The crystals are agitated to ensure thorough dispersion of the suspension. Bottles are dried with the caps loose for 14 days at 25°C until the silica gel crystals readily separate.

The viability is checked by sprinkling a few crystals on to a suitable medium and assessing the amount of growth from each crystal. Upon satisfactory growth, bottles are screwed down tightly and stored over indicator silica gel in an airtight container at 4°C. The indicator gel will require replacement once or twice a year. The used-up gel can be dried out by heating at 180°C for 2 hours or until the colour is fully restored. Repeated retrieval can result in contamination.

The silica gel technique was found successful for sporulating hyphomycetes, the coelomycetes and the ascomycetes but not for the discomycetes (Smith and Onions, 1983). Thin-walled spores, spores with appendages and mycelial cultures tend not to survive in this method. Apparently this technique is valuable for those groups that maintain fungi but have limited resources. Sporulating fungi can be maintained by this method for a period of 20 years or more. But it is recommended, following the experience at IMI that the majority of the cultures should be re-preserved before completion of 8 years as a large proportion of strains survive only for 8 - 11 years (Smith and Onions, 1994). This method is an alternate technique that has proved capable of maintaining genetic stability in fungi (Ogata, 1962; Perkins, 1962). Grivell and Jackson (1969) and Windles *et al.* (1988) used this method for the preservation of various groups of fungi. The pathogenicity of *Helminthosporium maydes* was maintained for one year using this method (Sleesman *et al.*, 1974).

SOIL STORAGE

Spore suspensions in sterile water are poured into a culture bottle containing twice autoclaved garden loam (moisture 20%). The fungus is allowed to grow for a few days and stored with loose caps in the refrigerator.

The revival of a culture maintained in soil is achieved by sprinkling a few grains of soil containing the fungus on a suitable medium and incubated under optimum growth conditions.

This method is cheap, needs no special equipment and is unlikely to be infected by mites. Some variations may occur but cultures are otherwise stable and the survival rate of upto 10 years is reported. Atkinson (1953) has obtained stability and good viability of *Rhizopus, Alternaria, Aspergillus, Circinella* and *Penicillium*. The successful preservation of *Fusarium* spp. was also done (Gordon,1952; Booth, 1971). *Septoria* spp and *Pseudocercosporella herpotricodes* have been maintained succesfully by this method without the loss of sporulation or pathogenicity (Shearer *et al.*, 1974; Reinecke and Fokkema, 1979).

PRESERVATION AND MAINTENANCE OF FUNGI BY FREEZE-DRYING

It is a convenient method for the preservation and long term storage of a wide variety of microorganisms. Freeze-drying is achieved by the sublimation of ice from the frozen state. It can be achieved by different means. The techniques of centrifugal freeze-drying, which rely on evaporative cooling, can be used successfully for the storage of many sporulating fungi, but a technique that allows the variation of the cooling rate to suit the organism being freeze dried is preferable. The sealing of the ampoules or vials is most important and heat-sealed glass is preferred to butyl rubber bungs in glass vials as these may leak over long-term storage and allow the deterioration of freeze-dried fungi. Some fungi may survive without a cryo-protectant but a correct choice of the suspending medium can improve viability of many strains.

Generally the cultures for lyophilization should be healthy and well sporulating to give the best results. The suspension medium gives protection to the spores from damage due to freezing. Commonly used suspension media are skimmed milk, serum, peptone, various sugars or a mixture of them.

The glass ampoules are acid-washed (by soaking in 2% hydrochloric acid), rinsed and dried.

The filter paper strips with respective accession number are put in the ampoules. These ampoules are then plugged and autoclaved.

A suspension of the respective organism is prepared in sterile 10% skimmed milk containing 3% meso-inositol by adding about 2 ml of the skimmed milk to the grown slant. 0.2 ml of the suspension is added into the ampoules with the help of Pasteur pipettes and cotton plugs are replaced with sterile lint caps under aseptic conditions.

These ampoules are then loaded on the spin-freeze rack of a suitable freeze dryer, covered with a chamber bell jar and centrifuged for 15 minutes. Drying is done under vacuum and continued for about 3 hours after which the primary drying is complete.

After three hours the vacuum is released. The ampoules are removed and plugged with sterile cotton plugs and constricted at about half the length of the ampoule using an air and gas flame. The bore of constriction should remain greater than one millimeter, and the outer diameter greater than 2.5 mm.

These ampoules are inserted into the ports of manifolds and placed under vacuum overnight (approx. 17 hours) for secondary drying. The ampoules are then sealed using an air and gas flame under vacuum and stored at 4°C. Storing the ampoule at low temperature is thought to give great longevity and a temperature of 4°C seems to be favored (Heckley, 1978). However, Smith (1983) reported that fungi survive over 15 years when the ampoules stored between 15°C and 20°C. Low temperature storage is thought to reduce the rate of deterioration.

For revival tips of the ampoules are opened by heating the tips and then adding a drop of water so that the glass cracks or are sawed with a file and then broken open. Sterile saline is added into the ampoules to obtain a suspension with the help of a Pasteur pipette or the dried inoculum is added directly onto a nutrient agar slant or plate.

This method is the most convenient and successful method of preserving sporulating fungi. It removes the possibility of contamination during storage and is ideal for distribution of the organisms. The organisms are kept very stable in storage. Sarbhoy (1974) found that 12 of their lyophilized cultures failed to grow after one year of storage. These results indicate that it is important to check the viability of stored ampoules frequently (very 1-2 years), at least until it is confirmed that the number of viable cells remain high. Freeze drying was used on a large scale for fungi by Raper and Alexander (1945) and the viability of their freeze-dried cultures after storage for 23 years was subsequently reported by Ellis and Robertson (1968). The rate of freezing is a very important factor. A slow rate of freezing i.e., 1°C/ min, has been successful with fungi (Hwang, 1966; Heckly, 1978). Over drying will kill the microorganisms; in other cases, mutation damages the DNA (Ashwood-Smith and Grant, 1976). A residual moisture content between 1 and 2 % proved to be successful (Smith, 1983). Dermatophyes have been preserved successfully by freeze drying for over 20 years (Stockdale *et al.*, 1989).

PRESERVATION AND MAINTENANCE OF FUNGI BY CRYOPRESERVATION

Lowering the temperature to a point where the organisms are frozen enables the preservation of fungi. The survival of fungal cultures depends upon the presence of a cryo-protectant, the rate of cooling, the temperature of storage and the rate of thawing. The fungal spores and mycelia survive if suitable conditions are employed.

Grow the isolate to maturity on slopes of a suitable agar medium, scrape the growth from the agar slopes and transfer to 2 ml plastic ampoules containing cryo-protectant (1.5 ml of 10 % glycerol) These ampoules are stored at -20 °C or they are cooled in a controlled cooler at -1°C / minute to -35 °C and stored in the freezer at -70 °C / -80 °C.

To test viability, place the ampoules in a heated water bath at +37°C and agitate rapidly until all the ice has melted. Pour the contents of the ampoules onto a suitable growth medium and incubate at the required growth temperature.

PRESERVATION AND MAINTENANCE OF FUNGI USING LIQUID NITROGEN

Preservation of microorganisms in the liquid or vapor phase of liquid nitrogen (-196°C) is the most universally applicable method of preservation. Storage in liquid nitrogen may be the only method for long-term preservation of fungi that do not survive freeze drying. Current knowledge suggests longevity and stability of cultures is higher in most organisms preserved in liquid nitrogen. The optimum conditions can be determined by the use of a cryogenic light microscope, where the effect of different protocol on the cells can be observed and the least stressful conditions are used (Smith, 1992). It is reported that longevity is indefinite if stored at temperature below -140°C, 0.5- 5 years at -20 °C, 1-7 years at -40°C, in excess of 10 years at -80 °C and approaching indefinite at -135 °C (Smith and Waller, 1992). It is a form of influence dormancy wherein the organism does not undergo any change either phenotypically or genotypically provided adequate care is taken during freezing and thawing. Both sporulating and non-sporulating cultures may be preserved by this method.

Prepare the spore suspension in 10% glycerol. Pipette 0.5 ml of the cells suspend into 2.0 ml sterile cryotubes. Cool in control rate freezer to -50°C. Transfer to a metal drawer rack in the liquid nitrogen storage freezer.

For revival thaw, the cryotube rapidly by placing it in a water bath at + 37°C or in the chamber of the controlled cooler on a warming cycle until the sample ampoule, monitored with a temperature probe, thaws. Slow thawing may cause damage due to re-crystallization of ice during warming, therefore rapid thawing in recommended. Slow freezing and rapid thawing generally gives the highest viability (Heckly, 1978).

Due to problems of space, propylene straws are also used as alternative to glass ampoules (Stalpers *et al.*, 1987). By their small size, the cheap polypropylene straws reduce space and the consumption of liquid nitrogen drops down drastically. Even though the plastic ampoules with screw caps may leak during storage, they are safer than glass ampoules that may explode on expansion of liquid nitrogen (Simione *et al.*, 1977). The method is as follows:

Sporulating fungi are grown on solid media until conidia develop. A heavy conidial suspension is prepared in glycerol (10 % w/v in water) and filled into a sterile straw (polyvinylchloride / polypropylene) sealed at one end, with a disposable syringe or Pasteur pipette. The straw may then be sealed completely and transferred aseptically to a sterile cryotube. Mycelial fungi are grown in media supplemented with 5% (w/v) glycerol. Strains that do not tolerate lower water activity caused by the cryo-protectent may be grown without glycerol and flooded with a 10% (w/ v) glycerol solution shortly before processing. A sterile straw open at both ends is now used to punch the mycelium with the agar near the margin of the colony. This process is repeated until the straw is filled completely. The straw is either left open at both the ends and transferred aseptically to a sterile cryotubes or it may be sealed. To obtain the freezing rate, that is the theoretical optimum of 1-10°C per minute, the cryotubes are either transferred to a mechanical deepfreezer at - 70°C for two hours in a Styrofoam box of 2 cm thickness or placed in the gas phase of a liquid nitrogen tank for above 40 minutes.

For revival, one straw at a time is removed from the frozen cryotube; the sealed straw are transferred into a 50ml glass beaker with warm water (30°C). Sealed straws may be surface-sterilized by immersion into 70% ethanol (v/v), before they are opened with sharp, sterile scissors or pincers. The cell suspension is withdrawn with a fine Pasteur pipette. Incubation is done at appropriate temperature until the growth is visible. Open straw filled with mycelial fungi are thawed directly on an agar slant at room temperature (22 to 25 °C).

The liquid nitrogen method is the technique that can be most widely applied to the storage of fungi. The viability of Zygomycetes, Ascomycetes, Basidiomycetes, Hyphomycetes and Coeliomycetes after freezing and storage are very high (Smith and Onions, 1994). The fungi that are difficult to grow in culture can be kept alive for long periods in liquid nitrogen, e.g., rust and smut spores (Loegering, 1965, Kilpatrick *et al.*, 1971) and *Sclerospora* spp (Smith, 1982). The main drawback of this method is that it is dependent on the supply of liquid nitrogen. Therefore, it should always be used as backup of some other preservation method. This method is the method of choice for all fungi if funds and facilities are available. The potential storage period and the stability of fungi stored are unequalled by any of the other techniques.

USE OF BLACK LIGHT TO INDUCE SPORULATION IN FUNGAL CULTURES

Successful preservation sometimes depends on the presence of spores. It is reported that light induces sporulation in fungal cultures (Leach, 1961, 1962a) and short wavelengths have been used to induce spore production. The wavelengths that appear to be most effective in inducing sporulation are mainly in the near range of the ultra violet region (300 - 380 nm) of the spectrum as opposed to the ultra violet range (200- 300 nm) which can be lethal or mutagenic. Near the range of ultra violet region or black light pigmentation, the gross morphology of the colony or even spore morphology may be affected, though the effects are not sufficient to interfere with identification.

For treatment the fungal cultures are grown in Polystyrene petri dishes for 3-4 days before irradiation and the edge sealed with clear tape to prevent rapid drying. They are illuminated on light benches that have three 122cm fluorescent lamp holder 13 cm apart. A black light tube (Philips TL 40 W /08) is held in the center holder and a cool white tube (Philips MCFE 40 W /33) is placed on either side. They are controlled by a time switch that is set at a 12 hour on and off cycle. The petri dishes are supported on the shelf 32 cm below the light source and illuminated until sporulation is induced.

Irradiation at 21°C has proved successful and at CMI the stimulation is carried out at room temperature. The media employed can have an effect on the stimulation and weak media should be used (Leach, 1962b). When growing on glucose casein hydrolysate medium and stimulated by near ultraviolet light, *Diaporthe phaseolorum var. batatis* produces many perithecia and ascospores. However, when grown on malt or potato glucose media, the number of perithecia is much lower (Timnick *et al.*, 1951). The formation of pycnidium is induced in *Septoria nodorum* when the culture is grown on minimal medium and exposed to black light 25°C. Similarly, long range UV induces the sporulation in *Pseudocercosprella herpotrichoides* when grown on wheat straw meal (wheat straw 20g/L, agar 15g/L pH 6.0) at 16°C to 20°C. Even less sporulating fungi sporulate well when they are inoculated on dried autoclaved wheat or rice leaves with a mycelium/spore suspension e.g. *Curvularia* (Deshmukh, unpublished data).

Present Status of Culture Collections in India

About 80 culture collections are there in India at various levels of which some culture collections are listed below:

1. CCDMBI	Culture Collection Department of Microbiology, Bose Institute, Calcutta, India.
2. CIPDE	Collection of Insect Pathogens, Department of Entomology, Marathwada Agricultural University, Parbhani, India.
3. DBV	Division of Standardisation, Indian Veterinary Research Institute, Izatnagar, India.
4. DFRM	Defence Research Laboratory (Materials), Culture Collection, R & D Organization, Ministry of Defense, Napier Road, Kanpur (Uttar Pradesh), India.
5. DMSRDE	DMSRDE Culture collection, DRDO, New Delhi.
6. DUM	Delhi University Mycological Herbarium, Delhi, India.
7. GPCK	Germplasm Centre for keratinophilic fungi, Department of Botany, Christ Church College Kanpur, India.
8. HACC	Hindustan Antibiotics Ltd., Pimpri, Pune, India
9. IJMARI	Indian Jute Mills Association Research Institute, Calcutta, India.
10. ICRISAT	International Crops Research Institute of Semi-Arid Tropics, Hyderabad, India
11. ITCC	Indian Type Culture Collection, New Delhi, India.
12. MCM	MACH Collection of Microorganisms, MACS – Agarkar Research Institute, Pune, India.
13. MTCC	Microbial Type Culture collection and Gene Bank, IMTECH Chandigarh, India.
14. MAC	MACS Collection of Microorgenisms, Pune, Maharashtra, India
15. MPKV	Biological Nitrogen Fixation Project, College of Agriculture, Mahatma Phule Agriculture University, Rahuri, India.
16. NCDC	National Collection of Dairy Cultures, Dairy Microbiology Division, National Dairy Research Institute, Karnal, India.
17. NCIM	National Collection of Industrial Micro-organisms, division of Biochemical Sciences NCL, Pune, India.
18. NTCC	National Type Culture Collection ,Forest Pathology Department, Forest Research Institute, Dehra Dun (U.P.), India.
19. NTCCI	Culture Collection Microbiology and Cell Biology Laboratory Indian Institute of Science, Bangalore, India.
20. RRL	Department of Microbiology, Regional Research Laboratory, Jammu, India.
21. RUBL	Department of Botany, University of Rajasthan, Jaipur, India.
22. UBFFTD	Food and Fermentation Technology Division, University of Mumbai: Department of Chemical Technology, India.
23. VPCI	Fungal Culture collection, Vallabhbhai Patel Chest Institute, University of Delhi, India.

The culture collections mentioned above have limited facilities and number of fungi. There is a need to make these collections diverse in all respects. Proper methods should be used for the preservation of fungi. Although freeze drying techniques are used in a few collections, cryopreservation using liquid nitrogen should be used as a backup. While using the liquid nitrogen method, proper cooling i.e. -1°C / minute should be monitored in the deep freezer. Cryomicroscopic observation should be undertaken for using this technique.

Human and animal pathogenic fungi are isolated from patients and also from soil and are maintained only in the center where they are isolated and their numbers are also very limited. These fungi require special attention for preservation. We should have a separate collection of these fungi at a single place keeping all safety precautions in mind.

Quite a few basidiomycetes are grown in forests and other localities during the rainy season. These fungi cannot be preserved easily for long terms. As so many reports suggest that these fungi can be preserved successfully in liquid nitrogen using polypropylene straws, we can make a good collection of this group of fungi.

As India is a large country with varied climatic conditions, we get varied groups of microorganisms. Knowing well the diversity and use of these organisms there is a need to have a regional culture collection with ultra modern techniques. These collections will help Indian scientists not only to obtain novel secondary metabolites for various pharmaceutical and agricultural uses but also for various food industries. These organisms can also be used for the biodegradation of various municipal waste and for the production of biogas.

Apart from these there should be a national collection for reference strains including a gene bank with identification services, where cultures can be deposited for patent purposes. It must be connected to the regional culture collections through data base.

ACKNOWLEDGEMENT

The authors are thankful to Dr. B. N. Ganguli, Emeritus Scientist, C. S. I. R., Govt. of India, U. D. C. T., Matunga, Mumbai for valuable suggestions and necessary help during preparation of this manuscript.

REFERENCES

Ashwood - Smith, M. J. and Grant, E. (1976) Mutation induction in bacteria by freeze drying. *Cryobiology*. 13: 206-213.

Atkinson, R.G. (1953) Survival and pathogenicity of *Alternaria raphini* after 5 years in dried soil culture. *Can. J. Bot.* 31: 542- 547.

Boeswinkel, H. J. (1976) Storage of fungal cultures in water. *Trans.Brit. mycol. Soc.* 66: 183-185.

Booth, C. (1971) *The genus Fusarium*. Kew; Common Wealth Mycological Institute pp. 237.

Buell, C. B. and Weston, W. H. (1947) Application of the mineral oil conservation method to maintaining collection of fungal cultures. *American Journal of Botany* 34: 555-561.

Castellani, A. (1939) Viability of some pathogenic fungi in distilled water. *J. Trop. Med. Hyg.* 42: 225-226.

Castellani, A. (1967) Maintenance and cultivation of common pathogenic fungi of man in sterile distilled water. Further researches. *J. Trop. Med. Hyg.* 70: 181-184.

Clark, G. and Dick, M.W. (1974) Long-term storage and viability of aquatic oomycetes. *Trans.Brit Mycol. Soc.* 63: 611-612.

Ellis, J. J. (1979) Preserving fungus strains in sterile water. *Mycologia* 71: 1072-1075.

Ellis, J. J. and Roberson, J. A. (1968) Viability of fungal cultures preserved by lyophilization *Mycologia.* 60: 399-405.

Figueiredo, M. B. and Pimentel, C. P. V. (1975) Metodos utilizados para conservacao de fungos na micoteca da Secao de Micologia Fitopatologica de Instituto Biologico. *Summa Phytopathogica*: 1: 299-302.

Gordon, W. L. (1952) The occurrence of *Fusarium* Species in Canada. *Can. J. Bot.* 30: 209-251.

Grivell, A. R. and Jackson, J.F. (1969) Microbial culture preservation with silica gel. *J. General Microbiol.* 58: 423-425.

Hartung de Caprieles, C. Mata S. and Middleveen, M (1989) Preservation of fungi in water (Castellani) 20 years. *Mycopathologia* 106: 73-79.

Hawksworth, D. L. (1991) The fungal dimention of biodiversity ; magnitude, significance and conservation. *Myco. Res.* 95: 641-655.

Heckly, R. J. (1978) Preservation of microorgenisms. *Advances in Applied Microbiology* 24: 1-53.

Heinonen-Tanski, H.(1989) Maintenance methods for ectomycorrizal fungi. *Agricultural Ecosystems and Environment* 28: 171-174.

Heinonen-Tanski, H. and Holopainen, T. (1994) Maintenance of Ectomycorrizal fungi. In *Techniques in Mycorrhizal Research, Methods in Microbiology* (*Ed.* Norris J. R. Read, D. J. and Varma A.) London, NewYork Acedemic Press, pp 413-422.

Hwang, S.W. (1966) Long term preservation of fungal cultures with liquid nitrogen refrigeration. *Applied Microbiology* 14: 784-788.

Kilpatrick, R. A., Harmon, D.L., Loegering, W. Q. and Clark, W. A. (1971) Viability of Uredospores of *Puccinia graminis* f. sp. *tritici* stored in liquid nitrogen. *Plant Disease Reporter* 55: 871-873.

Leach, C. M. (1961) The sporulation of *Helminthosporium oryzae* as affected by exposure to near ultraviolet radiation and dark periods. *Can. J. Bot.* 39: 706-715.

Leach, C. M. (1962a) The sporulation of diverse species of fungi under near-ultraviolet light radiation. *Can. J. Bot.* 40: 151-161.

Leach, C. M. (1962b) The quantitative and qualitative relationship of monochromatic radiation to the induction of reproduction in *Aschochyta pisi. Can. J. Bot.* 40:1577-1602.

Little, G.N. and Gordon, M. A. (1967) Survival of fungal cultures maintained under mineral oils for twelve years. *Mycologia* 59: 733-736.

Loegering W.Q. (1965) A type culture collection of plant rust fungi. Phytopathology. 55:247.

Marx, D. H. and Deniel, W. J. (1976). Maintaining cultures of ectomycorrhizal and plant pathogenic fungi in sterile water cold storage. *Can. J. Microbiol.* 22:338-381.

Ogata, W. N. (1962) Preservation of *Neurospora* stock cultures with anhydrous silica gel. *Neurospora News Letter.* 1:13.

Onion, A. H. S. (1971) Preservation of fungi. *In Methods in Microbiology* Vol 4. London, NewYork Acedemic Press, pp 131-151.

Perkins, D. D. (1962) Preservation of *Neurospora* stock cultures in anhydrous silica gel. Can. *J. Microbiol.* 8:591-594.

Raper, K. B. and Alexander, D. F. (1945) Preservation of mold by the lyophil process. *Mycologia.* 37: 499-525.

Reinecke, P. and Fokkema, N. J. (1979) *Pseudocercosporella herpotrichoides* : Storage and mass production of conidia. *Trans Brit Mycol Soc.* 72 : 329-331.

Sarbhoy, A. K. Ghosh, S. K. Lal , S. P. and Lall G. (1974) Investigation on the preservation of fungi by lyophilization technique. *Indian Phytopath.* 27: 361-363.

Shearer, B. L., Zeyen R. J. and Ooka J. J. (1974) Storage and behavior in soil of *Septoria* species. isolated from cereals. *Phytopathology* 64:163-167.

Simione, F.P., Daggett, P.M., McGrath, M. S. and Alexander, M. T. (1977) The use of plastic ampoules for freeze preservation of microorganism. *Cryobiology.* 14:500-502.

Singh S. (1995) Microbial culture collection - Their activities and importance. In "Microbes for Better living" (*Ed.* Sankaranand R.and Manja K. S.) The Bangalore Printing and Publishing Company Ltd. Bangalore, India, pp 143-151.

Sleesman, J. P., Larsen, P. O. and Safford, J. (1974) Maintenance of stock cultures of *Helminthosporium maydes* (race T and O). *Plant Disease Reporter* 58: 334-336.

Smith, D. (1982) Liquid nitrogen storage of fungi. *Trans Brit. mycol. Soc.* 79: 415-421.

Smith, D. (1983) A two stage centrifugal freeze drying method for the preservation of fungi. *Trans Brit. mycol. Soc.* 80: 333-337.

Smith, D. (1988) Culture and Maintenance : In Living Resources for Biotechnology : Filamentous fungi (*Ed.* Hawksworth, D. L. and Kirsop B. E.) Cambridge; Cambridge university press, pp 75-99.

Smith, D. (1992) Optimizing preservation. *Laboratory Practice.* 41: 25-28.

Smith, D. (1997). Sources of microorganisms and their preservation. In: Microbial Physiology - A practical approach (*Ed.* Rhoades M. and Stanbury P.) Oxford University Press. pp 1-22.

Smith, D. and Onions, A. H. S. (1983) A comparison of some preservation techniques for fungi. *Trans. Brit. Mycol. Soc.* 81: 535-540.

Smith, D. and Onions, A. H. S. (1994) *The preservation and maintenance of living fungi* (2nd Edition) IMI Technical Handbook, no 2 , International Mycological Institute , Egham UK.

Smith, D. and Waller, J. M. (1992) Culture collections of Microorganisms: Their importance in tropical plant pathology. *Fitopatol. bras.* 17: 1-8.

Smith, R. S. (1971) Maintenance of fungal cultures in Pre-sterilized disposable screwcap plastic tubes. *Mycologia* 63: 1218-1221.

Smith, R. S. (1978) A new lid closer for fungal culture vessels giving complete protection against mite infestation and microbiological contamination. *Mycologia* 70: 499-508.

Snyder, W. C. and Hansen, H. N. (1946) Control of mites by cigarette paper barriers. *Mycologia* 38: 455 - 462.

Stalpers, J. A., DeHoog, A. and Vlug, I. J. (1987) Improvement of the straw technique for the preservation of fungi in liquid nitrogen. *Mycologia.* 79:82-89.

Stockdale P. M ., Smith, D. and Campbell, C. K. (1989) The maintenance and preservation of fungi. In Medical Mycology, a practical approach (*Ed.* Evans E. V. G., and Richardson M. D.) IRL press Oxford, UK.

Timnick, M. B., Lilly, V. G. and Barnett, H. L. (1951). Factors affecting sporulation of *Diaporthe phaseolorum var. batatis* from soyabean. *Phytopathology.* 41:327-336.

Turner, W. B. (1971) Fungal metabolites.London Acedemic Press.

Turner W.B.and Aldridge, D.C. (1983) Fungal metabolites. II London Acedemic Press.

Windles, C. E., Burnes, P. M. and Kommedahl, T. (1988) Five years preservation of *Fusarium* spp. on silica gel and soils. *Phytopathology* 78:107-109.

Microbiology and Biotechnology for Sustainable Development (Ed. P.C. Jain),
CBS Publishers & Distributors, New Delhi (2004), pp. 84–90.

A-8

Rapid Diagnostic Tools for Typhoid Detection

G.P. Rai
Division of Microbiology, Defence R&D Estt.
Jhansi Road, Gwalior-474 002 (M.P.)

Abstract

Typhoid fever, caused by Salmonella typhi, is an important infectious disease especially in the third world countries. Laboratory diagnosis relies on culture isolation either from blood or urine of suspected patient or detection and demonstration of rising antibody titers against flageller (H) and somatic (O) antigens of S. typhi. In the present paper, many of the techniques commonly employed in the detection of either Salmonella typhi antigen or antibodies against it have been discussed with respect to their sensitivities, specificities, advantages and disadvantages.

Key Words: **Typhoid, PHA, LA, Co Ag, CIE, IFT, ELISA, DNA Probes, PCR**

INTRODUCTION

In our endeavor towards the economic development of the third world countries, a healthy population is of paramount importance. Infectious diseases continue to be the major health problem and important challenge to health authorities. According to an estimate the worldwide incidence to typhoid fever is a little over 12 million cases annually, of which Asia accounts for more than 62% cases. In some areas, typhoid fever is responsible for 2-5% of all deaths.

Typhoid fever continues to be a problem due to several factors, including increased urbanization, unsatisfactory water supply, poor sanitary conditions, malnutrition, emergence of antibiotic-resistant strains, problems in the identification and management of carriers, delays in definitive diagnosis, incomplete understanding of pathogenic mechanisms and virulence factors, and the unavailability of an universally effective, safe and cheap vaccine. Some of these problems have recently been studied by the newer approaches of immunology, molecular biology and biochemistry.

The causative agent of typhoid is *Salmonella typhi*. Its infection may be asymptomatic or cause overt disease in young children or adults. Laboratory diagnosis of typhoid fever is conventionally based on two methods: isolation of *S.typhi* from blood or urine by culture and demonstration of rising antibody titers to the 'H' and 'O' antigens of *S.typhi*, mainly by the widal test. An ideal diagnostic test for typhoid fever should be rapid, sensitive, specific and suitable for early diagnosis. It should be simple and inexpensive too because typhoid is endemic mainly in under developed areas of the world. Neither of the above two methods fulfill these requirements. During the last decade for rapid diagnosis of typhoid fever efforts have been devoted to the development of newer methods to detect elevated antibodies to antigens specific to *S.typhi* and to detect *S.typhi* specific antigens directly from blood or urine. Recent advances in hybridoma research and in the development of DNA technologies have provided two powerful tools to diagnostic microbiology. Detection of *S.typhi* specific antigens with monoclonal antibodies or *S.typhi* specific DNA sequence by polymerase chain reaction (PCR) for rapid diagnosis of typhoid fever became technically feasible.

In spite of many deficiencies, like low sensitivity, low specificity and time required to obtain the results, the Widal test remains most widely used method for serological diagnosis of typhoid fever. Other methods to detect antibodies are passive haemagglutination (PHA), counter immunoelectrophoresis (CIE), immunofluorescence test (IFT) enzyme-linked immunosorbent assay (ELISA) and Dot-ELISA using different types of purified antigen of *S.typhi*. In recent years ELISA has directed attention towards the detection of antibodies to the protein antigens of *S.typhi*. The main advantage of measuring these antibodies is that they can often be detected early in disease. In one study ELISA was used to measure serum antibodies in typhoid patients to different porins purified from *S.typhi*. In another study specific region of flagellin gene of *S.typhi* has been cloned and expressed as fusion protein. This fusion protein was used as specific antigen for detection of *S.typhi* antibodies by ELISA.

There are many reports on rapid diagnosis of *S.typhi* specific antigens directly from clinical specimens by latex agglutination (LA) test, coagglutination (COAg), CIE, ELISA etc., using polyclonal and monoclonal antibodies as probe. These techniques are being discussed below:

Haemagglutination assays (HA): A variety of antigens can be coupled to erythrocytes (RBCs) to provide the indicator system to detect antibodies. Target antigens such as polysaccharides readily adhere to RBCs, but protein antigens require pretreatment with tannic acid or with chromium chloride. Tanning the RBCs facilitates a high-density coating, which increases the sensitivity of the test system. Subsequent formalin or glutaraldehyde treatment of tanned RBCs coated with either protein or carbohydrate allows long-term storage. Tanned sheep or untanned human 'O' group RBCs coated either with whole cell lysate (WCL) antigens or lipopolysaccharide (LPS) have been used for serodiagnosis of typhoid (Zachariah and Rai, 1987; Petchclai *et al.*, 1987). For detection of Vi antibodies to typhoid organism in serum samples, a passive haemagglutination assay was developed using formalin fixed and chromium chloride treated sheep RBCs sensitized with Vi antigen of *S.typhi*. The test had a sensitivity of 83.3% while its specificity was 94% (Kang *et al.*, 1992). Kalhan *et al.* (1998) designed a reverse passive haemagglutination test for *S.typhi* antigen detection. In this test fresh sheep RBCs were coated with anti *S.typhi* immunoglobulin. The sensitivity and specificity of this assay was 70% and 92%, respectively.

Latex agglutination (LA): Latex particles are spheres of polystyrene, which readily bind IgG molecules by the Fc region at pH 9.0 when a low ionic-strength buffer is used. When antibodies are bound by their Fc region, the antibody-combining site [F (ab) regions] remain exposed and are capable of binding antigens. When the target antigens have repetitive antigenic structures (e.g., polysaccharide), multivalent antibodies coupled to multiple latex particles can bind antigen molecules and cross-link the latex particles, resulting in agglutination. The latex particles serve as the indicator system to detect the antigen-antibody reaction. LA has been used extensively for detection of Vi, O and Barber protein antigens of *S.typhi* in serum samples of typhoid patients with sensitivity varied from 39.5% to 93.3% and specificity varied from 95.8% to 100% (Jesudason *et al.*, 1994; Abdurakhmanov *et al.*, 1995 and Pandya *et al.*, 1995). LA has not been deployed to a greater extent for detection of typhoid antibodies in serum samples owing to its comparable sensitivity and specificity with that of widal test except in one report where authors have indicated that LA system is better than conventional widal test (Tantivanich *et al.*, 1984).

Coagglutination (CoAg): *Staphylococcus aureus* (Cowan strain I) contains protein A distributed evenly on the outermost layer of the cell wall. Protein A binds the Fc region of IgG subclasses 1,2 and 4 (which constitute 95% of the total IgG), analogous to the binding of IgG to latex particles. Formalin treatment stabilizes the *staphylococcus* cells. The antibody-coated *Staphylococcus* becomes the indicator reagent to detect the presence of antigens corresponding to the specificity of the coupled antibody. The reaction is observed in the form of a visible clumping i.e. agglutination of the particles.

Since protein A is an effective cross-linking reagent for most IgG subclasses, any other preformed complexes containing IgG and antigen would also cause agglutination of the sensitized *Staphylococcus* reagent. Nonspecific agglutination is prevented by treating the body fluid (serum, urine etc.) to be tested with soluble protein A to block binding of pre-formed complexes or by heating the body fluid to 65°C for 5 minutes to denature patient IgG molecules before testing.

CoAg must be well controlled to detect non-specific agglutination in the body fluid, using unsensitized *Staphylococcus* particles and particles sensitized with an irrelevant, but species specific antibody.

Many investigators have adapted the method of CoAg to detect O (somatic), d (flagellar) and Vi (Capsular) antigens in serum or urine or blood clot cultures of patients with typhoid fever with varying degree of sensitivity (83-97%) and specificity (97-98.5%) (Rockhill *et al.*,1980; Sarvamangala Devi and Shivananda, 1985 and Pandya *et al.*, 1995).

Counterimmunoelectrophoresis (CIE): CIE, one-dimensional double-electrophoresis, specifically directs the movement of antigen and antibody toward each other in an electric field. The buffer pH is selected to optimize the electroendosmotic effects of antibody toward the cathode (negative pole) while the antigen moves toward the anode (positive pole). This electrophic movement rapidly (30 min) concentrates the antigen and antibody in the zone between the adjacent wells. Depending on the sensitivity and specificity of the antibody used, minimal detectable concentrations of bacterial antigen range from 50 to 10 ng/ml (Fung and Tillton, 1985).

CIE has been widely used for detection of antigen or antibody of *S.typhi* in sera of typhoid patients (Gupta and Rao 1980; Sundararaj *et al.*, 1983). The antigen detection sensitivity has been reported in the range of 25-92% while specificity was in order of 95-100%. Simultaneous detection of typhoid antigen and antibody in serum samples by CIE has also been reported for early and rapid diagnosis of typhoid fever during the acute as well as in the chronic or late stages of the disease (Gupta and Rao, 1979). A radial CIE has also been developed for detection of typhoid antibodies within 4 minutes in serum samples of typhoid patients during acute stage of disease (Gupta and Rao, 1981).

Immunofluorescence assays (IFAs): IFA is most widely used technique in diagnosis of microbial infections. It uses bacterial cells as source of antigen affixed to a glass slide and a fluorochrome conjugated antibody as detection system. IFA remains the "gold standard" for many infectious disease serology test systems. The advantage of IFA are that (i) the antigen can be visualized, ensuring specificity of the reaction; (ii) it is significantly less cumbersome (iii) it is highly reproducible when performed by well trained technologists, and (iv) in indirect IFA; the same conjugate and dilution of patient sera can be used to detect antibody to many different organisms or antigens.

The disadvantage of IFA are that it (i) requires fresh cells; (ii) requires special equipment and conditions (a fluorescence microscope and a dark room for reading); (iii) is labour intensive, even when the substrate for indirect IFAs can be purchased (reagent dilution, multiple incubation and wash steps, and cover slips are required) (iv) is subjective, requiring extensive training to read the reactions and multiple controls to ensure test specificity and sensitivity and (v) has not been successfully automated.

IFA has been performed in two forms, namely; direct IFA and indirect IFA. Direct IFA is used to detect antigens or organisms present in cells or tissues, using fluorochrome conjugated antisera (conjugate) specific for the antigen(s) in question. IFA is used to detect antibodies in patient sera. Standardized antigens are fixed to glass slide. Patient serum is diluted, layered over the antigen, and incubated to allow the antigen - antibody complex to form. Unbound antibody is washed away, leaving only bound antibody, which is then incubated with the fluorescent conjugate. When antibodies are present in the patient's serum, a second antigen-antibody reaction will take place, with the conjugate becoming the third layer on the slide.

For general testing, fluorescein - conjugated anti-human immunoglobulin is usually anti-IgG with reactivity to both kappa and lambda light chains. This light chain reactivity also detects antibodies of the IgA or IgM class or both, which would be advantageous to detect all classes of antibody reactive with microorganisms.

Indirect fluorescent antibody test has been used for, serodiagnosis of typhoid by various workers (Chitkara and Urquhart, 1979; Rai *et al.*, 1989). For detection of typhoid carrier state Vi indirect fluorescent antibody test was developed (Doshi and Taylor, 1984) with a sensitivity and specificity of 98% and 99%, respectively. This test was found to be more sensitive than widal test.

Enzyme-linked immunosorbent assay (ELISA): The enzyme immunoassay, in which enzyme-labeled antibodies and antigens are used, is the most recent labeled reagent method and has been used extensively in typhoid diagnosis. In the enzyme immunoassays the antigen or antibody is usually attached to a solid-phase support to allow for easy separation of bound and free reagents. It has been found that both antigens and antibodies can be covalently attached to particulate materials, such as cellulose and polyacrylamide, and that satisfactory passive adsorption can also be obtained to tubes, beads, disks, or microplates, made of nylon, polystyrene, polyvinyl or polypropylene. Besides an essential part of an enzyme immunoassay is the conjugate of antibody (or antigen) linked to an enzyme. To reveal the reaction in enzyme immunoassays, the choice of substrate is critical. The substrates should be stable and should be soluble before and after degradation. Chromogenic substrates should be colorless initially and strongly colored after degradation.

Like IFA, ELISA can also be performed in direct (antigen detection) and indirect forms (antibody detection). Direct and indirect ELISA can further be performed in different formats such as competitive, sandwich ELISA etc. (Voller *et al.*, 1980).

ELISA has been widely used for serodiagnosis of typhoid. IgG, IgM and IgA antibodies to Vi capsular polysaccharide antigen of *S.typhi* has been measured by ELISA and results were compared with PHA. The IgG ELISA was as sensitive as the PHA (86 versus 76%) and as specific (95 versus 95%) in screening for chronic carriers (Losonsky *et al.*, 1987). Similarly IgA, IgG and IgM anti *S.typhi* lipopolysaccharide antibodies were measured by ELISA and gave the best discrimination between typhoid and nontyphoidal sera (Nardiello *et al.*, 1984). Anti-flagellin antibodies in typhoid sera have been determined, by ELISA with sensitivity and specificity of 93.6% and 94.9%, respectively (Jesudason *et al.*, 1998). A sandwich ELISA has also been developed for detection of *S.typhi* protein antigen in typhoid sera with sensitivity of 83.87% and specificity of 89.04% (Appassakiz *et al*, 1987).

Polymerase chain reaction (PCR): It results in the selective amplification of a chosen region of a DNA molecule to many folds. Any region of any DNA molecule can be chosen, so long as the sequences at the borders of the region are known. This is because in order to carry out DNA amplification by PCR, two short oligonucleotides must be annealed to the DNA molecule, one to each strand of the double helix. These oligonucleotides delimit the region that will be amplified. Amplification is carried out by DNA polymerase enzyme. The size of the amplified molecule can be determined by gel electrophoresis.

Though PCR fulfills the needs from the clinical microbiology laboratory: extreme specificity; high sensitivity and sufficient rapidity but it does have some shortcomings: it continues to require specialized equipment and personnel and its costs have yet to be lowered, which is an essential condition for its implementation in small, low budget laboratories. In turn PCRs are susceptible to contamination with extraneous DNA fragments that can be coamplified and carried over through successive amplification rounds. Overall these assays remain somewhat insensitive when applied to clinical specimens because of difficulties in sampling and purifying the target nucleic acid, the presence of polymerase inhibitors in samples or degradation of DNA.

A large number of reports are available in literature on the deployment of PCR for rapid detection of *S. typhi* in clinical samples. A polymerase chain reaction-microtitre plate hybridization technique was developed using 389 bp PCR product from the inv A gene of *S. typhi* for diagnosis of typhoid fever (Cocolin *et al.*, 1998). Similarly flagellin gene (d-H) was also amplified by PCR for diagnosis of typhoid (Song *et al.*, 1993; Chaudhry *et al.*, 1997).

Any of the above techniques can be adapted by clinical laboratories depending upon their capabilities and expertise.

REFERENCES

Abdurakhmanov, A.G., Iushchuk, N.D., Abdurakhmanova, E.G., Tendetnik, IuIa. and Shabalina, S.V. (1995) The demonstration of specific *Salmonella typhi* antigens by the latex agglutination method. Zh. Microbiol. Epidemiol. Immunobiol., 4, 86-87.

Appassakiz, H., Bunchuin, N., Sarasombath, S., Rungpitarangsi, B., Manatsathit, S., Komolpit, P. and Sukosol, T. (1987) Enzyme - linked immunosorbent assay for detection of *Salmonella typhi* protein antigen. J. Clin. Microbiol., 25, 273-277.

Chaudhry, R., Laxmi, B.V., Nisar, N., Ray, K. and Kumar, D. (1997) Standardisation of polymerase chain reaction for the detection of *Salmonella typhi* in typhoid fever. J. Clin. Pathol., 50, 437-439.

Chitkara, Y.K. and Urquhart, A.E. (1979) Fluorescent Vi antibody test in the screening of typhoid carriers. Am. J. Clin. Pathol., 72, 87-89.

Cocolin, L., Manzano, M., Astori, G., Botla, G.A., Cantoni, C.and Comi, G. (1998) A highly sensitive and fast non - radioactive method for the detection of PCR products from *Salmonella* serovars, such as *Salmonella typhi*,in blood specimens. FEMS Immunol. Med. Microbiol., 22, 233-239.

Doshi, N. and Taylor, A.G. (1984) Comparison of the Vi indirect fluorescent antibody test with the widal agglutination method in the serodiagnosis of typhoid fever. J. Clin. Pathol., 37, 805-808.

Fung, J.C. and Tilton, R.C. (1985) Detection of bacterial antigens by counterimmunoelectrophoresis, coagglutination and latex agglutination. *In:* Manual of Clinical Microbiology, 4th ed. (*Ed.* E.H. Lennette, A. Balows, W.J.Hausler, Jr. and H.J. Shadomy) Am. Soc. Microbiol., Washington, D.C. pp. 833-890.

Gupta, A.K. and Rao, K.M. (1979) Simultaneous detection of *Salmonella typhi* antigen and antibody in serum by counter – immunoelectrophoresis for an early and rapid diagnosis of typhoid fever. J. Immunol. Meth., 30, 349-353.

Gupta, A.K. and Rao, K.M. (1980) Antigen detection in serum by counter-immunoelectrophoresis for an early diagnosis of typhoid fever . J. Ind. Inst. Sci., 62, 105-109.

Gupta, A.K. and Rao, K.M. (1981) Radial counter-immunoelectrophoresis for rapid serodiagnosis of typhoid fever. J. Immunol. Meth., 40, 373-376.

Jesudason, M.V., Sridharan, G., Mukundan, S. and John, T.J. (1994) Vi - specific latex agglutination for early and rapid detection of *Salmonella* serotype *typhi* in blood cultures. Diagn. Microbiol. Infect. Dis., 18, 75-78.

Jesudason, M.V., Sridharan, G., Arulselvan, R., Babu, G.P. and John, T.J. (1998) Diagnosis of typhoid fever by the detection of anti - LPS and anti - flagellin antibodies by ELISA. Ind. J. Med. Res., 107, 204-207.

Kang, G., Sridharan, G., Jesudason, M.V. and John, T.J. (1992) Evaluation of modified passive haemagglutination assay for Vi antibody estimation in *salmonella typhi* infections. J. Clin. Pathol., 45, 740-741.

Kalhan, R., Kaur, I., Singh, R.P. and Gupta, R.C. (1998) Rapid diagnosis of typhoid fever. Ind. J. Pediatr., 65, 561-564.

Losonsky, G.A., Ferreccio, C., Kotloff, K.L., Kaintuck, S., Robbins, J.B. and Levine, M.M. (1987) Development and evaluation of an enzyme – linked immunosorbent assay for serum Vi antibodies for detection of chronic *Salmonella typhi* carriers. J. Clin. Microbiol., 25, 2266-2269.

Nardiello, S., Pizzella, T., Russo, M. and Galanti, B. (1984) Serodiagnosis of typhoid fever by enzyme-linked immunosorbent assay determination of anti - *Salmonella typhi* lipopolysaccharide antibodies. J. Clin. Microbiol., 20, 718-721.

Pandya, M., Pillai, P. and Deb, M. (1995) Rapid diagnosis of typhoid fever by detection of Barber protein and Vi antigens of *Salmonella* serotype *typhi*. J. Med. Microbiol., 43, 185-188.

Petchclai, B., Ausavarungnirun R. and Manatsathit, S. (1987) Passive haemagglutination test for enteric fever. J. Clin. Microbiol., 25, 138-141.

Rai, G.P., Zachariah, K. and Shrivastava, S. (1989) Comparative efficacy of indirect haemagglutination test, indirect fluorescent antibody test and enzyme linked immunosorbent assay in serodiagnosis of typhoid fever . J. Trop. Med. Hyg., 92, 431-434.

Rockhill, R.C., Rumans, L.W., Lesmann, M. and Denis, D.T. (1980) Detection of *Salmonella typhi* D, Vi and d antigens by slide coagglutination in urine of patients with typhoid fever. J. Clin. Microbiol., 11, 213-216.

Sarvamangala Devi, J.N. and Shivananda, P.G. (1985) Coagglutination for diagnosis of enteric fever. Ind. J. Pathol. Microbiol., 28, 349-353.

Song, J.H., Cho, H., Park, M.Y., Na, D.S., Moon, H.B. and Pai, C.H. (1993) Detection of *Salmonella typhi* in the blood of patients with typhoid fever by polymerase chain reaction. J. Clin. Microbiol., 31, 1439-1443.

Sundararaj, T., Ilango, B. and Subramanian, S. (1983) A study on the usefulness of counter immunoelectrophoresis for the detection of *salmonella typhi* antigen in sera of suspected cases of enteric fever. Trans..Roy. Soc. Trop. Med. Hyg., 77, 194-197.

Tantivanich, S., Chongsanguan, M., Sangpetchsong, V. and Tharavanij, S. (1984) Simple and rapid diagnosis test for typhoid fever. Southeast Asian J. Trop. Med. Publ. Hlth., 15, 317-322.

Voller, A., Bidwell, D. and Bartlett, A. (1980) Enzyme linked immunosorbent assay. *In*:Manual of Clinical Microbiology, (*Ed.* N.R. Rose and H. Friedman) 2nd ed. Am. Soc. Microbiol., Washington, D.C. pp 359-371

Zachariah, K. and Rai, G.P. (1987) Serodiagnosis of typhoid fever by indirect haemagglutination using lysate antigen. Curr. Sci., 56, 1118-1119.

Microbiology and Biotechnology for Sustainable Development (Ed. P.C. Jain),
CBS Publishers & Distributors, New Delhi (2004), pp. 91–109.

A-9

Biotechnology, Human Health and Microbes

A. Basu and S.K. Jain
Center for Biotechnology, Hamdard University, New Delhi-110 062

Abstract

The modern biotechnology has been revolutionized by a series of new developments in molecular biology during last two decades. Advances in recombinant DNA technology have made it possible to modify the genetic constitution of a cell in desired manner. Consequently a new discipline, namely the genetic engineering, has evolved which has opened new vistas in biotechnology. A number of diseases which were major killer just a few years back can be successfully treated today. The list of commercially available recombinant DNA products of biomedical importance is ever growing. Improved techniques for mass production of traditional vaccines and formulation of new generation of vaccines are major achievements of gene cloning technology. Based on the information obtained by human genome project, an entirely new concept of proteomics has evolved. Major advances have been also made in both gene replacement and gene augmentation therapy. Using proteomics it is possible to identify the cause of many diseases. The applications, implications and advantage of biotechnology are too many. Modern biotechnology and genetic engineering has opened a new era in human health management

Keywords: Human health, Microbes, Biotechnology, Recombinant DNA Techno-logy, Vaccines, Monoclonal antibodies and Diagnostics.

INTRODUCTION

Biotechnology can be defined as the use of microorganisms, plant and animal cells to produce materials such as food, medicine and chemicals that are useful to mankind or the applications of scientific and engineering principles for the processing of materials produced by living organisms to provide goods and services to human being. The science of biotechnology started about 6000 years back with the onset of civilization and with the use of yeast for brewerages and bread formation. However, the modern biotechnology has been revolutionized by a series of new developments in molecular biology during last two decades. Advances in recombinant DNA technology have made it possible to modify the genetic constitution of a cell in desired manner. Consequently a new discipline, namely the genetic engineering, has evolved which has opened new vistas in biotechnology. Today biotechnology and genetic engineering have almost become synonyms for each other. Genetic engineering is a very powerful technique with applications in various fields. It has numerous applications in the field of health management. A number of diseases which were major killer just a few years back can be treated today. A human gene can easily be cloned in bacteria and expressed in bacterial or other hetrologous systems to produce bioactive proteins. Today, a number of biomolecules, therapeutic agents and medicines can be produced by alternate route. The bacteria, yeast and other microorganisms can produce hormones such as insulin, growth hormone and gonadotropins; various growth factors such as cytokines and interleukins; interferon, blood product substitutes and many other useful proteins. The bacteria can be used as a biofactory for the production of therapeutic agents and other proteins of biomedical importance. The list of commercially available recombinant DNA products of biomedical importance is ever growing. Improved techniques for mass production of traditional vaccines and formulation of new generation of vaccines are major achievements of gene cloning technology.

Antigens such as HBsAg, HIV envelope proteins, influenza virus proteins, filarial antigens, malaria antigens etc. are been synthesized by gene cloning techniques. Similarly a number of multivalent vaccine constructs made by the integration of more then one genes are under development. The above process creates novel protein molecules with multiple antigenic epitopes and a single vaccination with such molecules can protect the recipient against a number of diseases. Subunit vaccines reduce the non-specific cross reactivity and ensure safety as well as enhance its specificity. The concept of DNA vaccine is a very novel idea. It provides a way to introduce genetic information for continuous production of immunizing agents by the recipient individual, thereby eliminating the need for repeated vaccination. The construction of live recombinant vaccine, using vaccinia virus as a vector has given a new dimension to immunization. The technology also has implications in discovery of new and novel drugs as well as in their better utilization.

Traditional methods for diagnostics of diseases are based primarily on immunological detection of specific antigens or the antibodies produced in the body as the result of infection. Their detection is possible only after the manifestation of the diseases. Often this late detection of the disease makes the treatment difficult and in some cases it could also be fatal. However, the advent of DNA diagnostics probes has made the early detection possible. These probes are highly specific and very sensitive. When combined with PCR, the nucleic acid probes can detect the presence of a single virus particle in a blood sample or a single malignant cell in a tissue biopsy sample. Having the capability to detect a pathogen much earlier than the manifestation of disease, these probes act as arsenals in fighting against the diseases and are very helpful in diagnosis and treatment of otherwise fatal diseases such as cancer, AIDS, etc.

Gene therapy has been the ultimate dream of biomedical scientists. Using plasmid and virus based vectors a great deal of progress has been made in this field and it is now possible to cure many genetic disorders by manipulating these defective genes. Major advances have been made in both gene replacement and gene augmentation therapy. Clinical trials of gene therapy for diseases like SCID, ADA deficiency, Parkinson's disease, and Citrullinemia etc. have been successful. In the foreseeable future, a diabetic patient will no longer require the daily dose of insulin rather, a simple augmentation of pancreatic cells with copies of functional insulin gene will render him disease free. By employing the germ cell therapy, it will be possible for the carriers of genetic diseases to have normal offsprings. Hopefully the other benefits of gene therapy will soon be available. By using the transgene technology it is possible to provide new traits and novel characters to animals and plants. The production of edible vaccines by transgenic plants will be a great revolution in field of mass immunization against many diseases.

The genetic improvement of livestock by embryo transfer technology (ETT) and other biotechnological means will help in achieving more milk, meat and other nutritionally important products from these animals. Along with quantity, the nutritional value of foods can also be increased. The production of single cell protein from fungi can go a long way in providing better nutrition to the ever-growing population.

The hybridoma technology and the production of monoclonal antibodies have provided a new vista for immuno-diagnostic and therapy. The monoclonal antibodies are highly specific and can be used both for diagnosis and therapeutic purposes. Raised in mouse, these antibodies may have certain undesirable effects. However recent advances have made it possible to humanize these antibodies. The humanization of monoclonal antibodies reduces undesirable complications, making them much more useful. The engineered antibodies can produce a number of useful and novel features. These can be used for targeting the delivery of therapeutic agents as well as the natural killer cells in human being. It is now possible to produce multivalent antibodies to combat against complex diseases. The anti-idiotype antibodies and antisense RNA therapy are new biotechnological means for the health management.

The completion of first phase of human genome project has recently been reported. It is a major achievement with far reaching applications. The mapping of human genome has opened new avenues. The day is not far when we will carry our gene profile in form of a biochip and any pathological condition will be treated at the gene level. It will be possible for the physician to tailor drugs to suit and provide maximum benefits to individual patients. Based on the information obtained by human genome project, a new concept of proteomics has been developed. Using proteomics it is possible to identify the cause of many diseases. The applications, implications and advantage of biotechnology are too many. Modern biotechnology and genetic engineering has opened a new era in human health management

Gene cloning

Decades ago Paul Berg, Herbert Boyer and Stanley Cohen shared their hands to work upon small segments of DNA derived from much larger chromosome by a technique called as DNA cloning. Today the same is named as recombinant DNA technology, which is also called gene cloning or molecular cloning and which has opened opportunities unimaginable just a few decades ago. It includes the identification and study of genes involved in almost every known biological process. These new methods are transforming basic research in agriculture, forensics, medicine, ecology and many other fields, while at the same time presenting society with bewildering choices for better life.

In a layman term "clone" means to make identical copies. Gene cloning involves separating a specific gene or a gene segment of DNA from a larger chromosome and attaching it to a small carrier DNA, then replicating this modified DNA thousands or even millions of times, a process which is called gene amplification. (Fig. 1). Cloning a segment of DNA either prokaryotic or eukaryotic includes five essential steps.

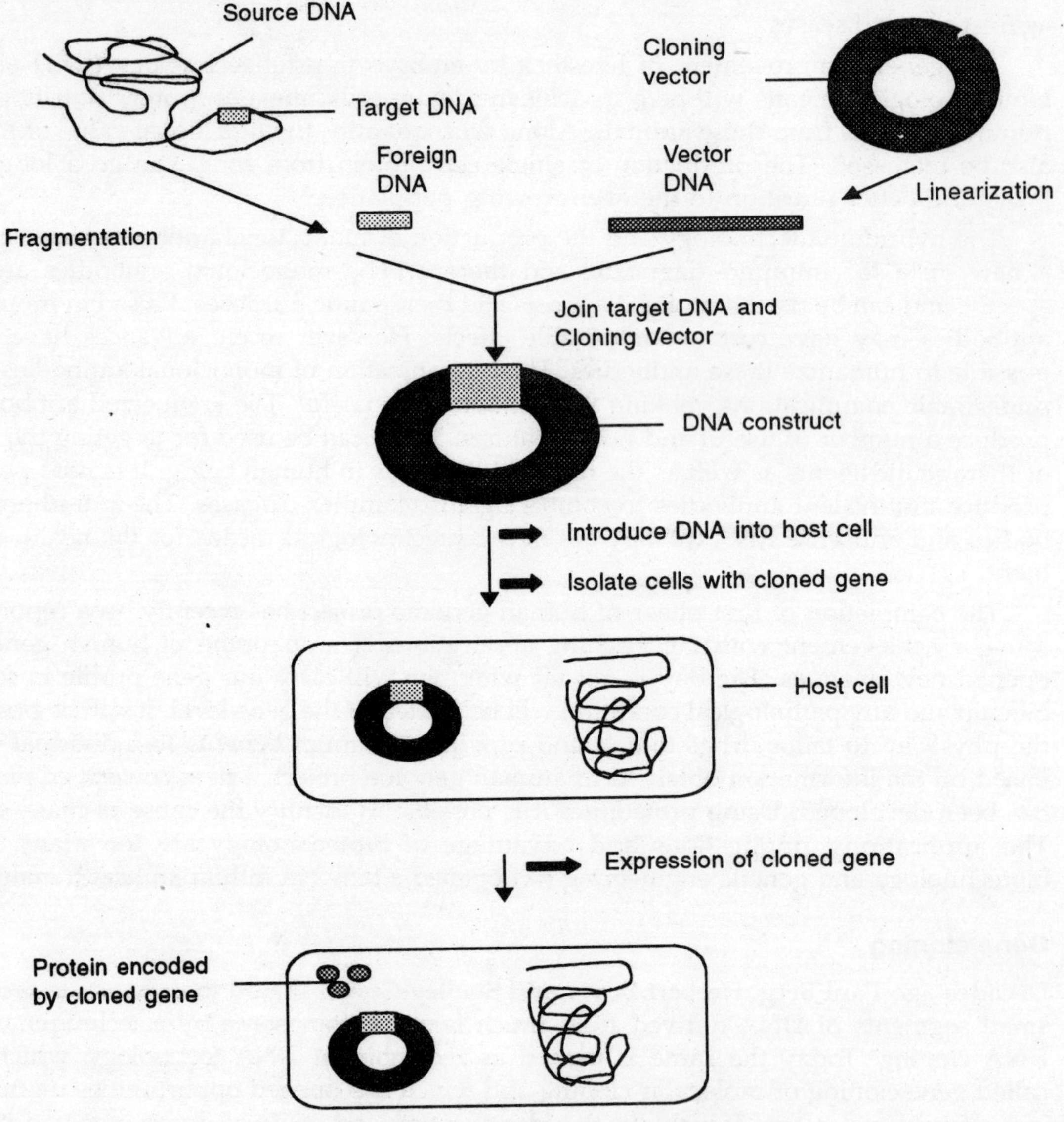

Fig. 1. Steps involved in gene cloning

1. The DNA should be cut at precise location. The discovery of sequence-specific type II restriction endonucleases has provided the necessary molecular scissors.
2. After selection of a small molecule of DNA capable of self-replication (the vector DNA), segment of the desired DNA to be cloned (the insert) is joined to plasmids or viral vector. These composite DNA molecules containing covalently linked segments derived from two or more sources are called the recombinant DNAs.
3. The two fragments DNAs, namely the insert DNA and the vector DNA must be joined covalently. The enzyme DNA ligase is used for this purpose.
4. The recombinant DNA should be moved from the test tube into a cell that can provide the necessary biological machinery for its replication. This process is known as the transformation. The transformation of the cells and the amplification of the transformants result in the creation of a battery of clones, which are referred as the gene library.
5. A method should be devised to select or identify those cells that contain the desired recombinant DNA. This is achieved by the screening of the gene library.

The foreign DNA and the vector DNA segments are often cut with same type of restriction endonucleases resulting into either blunt ends or cohesive (or sticky) ends. The commonly used cloning vectors are plasmids (bacterial extranuclear DNA), bacteriophages (the bacterial viruses), or the cosmids (an artificially made hybrid between a plasmid and the phage gene having cos sites). The choice of vector depends on the size of foreign gene to be cloned. Recombinant plasmids are introduced into the host bacterial cells by transformation technique, which involves heat and cold shock treatment to the cells (so called competent cells) so that the membrane structure is disturbed and the uptake of DNA becomes possible. Propagation of bacterial cell results in creation of a DNA library. Screening is an important aspect of gene cloning, which is similar to fishing out a needle from a haystack. This is done with the help of a specific tool, the probe. A probe can be a DNA fragments complementary to the desired foreign DNA of interest (nucleic acid probe), an immunologocial assay (using antibodies) or detection of the protein activity (using enzymes). A suitable probe and the hybridization methods are used for the selection of the clones containing the gene of interest from the gene library.

Following are some of the applications of gene cloning:

- DNA sequencing and hence derivation of protein sequence.
- Isolation and analysis of genes to identify the sequences of promoters and other regulatory elements.
- Investigation of functions of protein/enzyme/RNA by large-scale production and also with their altered forms.
- Identification of mutants with defects in genes leading to genetic diseases.
- Large scale commercial production of proteins and other molecules of biological importance.
- Engineering of plants and animals for transgenics and also for gene therapy.
- Engineering of proteins to alter their properties.

Table 1: Some of the commercially available products of Rec. DNA technology and their uses.

Product Category	Uses
Anticoagulants	Tissue plasminogen activator (TPA) activates plasmin, an nzyme involved in dissolving blood clots, effective in treating heart attacks victims.
Blood factors	Factor VII promotes clotting and is deficient in hemophiliacs. Use of factor VII produces by Rec. DNA technology eliminates the risk associated with blood transfusion.
Colony stimulating factors	Immune system growth factors that stimulate leukocyte production; used to treat immune deficiencies and fight infections.
Erythroprotein	Stimulates erythrocyte production; use to treat patients with anemia with kidney disease.
Growth factors	Stimulates differentiation and growth of various cell types; use to promote wound healing.
Human growth hormone	Use to treat dwarfisms.
Human insulin	Use to treat diabetic patients.
Interferon (alpha2-b, beta, gamma)	Interfere with viral reproduction also used in some type of cancer.
Monoclonal antibodies	Extraordinary binding specificity and used in diagnostic tests. Also used to transport drugs, toxins and radioactive compounds to tumors as a cancer therapy.
Superoxide dismutase	Prevents tissue damage from reactive oxygen species when tissues deprived of oxygen for short period during surgery suddenly have blood flow restored.
Vaccines	Proteins derived from viral coat are as effective in "priming" an immune system as the killed
	Virus more traditionally used for vaccines, but is safer. First of this kind was hepatitis B vaccine
Procollagen	Used as a gelling agent in food industry and as a bulking agent in corrective plastic surgery.
Interleukins	Activates and stimulates different classes of leukocyte; possibly used in wound healing, HIV infection, cancer, immune deficiencies.
Tumor necrosis factor	Used in treatment of various type of cancers.
Epidermal growth factor	Used in artificial skin growth in culture banks.

Using the cloning tool, in February 1997, "Dolly" the sheep was engineered from the genome of an adult somatic cell. The experiment for the first time showed that animal cells can have totipotency. Now scientists have moved from Dolly and Polly to other species, and the day is not far, when the cloning of human being will be possible. On the other hand, the transgenic animals have been produced whose milk could be used to make drugs and oral vaccines. The developments in gene cloning technology have thus opened a new era of recombinant products and biomolecules. Today a large number of recombinant products are commercially available. Some of the commercially available Rec. DNA products have been given in Table 1.

Gene therapy

Gene therapy may be defined as the correction of a diseased phenotype through the introduction of correct genetic information into the affected individual. This 'foreign' genetic information may either restore or supplement defective functions or alternatively interfere with the expression of a mutagenic genetic function. Currently the gene therapy is being targeted primarily at somatic cells. Gene therapy has now been successful in treating severe combined immunodeficiency syndrome (SCID) disease. Other genetic disorders that are candidates for gene therapy are cystic fibrosis, Duchenne's muscular dystrophy, familial hypercholesterolemia, hemoglobin defects, hemophilia and a number of other genetic diseases. Various strategies for implementation of somatic cell gene therapy now available can be broadly classified under three categories. The *ex-vivo* gene therapy, the *in-vivo* gene therapy and the antisense therapy.

Ex-vivo gene therapy:

It involves following steps.

1. Collection of autologous cells from the affected individual (Ennist, 1999).
2. Correction of genetic defect by gene transfer.
3. Selection and growth of genetically corrected cells.
4. Infusion and transplantation of these corrected cells back into the patients.

While a number of different cell types can be used for this purpose, the bone marrow cells provide great potential for the purpose. Similarly a number of different vectors can be used for the introduction of corrected gene. However, the adenoviral vectors seems to be the vector of choice for future.

In-vivo gene therapy:

The *in vivo* gene therapy is envisioned as the direct administration of a vector carrying the therapeutic gene to a patient. In this approach the vector is delivered either intravenously or directly to the lungs by instillation or by nebulization. The vectors in use can be non-viral [such as plasmids, catonic lipids (Lee and Huang 1996) and ligand-polylysine-DNA complexes (Cristiano and Roth, 1996)] or viral [adenovirus (Bartlett *et al.*, 1999), adeno-associated virus (Laquerre *et al.*, 1998) and retrovirus (Perrricone *et al.*, 2001)]. A gene therapy vector must meet three important criteria: safety; high gene transfer efficiency and stable and reliable expression of the transgene. The use of adenoviral vector system was a major achievement when the retroviral based vector system had to be terminated due to many reasons. The tissues under treatment are generally quiescent whereas the retroviral vectors acts only on tissues that are dividing. Unfortunately it integrates their genes into the host genome randomly making it possible that indispensable genes may be inactivated or oncogenes (cancer-causing genes) may be activated. Looking at the above scenario non-pathogenic adenoviruses, are now being used to treat disorders because they do not integrate into the genome. Studies in rodents using adenoviral vector system demonstrated successful gene transfer to the lungs via trachea (Vile, 1994; Dong *et al.*, 1996). The accessibility of the pulmonary epithelium, combined with the ability to use adenoviral vector system and synthetic vector system to transfer gene to the lungs, have made *in-vivo* gene therapy of the lungs a main focus in many worldwide labs. Expression of the gene is one of the important aspects of gene therapy. There are two methods to ensure targeted gene expression. First method is to engineer an expression cassette that contains the gene of interest so that the transgene is expressed only in the specific cell type. Different types of tissue or tumor specific promoters can be used in the cassette to restrict the gene expression (Vile, 1994;Walter and Stein, 1996; Miller and Whelan 1997). The second category of methods, include targeted gene delivery by using targeted vectors. The success of gene therapy for human SCID is like a dream becoming reality. SCID, commonly known as the bubble boy disease, is caused by defects in adenosine deaminase (ADA), a purine salvage pathway enzyme. SCID is due to diverse genetic syndromes, which result in absence of functional T cells, B cells and the natural killer cells (NK). All forms of SCID can be mitigated by transplantation of haemopoetic stem cells, suggesting that the stem cell gene therapy can be exploited as a possible cure of SCID (Kohn *et al.*, 1998). The bone growth factors are widely used today after its successful production using recombinant DNA technology to treat diverse orthopedic applications as the healing of broken bones, increasing bone density lost naturally as the result of aging and the strengthening of spines (Rebecca and Wozney, 2001).

Anti-sense therapy:

Antisense therapy entails the introduction of antisense RNA (or DNA) molecules, which are stretches of single stranded nucleic acid that target and bind with a specific messenger RNA, interfering with and even preventing its translation or over expression of the protein encoded by the mRNA. These are referred as antisense because the sense sequence and orientation of the mRNA is the one that directly translate itself into protein, whereas antisense is the complimentary stand that hybridizes with the mRNA and prevents it from carrying out its function. The ability to interfere at a critical point in the gene expression and protein synthesis pathway is what makes antisense such an attractive molecular therapeutic platform. After the two RNA sequences namely the endogenous mRNA and the exogenous antisense RNA hybridize, none or only a smaller amount of the target protein is synthesized (Aris, 1999). In principle antisense molecules can be applied to any disease in which protein over expression or even gene activation is detrimental. They are now being used to dissect gene functions (Knipple *et al.*, 1985) as well as to develop therapeutic procedures for a wide variety of diseases. In case of certain cancers, where the diseased state is not due to faulty gene but due to the faulty expression of growth factors, the defective regulation may be overcome by the limiting the amount of translation of mRNA into proteins from an over producing gene. The antisense molecules are also used as probe for gene transcription, one such example is globin gene, the expression of which is studied in cell free system (Orkin *et al.*, 1980). Vitravine was the first antisense molecule to come in the market, which was approved by FDA for the treatment of cytomegalovirus (CMV) retinisis in AIDS patients. Its applications range from cancer therapeutics to viral infection in human and also in treatment of plant diseases, illustrating the wide potential of this approach. Antisense WNT1 molecule was developed against mammary cancer (Hennighaunen, 2000). Antisense human telomerase template RNA (ahTR) has been shown to have growth inhibitory effect on gastric cancer cell line model (Naka *et al.*, 1999). HTGV-43 is used as an antisense molecule against HIV-1 infection. Today vectors are no longer in use with antisense molecules bearing antigenic construct but peptide nucleic acid (PNA) whose drug like properties are easier to manipulate than those of vectors (Von Wintzingerode *et al.*, 2000) serve as the method of choice.

The new vistas of nonviral delivery systems are much safer. These delivery systems include: liposome transfer, microinjection, microinjectile bombardment and electroporation. These systems do not awake an immune response and the vectors are able to survive and travel through the body to reach target cells

Embryonic stem cell therapy

The embryonic stem cells (ESC) are the mother of all type of cells in the body. Arising from the inner side of the bloastocyst, these cells divide rapidly and progressively becoming more specialized and finally can result into any type of specialized cells. Under normal physiological conditions ESCs do not persist till birth but their legacy shapes the body during pre-natal state. Researchers today have been with much less cajoling able to destine a mouse neuron to be metamorphosed into muscle cells or a human marrow cell may be coaxed to become a nerve cell. These cells are today grown in laboratories in a state of permanent infancy. They are coax under various conditions to grow them into mature tissue resembling gut, neuron and cartilage etc suggesting the pleuripotency of the ESCs. Time perhaps have to rewrite the rules of the game when in near future Alzheimer's and Parkinson's disease could be treated, spinal cord injury could be repaired and the paralysis due to strokes or accidents could be reverted because healthy tissue of the required type could be made to replace those dead or malfunctioning. A single substitute of ESC could revert the requirement of bone marrow transplantation in thalesemic patients (Datta, 1999). ESC research is a cutting edge technology representing a territory where no one has ventured before. There are few speed breakers and pitfalls. The lingering of the ESC during the process of maturation could lead to the development of teratocarcinomas, a deadly type of cancer (Lanza *et al.*, 1997).

Xenografting or xenotransplantation

Even before the emergence of the new fields of cell transplantation and tissue engineering, there was a serious shortage of human donor organs and tissues (Kahan, 1989). Diabetes alone affects an estimated 100 million people worldwide, whereas only a few thousand pancreases become available each year. With the advent of technology like xenografting, scientist and doctors could handle the above situation. Xenografting is the art of replacing a malfunctioning or weak organ of a species with the organ of another species. Unfortunately, isolated organ cells are exquisitely sensitive both to conventional rejection and to damage by autoimmune activity directed specifically against them. Now the patients will not require to use pigs or dacron made organs. In future it may not be necessary to use huge doses of immunosuppresent drugs as a post surgical measure, which exposes these patients to wide variety of serious complication, including cancer, kidney failure etc. Steroidal drugs as well as cyclosporin have deleterious effects on islet cell function and glucose homeostasis (Gunnarsson *et al.*, 1983; Hunkeler, 1999). Above complications could be handled with the advent of cell encapsulation technique, which presents significant advantages over cellular or whole organ replacement methods, when used without the use of immunomodulatory drugs. Cell encapsulation strategies differ from conventional xenotransplantation approaches by using cells or cell clusters, sterically isolated from host immune system by synthetic membranes made of hydroxyethyl methacrylatemethyl methacrylate (HEMA-MMA)(25,26). Not only encapsulation technologies appear to be working well as compared to conventional xenotransplants but also they are safer against the older methods of transplantation, in terms of infectious agent transmission. Pancreatic cell encapsulation is one of the leading events in the short history of xenograft technology (Sutherland *et al.*, 1994; Colton, 1995; Hering *et al.*, 1996; Zielinski *et al.*, 1997). A minute quantity of pancreatic tissues were obtained from pigs and treated with the enzyme liberase by Roche Boehringer Mannheim's scientists to segregate these tissues. Keeping the diameter within critical limits (350-450 ìm), maximal transfer of oxygen and nutrients from the blood to these encapsulated islets cells is maintained while the entry of large molecules such as antibodies and immune cells is blocked, hence preventing cell necrosis (Aebischer *et al.*, 1994). The pancreas is not the only organ in which encapsulation approaches are being developed; it is now being extended to artificial cartilage, liver and skin (Andre, 1990; Aebischer and Kato, 1995; Eguchi *et al.*, 1996; Jauregui *et al.*, 1997). This has been summarized in Table 2. In the coming years such therapies will become more accessible, inexpensive, and will be widely adopted in clinical practice.

Table 2: Treatment of some of the disorders by cell transplantation.

Disorder	Cells transplanted
Diabetes	Islets of Langerhans
Liver failure	Hepatocytes
Chronic pain	Adrenal chromaffin cells
Parkinson's disorder	Fetal nerve cells
Alzheimer's disease	Cells producing trophic factors
Amylotrophic lateral sclerosis	Cells producing trophic factors
Huntington's disorder	Cells producing trophic factors
AIDS	Bone marrow cells
Hypocalcemia	Parathyroid cells
Hypercholesterolemia	Hepatocytes
Lysosomal storage disorder	Cells producing deficient enzymes
Hemophilia	Cells producing clotting factors
Spinal cord injury	Fetal nerve cells
Anemia	Erythropoietin
Dwarfisms	Cells producing growth hormone

Embryo banking

In the present day hectic life style often the professional settlement takes long time and could be as late as in the age groups of late thirties or even forties. Unfortunately for women it is the age when early menopause starts knocking the door or late conceiving results in a number of genetical disorders. Fortunately advances in biotechnology now have the answer to their dilemma. The answer lies in frozen embryo banking. Ovarian banking is often synonymically used, for egg farming and *in vitro* fertilization (IVF), however, these are actually quite different. In IVF, the hormonal treatment is given so that many ova are ripened causing super ovulation. These ova are then collected and fertilized outside the body. Ovarian banking on the other hand stores the ovary (or a bit of it) for future use as and when required. A small slice of ovarian tissue contains thousands of immature eggs. They are retransplanted into the donor to restore the fertility after menopause or radiation treatment. Egg farming are eggs extracted from the thawed tissue, ripened in petri dish while still in their nest of follicle cells. It is used in cases where women have to undergo chemotherapy, which might make them infertile. Many young patients with Hodgkin's disease, or cervical tumors often have embryo banking as the soul savior.

Vaccines

The spine chilling epidemics of killer diseases of yester years such as small pox, polio and plague, to name a few, are today's forgotten stories. Biotechnology has helped in development of new vaccines. A large portion of currently available vaccine falls into three categories: (a) attenuated or killed microorganism; (b) bacterial toxins; and (c) polysaccharide-carrier protein conjugates. Conventional vaccines used weakened or killed forms of a virus or bacteria to introduce antigens (such as surface proteins) that the immune system uses to identify a pathogen. The body then produces antibodies against and develops resistance to that disease. A subunit vaccine consists only of the antigen and not the complete microbe. By isolating antigens and producing them in the laboratory, it is possible to make new subunit vaccines. As no pathogen is used in these vaccines, there are not even remote chances of developing the disease by immunization with subunit vaccines. Currently, the FDA has approved the use of anti-HBV (Greco, 1996) and anti-*Bordella pertusis* vaccine (Chawla, 2000) developed through recombinant DNA technology. Anti-HBV is developed, by inserting the gene that produces the hepatitis B surface antigen into yeast cells. These cells are cultured and antigen is later purified. Research is under way on vaccines for influenza, AIDS, herpes viruses, cholera, Rocky Mountain spotted fever and several diarrheal diseases. The different approaches for vaccine production by Rec. DNA technology have been illustrated in Fig. 2.

Genetically Modified Organisms:

It involves attenuation of the live virus so that it looses the pathogenesity but evokes the immune response. Vaccines of such kind was developed against the herpes virus in which thymidine kinase gene which is necessary for replication in non dividing cells such as neuron was deleted. Hence the virus can infect the cells but cannot replicate. Other approaches include gene segment reassortment in organisms with segmented genomes such as in rotavirus and influenza. Gene deletion was a technique used in *Vibrio cholera* where the toxin gene was removed. Use of insertion of missense gene is another method of choice.

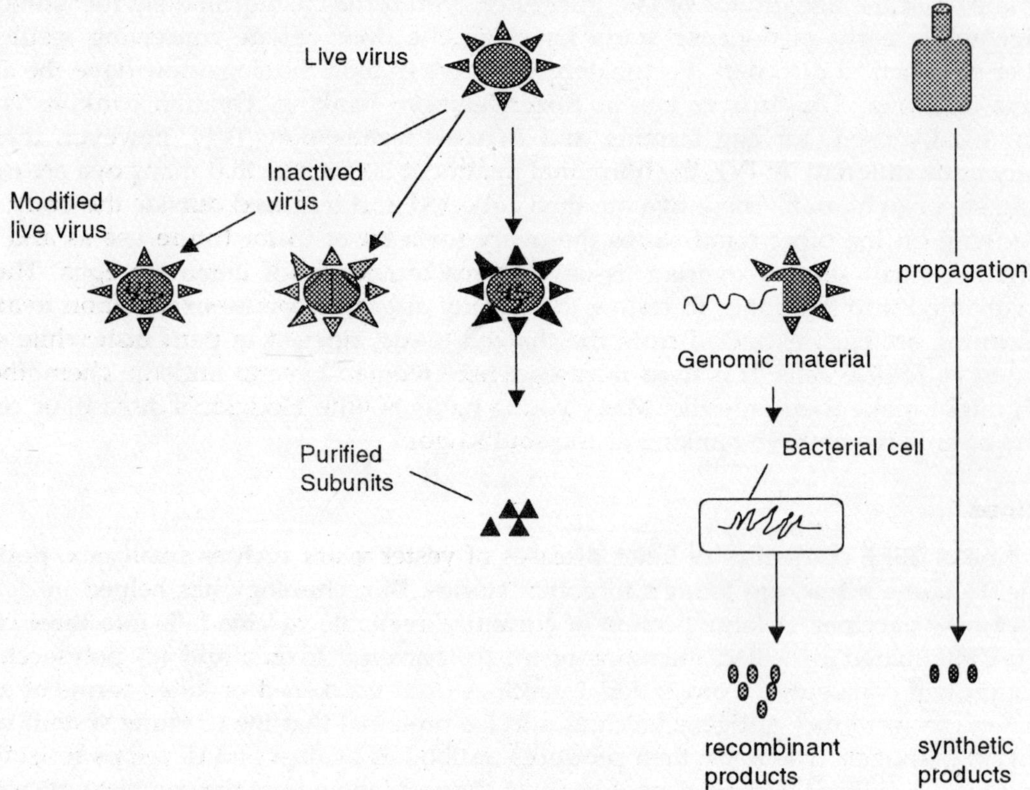

Fig. 2. Strategies for vaccine development.

Recombinant Vaccines:

In recombinant vaccine the genetic material coding for the protein of interest is isolated and cloned in vectors such as bacterium, yeast or other systems. The first vaccine of its kind to be developed was against foot and mouth disease virus. The process is highly efficient as $4X10^7$ doses of vaccine for foot and mouth disease can be obtained from 10 liters of *E. coli* culture with concentration of 10^{12} organism/ml. Today hepatitis B vaccine has been developed successfully through Rec. DNA technology in transfected yeast.

Synthetic peptides:

Although globular protein molecules may be large but, they have a limited number of immunogenic epitopes on their surface. Only a few of these epitopes induce protective immunity. Thus if the structure of the protective epitope is known, it may be chemically synthesized and used as vaccine. Through the sequencing entire antigen is possible, with molecular modeling technique different epitopes are predicted and tested. Experimental synthetic vaccines have been developed against several viruses including hepatitis B, influenza A and many others.

DNA Vaccines:

DNA vaccines are created from genetic material of a particular pathogen. The aim is to introduce the specific genes of a pathogen into human body, which code for the antigens, which evoke protective response. This prompts the immune machinery to attack that pathogen if it invades the body in future (Fig. 3).

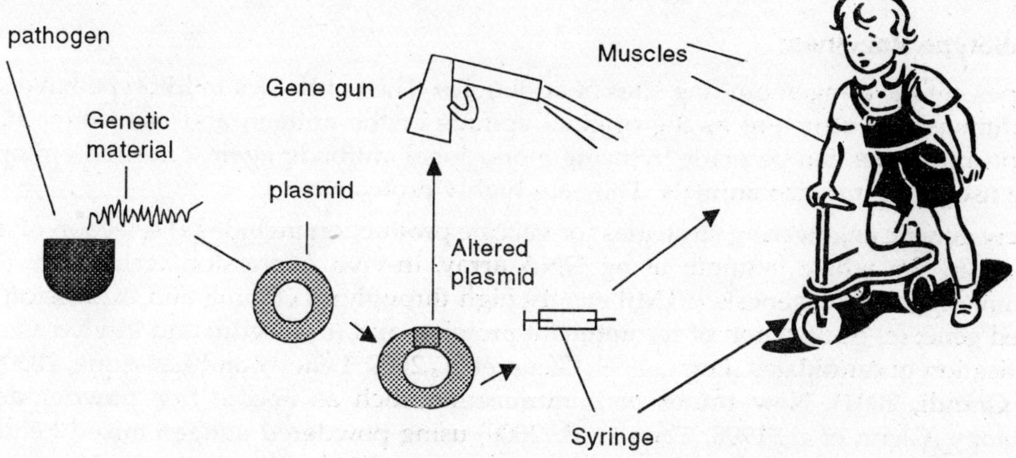

Fig. 3. Methods used for transfer of recombinant gene to recipient cells for gene therapy.

The genes are incorporated into plasmids under proper regulatory elements and the resultant recombinant plasmid constitutes the DNA vaccine. A DNA vaccine can be administered by injecting into muscle cells or alternatively the vaccine could be coated into gold particles and delivered by a gene gun, which propels the plasmid in the epidermal cells and mucous membranes. A conventional vaccine, which consists of killed pathogen, cannot make its way into the cell resulting in awakening of only humoral response. The cell mediated immune response does not get activated and the natural killer T-cells are not put into action. On the other hand the DNA vaccines activates T-cells, do not require boosting and there is no chance of reversion from non-pathogenic form to pathogenic form. These can therefore, be used against cancer and AIDS (Carter *et al.*, 2000). Since DNA vaccine can also offer protection against different strains of pathogens, it could be highly effective against pathogens like the influenza virus, which are highly variable due to presence of several strains. Plasmids can be engineered to carry specific genes of different strains of such pathogen to make DNA vaccine extremely effective. DNA vaccines are often more stable than traditional vaccines as DNA remains unaltered even under extreme conditions. In case of malarial parasite (Kaslow, 1997) the stages that cause disease is different from the stages that transmit the parasite from the mosquito vector to the human host, the vaccines are therefore, developed against different infective stages and strains to achieve desired efficacy. Vaccines against the stages that make mosquito a carrier can prevent the spread of malaria. Such vaccines are called malaria transmission blocking vaccines (TBVs) (Engers and Goldal, 1998). TBVs prevent the transmission of malaria by inducing antibodies against antigens present on the sexual stages of parasite, which develops in the mosquito midgut, and thus blocks their development (Chiang, 1999). Another important property of TBVs is that they would reduce the emergence and spread of parasites resistant to other malarial vaccine components, and even anti malarial drugs. For making DNA vaccine more effective, scientists are also including the genes for signaling cytokines. The cytokines regulate the activities of various cells of defense machinery. In 1999 with the outbreak of Ebola epidemic, Ebola virus membrane glycoprotein was used to develop DNA vaccine, which was highly effective.

Anti-Idiotype Vaccines:

Idiotypes are the antigen binding sites of antibodies. The antibodies to idiotype have similar three-dimensional structure as the original epitope of the antigen and can mimic it. Anti-idiotype antibodies can be made by using monoclonal antibody against desired epitope and can be used to immunize animals. They are highly protective.

New genetic engineering strategies for vaccine production include (a) selection of a set of genes from the whole genome using DNA array, in-vivo expression technology (IVET), signature-tagged mutagenesis (STM]) etc; (b) high throughput cloning and expression of the selected gene; (c) purification of recombinant proteins; and (d) in-vitro and in-vivo assays for identification of candidates (Perry, 1999; Glenn *et al.*, 2000; Lehoux and Levesque, 2000; Shea, 2000; Grandi, 2001). New routes of immunization such as needle free powder delivery technology (Glenn *et al.*, 1998; Chen *et al.*, 2000) using powdered antigen mixed helium gas at high pressure and transcutaneous immunization technology using a patch mixed with antigen and adjuvant have made syringes or gene guns obsolete thus preventing risk of needle contaminated diseases and also causing the activation of Langerhan cells which constitute the 25% of immune cells and are in close proximity to the superficial layer of the skin (Nishimura *et al.*, 1987; Snider, 1995).

Monoclonal antibodies

Monoclonal antibodies have revolutionized the diagnosis of bacterial and viral infections. Being highly specific, the monoclonal antibody bind to a bacterium or virus, and this antibody-antigen combination can easily be detected. A number of antibodies have been developed for diseases like asthma, psoriasis, vision deterioration, bacterial infections, heart attacks, stroke and rejection of transplanted organs. Improved techniques of antibody production are being developed. Being produced in mice, the monoclonal antibodies can be recognized as foreign molecules and elicit immune response in human, which prevented their use for therapeutic purposes. However, the humanization of the antibodies eliminates this problem. This is achieved by replacing the constant region of murine antibody with those of human antibody, yielding a chimeric antibody. Recently the antibodies have also been engineered where the complementarity determining regions (CDRs) of a human antibody is replaced with those of a clinically useful murine antibody (CDR grafting) thus increasing the usefulness of antibodies for therapeutic purposes. Another development in this field is the use of phage display techniques where the human antibody genes are inserted into the phage, which displays it on its surface. Each phage produces a different antibody.

Chimeric antibodies:

For the creation of a chimeric antibody, the DNA sequences encoding the mouse variable regions (specific for any given antigen) are joined to sequence of DNA encoding human constant region, thus forming a new gene. To introduce the chimeric gene into cells, plasmid vector such as pSVgpt and pSVneo are used to transform mouse myeloma cell line (X63Ag8 and X63Ag653, respectively). The transformants have been shown to produce high amounts (upto10-30ìg/ml) of chimeric antibody. A chimeric antibodies generated to acute lymphoblastic leukemia antigen (Sun *et al.*, 1987), carcinoma associated antigen (Lue *et al.*, 1987), colorectal carcinoma antigen (Skerra and Pluckthun, 1988), are now commercially available. The advantages of chimeric antibodies are that these are stable in mouse myeloma cell lines, can be used to produce the transformants (transfectomas) and the chimeric antibodies have tumoricidal activity in the presence of human effector cell due to CDC and antibody dependent cell cytotoxicity (ADCC) by virtue of the presence of human constant region.

CDR Grafting:

Light chain and heavy chain of the immunoglobin molecules consist of three complimentarity determining region in each domain, which are flanked by four relatively conserved regions known as framework regions. These framework regions form the majority of â-sheets, which along with CDRs form the antigen-binding site. Using crystallography these CDRs can be exchanged from the heavy chain of variable region of a human myeloma antibody NEWM with the CDRs of Mumab B1-8. Later an approach was made to replace all the six CDRs from both light and heavy change by Reichmann.

One of the main disadvantages of human monoclonal antibody is relatively low stability of the mammalian cell expressing the immunoglobulins and the drop in the level of secreted product with time. A recent approach has been proposed with the potential to bypass hybridoma technology. This advancement in biotechnology, called antibody engineering, involves the cloning of antibody gene directly from hybridomas or lymphocytes expressing antibody of desired specificity into suitable vector such as phage to add more shelf life and also enhance its productivity. Antibody engineering had enabled the construction of wide range of antibody fragments, all of which can be expressed in active form when introduced into mammals or other recipients (Chee, 1996).

Diagnostics

Diagnostic agents are used to detect a wide variety of diseases and genetic disorders. Donated blood in Blood Banks is screened for HIV and hepatitis. Home pregnancy test kit is a regular biotech diagnostic product. A new blood test has been developed through biotechnology to measure the amount of low-density lipoprotein (LDL) in blood. As compared to conventional tests requiring a total lipid profile, including expensive tests for total cholesterol, triglycerides and high-density lipoprotein cholesterol and inconvenience to patient as they have to fast 12 hours before a blood sample could be drawn, the new test allows patients to be tested with one simple test that can measure LDL directly without the need to fast. Gene probes, which chemically label specific segments of DNA within the chromosomes are valuable diagnostic tool. These are being used to test fetuses for possible genetic disorders as early as four weeks. A wide range of genetic diseases including Down's syndrome can be tested. They can also be used to determine an individual's susceptibility to autoimmune diseases such as insulin-dependent diabetes, certain forms of arthritis and anemia, and chronic diseases of the liver, kidney, and nervous system. The DNA chip or DNA microarray technology has made it possible to get information regarding the expression of specific mRNAs from complex cellular systems (Shena, 1995; Wen, 1998). A typical microarray data set includes expression levels for thousands of genes across hundreds of conditions such as internal cellular physiology from different cell line, diverse physiological conditions in an intact organism, pathological tissue specimens from patients etc. (Eisen, 1998; Golub, 1999; Brown and Botstein, 1999; Alizadeh, 2000). DNA chips are single stranded DNA array accessible to proteins. Their system could allow the systemic study of DNA-protein interactions, transforming the analysis of eukaryotic transcriptional control. These are synthetic oligonucleotide arrays consisting of single stranded 20-30mers affixed to glass surface by oligoethylene glycol linkers. These are used for monitoring the presence and abundance of specific mRNAs in a population (Lockhart and Winzeler, 2000), assessing the sequence variations in HIV-1 (Duggan, 1999), understanding the functional relationship between the large set of genes population and various genome databases (Cheung, 1999; Lipshutz, 1999; Eckmann, 2000). The protein array is more powerful than DNA array. DNA array gives little information about the final concentrations of gene product in a cell, reveals nothing about the post-translation modification, protein activity and protein-protein interactions. Protein arrays are composed of approximately 19,000 bacterial clones, each expressing a different single chain antibody, double spotted on a palm size filter paper. The approach is useful in screening different antibodies against various antigens, elimination of false positive clones in early stages of screening process and as a general approach to proteomics.

Future prospects

At the beginning of the new millennium, infection diseases still pose increasing threats to human health. This is true for developing countries as well as for developed countries and the mortality rate from infectious diseases has increased by 58% between 1980 to 1992. New diseases have emerged over the past two decades and at the same time diseases, which, were thought to be controlled such as tuberculosis, have re-emerged. Furthermore, the development of resistance to anti-microbial agents has rendered the management of variety of illnesses more difficult and expensive. Genomic technologies are expected to play a key role in vaccine research, offering revolutionary tools for identification of surface associated proteins and virulence factors. With the successful completion of human genome project, it has now become possible to foresee major new steps in the understanding of the molecular basis of disease, both from attack by external pathogens and internally from variations within the human genome resulting in a plethora of new molecular therapeutics targets for drug design and discovery. New technologies have sprung up to cope with the avalanche of genomic data. As a consequence of these exciting developments, the research process of drug discovery is beginning industrialized with research impetus taken out of academic institutes and put into cutting-edge niche of biotechnology companies with better funding and significant commercial opportunities. The advent of technologies like IVET, STM and DNA microarray has opened new avenues for diagnostics and are also useful for addressing a broad range of biological problems. The ultimate power to manipulate all biological processes is now getting into private hands. The health benefits deriving from stem cell research are likely to be tremendous but arcane and expensive. With a lot of promises in the coming decades these technologies are bound to revolutionize the health management and disease prevention.

REFERENCES

Aebischer, P. and Kato, A.C. (1995). Treatment of amyotrophic lateral sclerosis using a gene therapy approach, *Eur. Neurol.* 35: 65-69.

Aebischer, P. *et al.* (1994). Transplantation in humans of encapsulated xenogenic cells without immunosuppression, *Transplantation* 58: 1275-1277.

Alizadeh, A.A. (2000). Distinct types of diffuse large B-cell lymphoma identified by gene expression profiling, *Nature.* 403: 503-511.

Andre, F.F. (1990). Overview of a 5-yr clinical experience with a yeast derived hepatitis B vaccine, Vaccine 8 (suppl.) S74-S78.

Aris, P. (1999). Antisence therapeutics, *Nature. Biotechnol.* 17: 403-404.

Bartlett, J.S., Kleinschmidt, J., Boucher, R.C. and Samulski, R.J. (1999). Targeted adeno-associated virus vector transduction of non-permissive cell mediated by a bispecific F (ab' gamma) 2 antibodies, *Natl. Biotechnol.* 17: 181-186.

Bretzel, R.G. *et al.* (1996). International Islet Transplant Registry report, in 1996/97 *Yearbook Of Cell And Tissue Transplantation* (Ed. Lanza R.P. and Chick W.L.), Kluwer, pp. 153-160.

Brown, P.O. and Botstein, D. (1999). Exploring the new world of the genome with DNA microarrays, *Nature. Genet.* 21: 33-37.

Carter, R., Mendis K.N., Miller L.H., Molineaux L. and Saul A. (2000). Malaria transmission blocking Vaccines-how can their development be supported? , *Nature. Med.* 6: 241-244.

Chawla, P. (2000). DNA Vaccines, *Science Reporter.* Nov. 46-47.

Chee, M. (1996). Accessing genetic information with high-density DNA arrays, *Science*. 274: 610-614.

Chen, D., Endres, R.L., Erickson, C.A., Weis, K.F., McGregor, M.W., Kawaoka, Y. and Payne, L.G. (2000). Epidermal immunization by a needle-free powder delivery technology: Immunogenecity of influenza vaccine and protection in mice, *Nature. Med.* 6(10): 1187-1190.

Cheung, V.G. (1999). Making and reading microarrays, *Nature. Genet.* 21: 15-19.

Chiang, S.L. (1999). *In vivo* genetic analysis of bacterial virulence, *Ann. Rev. Microbiol.* 53: 129-134.

Colton, G.K. (1995). Implantable biohybrid artificial organs, *Cell Transplant.* 4: 415-436.

Cristiano, R.J. and Roth, J.A. (1996) Epidermal growth factor mediate DNA delivery into lung cancer cell via the epidermal growth factors receptor, *Cancer Gene Ther.* 3: 4-10.

Datta, S. (1999). Stemming Forth, *Science Reporter*, Aug 14-15.

Dong, J.Y., Wang, D., Van Grinkel, F.W., Pascual, D.W. and Frizzell, R.A. (1996). Systematic analysis of repeated gene delivery into animal lungs with recombinant adenoviral vector, 10; 7(3): 319-331.

Duggan, D.J. (1999). Expression profiling using cDNA microarrays, *Nature. Genet.* 21: 10-14.

Eckmann, L. (2000). Analysis of high-density cDNA arrays of altered gene expression in human intestinal epithelial cells in response to infection with invasive enteric bacteria *Salmonella*, *J. Biol. Chem.* 275: 14084-14094.

Eguchi, S., Chen, S., Rozga, J. and Demetrion, A.A. (1996). Tissue engineering; Liver, in 1996/97 *Yearbook Of Cell And Tissue Transplantation* (*Ed.* Lanza, R.P. and Chick, W.L.), Kluwer, pp. 145-152.

Eisen, M.B. (1998). Cluster analysis and display of genome-wide expression patterns, *Proc. Natl. Acad. Sci.* USA. 95: 14863-14868

Engers, H.D. & Goldal, T. (1998). Malaria vaccine development current status, *Parasitol. Today*. 14: 54-56.

Ennist, D.L. (1999). Gene therapy for lung diseases, *TiPS* 20: 260-265.

Glenn, G.M., Rao, M., Matyas, G.R. and Aliving, C.R. (1998). Skin immunization made possible by cholera toxin, *Nature*. 391: 851.

Glenn, G.M., Taylor, D.N., Li X., Frankel, S., Montemarano, A. and Aliving, C.R. (2000). Transcutaneous immunization: A human vaccine delivery using a patch, *Nature. Med.* 6(12): 1403-1405.

Golub, T.R. (1999). Molecular classification of cancer class discovery and class prediction by gene expression monitoring, *Science*. 286: 531-537.

Grandi, G. (2001). Antibacterial Vaccine design using genomics and proteomics, *TRENDS* in Biotechnology 19(5): 181-188.

Greco, D. (1996). A controlled trail of two cellular vaccines and one whole cell vaccine against pertusis, *N. Engl. J. Med.* 334: 341-348.

Gunnarsson, R *et al.* (1983). Detoriation in glucose metabolism in pancreatic transplant recipients given cyclosporin, *Lancet* 2: 571.

Hennighaunen, L. (2000). Mouse models for breast cancer, *Breast. Cancer. Res.* 2: 2-7.

Hering, B.J., Wahoff D.C. and Sutherland D.E.R. (1996). Clinical islets transplantation, in 1996/97 *Yearbook of Cell and Tissue Transplantation* (Ed. Lanza R.P. and Chick W.L.), Kluwer pp. 145-152.

Hunkeler, D. (1999). Bioartificial organs transplanted from research to reality, *Nature. Biotechnol.*17: 335-336.

Jauregui, H.O., Muilon, C.P.J. and Solomon, B.A. (1997). Extra corporeal artificial liver support, in *Principles of Tissue Engineering* (*Ed.* Lanza R.P., Langer R. and Chick W.L.), Academic Press, pp 463-479.

Kahan, B.D. (1989). Cyclosporine, *New Engl. J. Med.* 321: 1725-1738.

Kaslow, D.C. (1997). Transmission blocking Vaccines: uses and current status of development, *Int. J. Parasitol.* 27: 183-189.

Knipple, D.C., Seifert, E., Rosenberg, U., Preiss, A. and Jackle, H. (1985). Spatial and temporal patterns of kruppel gene expression in early drosophila embryos. *Nature*. 317: 40-44.

Kohn, D.B. *et al.* (1998). T lymphocytes with a normal ADA gene accumulate after transplantation of transduced autologous umbilical cord blood CD34+ cells in ADA deficient SCID neonates, *Nature. Med.* 4: 775-780.

Lanza, R.P., Cooper, D.K.C. and Chick, W.L. (1997). Xenotransplantation, *Sci. Am.*277: 54-59.

Laquerre, S., Anderson, D.B., Stolz, D.B., and Glorioso, J.C. (1998). Recombinant herpes simplex virus type 1 engineered for targeted binding to erythropoietin receptor binding to receptor binding cells, *J.Virol.* 72: 9683-9687.

Lee, R.J. and Huang, L. (1996). Folate targeted anionic liposome-entrapped polylysine-condense DNA for tumor cell-specific gene transfer, *J Biol. Chem.* 271: 8481-8487.

Lehoux, D.E and Levesque, R.C. (2000). Detection of genes in specific niches by signature-tagged mutagenesis, *Curr. Opin. Biotechnol.* 11: 434-439.

Lipshutz, R.J. (1999). High-density synthetic oligonucleotide arrays, *Nature. Genet* 21: 20-24.

Lockhart, D.J. and Winzeler, E.A. (2000). Genomics, gene expression and DNA arrays, *Nature*. 405: 827-837.

Lue, A.Y., Robinson, R.R., Hellstrom, K.E., Murray, E.D., Chang, C.P., and Hellstrom, I (1987). Chimeric mouse human IgG1 antibody that can mediate lysis of cancer cells, *Proc. Natl. Acad. Sci.* USA. 84: 3439-3443.

Margulis, M.S. (1989). Temporary organ substitution by hemoperfusion through suspension of active donor hepatocytes in a total complex of intensive therapy in-patients with acute hepatic insufficiency, *Resuscitation* 18: 85-94.

Miller, N. and Whelan, J. (1997). Progress in transcriptional targeted and regulatable vectors for genetic therapy, *Hum. Gene. Ther.* 8: 803-815.

Naka, K. Yakosaki, H., Yasui, W., Tahara, H. and Tahara, E. (1999). Effect of antisence human telomeraes RNA transfection on the growth of human gastric cancer cell line, *Biochem. Biophys. Res. Commun.* 255: 753-758.

Nishimura, Y., Yokoyama, M., Araki, K. and Ueda, R. (1987). Recombinant human-mouse chimeric monoclonal antibody specific for common acute lymphocyte leukemia antigen cancer research, 47: 999-1005.

Orkin, S.H., Kolodner, R., Michelson, A. and Husson, R. (1980) cloning and direct examination of a structurally human beta o-thalesemia globin gene, *Proc. Natl. Acad. Sci.* USA. 77(6). 585-562.

Perricone, M.A., Morris, J.E., Pavelka, K., Plog, M.S., O' Sullivan, B.P., Joseph, P.M., Dorkin, H., Lapey, A., Balfour, R., Meeker, D.P., Smith, A.E., Wadsworth, S.C. and St George, J.A. (2001). Aerosol and lobar administration of recombinant adenovirus to individuals with cystic fibrosis and transfection efficiency with in airway epithelium, *Hum. Gene. Ther.* 20; 12(11): 1383-1394.

Perry, R.D. (1999). Signature-tagged mutagenesis and the hunt for virulence factors, *Trends. Microbiol.* 7: 385-388.

Rebecca, H. Li. and Wozney, J.M. (2001). Delivering on the promise of bone morphogenetic proteins, *TRENDS in Biotechnology* 19(7): 255-265.

Shea, J.E (2000). Signature-tagged mutagenesis in the identification of virulence genes in pathogens, *Curr. Opin. Microbiol.* 3: 451-458.

Shena, M. (1995). Quantitative monitoring of gene expression patterns of central expression system with a complementary DNA microarray, *Science*. 270: 467-470.

Skerra, A. and Pluckthun, A. (1988). Assembly of functional immunoglobin Fv fragment in E.coli, *Science*. 240: 1035-1040.

Snider, D.P. (1995). The mucosal adjuvant activities of ADP-ribosylating bacterial enterotoxins, *Crit. Rev. Immunol.* 15: 317-348.

Sun, L.K., Cutis, P., Rakoulez-Szulezynska, E., Ghrayels, J., Chang, N., Mannson, S.L. and Prowski, H. (1987). Chimeric antibody with human constant regions and mouse variable regions directed against carcinoma-associated antigen 17-1A, *Proc. Natl. Acad. Sci.* USA. 84: 214-218.

Sutherland, D.E.R., Grnessner, R.W.G. and Gores, P.R. (1994). Pancreas and islet transplantation, *Transplantation. Rev.* 8: 185-206.

Vile, R.G. (1994). Tumor-specific gene expression, *Semin. Cancer. Biol.* 5: 429-436.

Von Wintzingerode, F., Landt, O., Ehrlich, H. and Gobel, U.B. (2000). Peptide nucleic acid mediated PCR clamping as a useful suppliment in the determination of microbial diversity. *Appl. Environ. Microbiol.* 66(2): 549-557.

Wen, K. (1998). Large-scale temporal gene expression mapping of central nervous system development, *Proc. Natl. Acad. Sci.* USA. 95: 334-339.

Walter, W. and Stein, U. (1996). Cell type specific and inducible promoters for vectors in gene therapy as an approach for cell targeting, *J. Mol. Med.* 74: 379-392.

Zielinski, B.A., Goddard, M.R. and Lysaght, M.J. (1997). Immunoisolation, in *Principles Of tissue Engineering*. (Ed. Lanza, R.P., Langer, R. and Chick, W.L.) Academic Press, pp 321-326.

Microbiology and Biotechnology for Sustainable Development (*Ed.* P.C. Jain),
CBS Publishers & Distributors, New Delhi (2004), pp. 110–120.

A-10

Production and Characterization of Thermostable Starch-Hydrolysing α-Amylase and Amylopullulanase of *Geobacillus thermoleovorans*

S. M. Noorvez, M. Ezhilvannan and T. Satyanarayana
*Department of Microbiology, University of Delhi South Campus,
New Delhi – 110 021.*

Abstract

Starch, a mixture of linear and branched glucose polymers, is hydrolyzed by endo- and exo- amylases, as well as by debranching enzymes. Most industrial starch applications require its hydrolysis into glucose, maltose or oligosaccharides. Because of its insolubility in water and the risk of side-reactions, starch processing is best performed at high temperatures. In addition, the currently used amylolytic enzymes as well as most of the others reported are dependent on the presence of calcium ions for their action. The use of thermostable and calcium-independent enzymes would increase starch processing yields and decrease costs. Recently isolated strains of Geobacillus thermoleovorans produced a thermostable, calcium-independent α- amylase, and an amylopullulanase that cleaves α-1,4 as well as α-1,6-glycosidic linkages of starch. These intrinsically thermostable and calcium-independent enzymes will serve as a model of starch-degrading enzymes to design new enzyme activities including an improved starch solublizing (α-amylase) activity, an improved debranching activity, and a transglycosylation activity for the synthesis of high value glycosides.

Key words: *Geobacillus thermoleovorans*, starch, starch-hydrolyzing enzymes thermostable, α-amylase, amylopullulanase.

INTRODUCTION

Starch is a carbohydrate occurring in granular form in different parts of plants. After cellulose, starch is the next most abundant compound that is synthesized by plant cells. While starch is generated in the chloroplasts of every growing green leaf, major practical sources of starch are amyloplasts of cereal grains, roots and tubers. Under the microscope, the appearance of the granules of starch from these different sources varies both in shape and size. Chemically, however, they are similar (Zobel and Stephen, 1995).

Starch, a homopolymer of D-glucose subunits, comprises two components: amylose and amylopectin. Amylose, the minor component, constitutes about 15-25% of starch and it is an unbranched, straight chain (linear) polymer of glucose subunits linked by α-1,4-glycosidic bonds. The chain length varies from few hundreds to 6,000 residues. Amylopectin, although essentially linear, exhibits branching at the α-1,6 position and contains both α-1,6-glycosidic linkages (of every 17-26 glucose residues) plus the α-1,4 glycosidic linkages as in amylose (Hermansson and Svegmark, 1996).

Starchy substances constitute the major part of the human diet for most of the people in the world, as well as many other animals. Starch is the cheap and reliable source of energy for the biochemical manufacturing of alcohol, enzymes and fine chemicals. Starch is used in food industry as a thickener, binder, stabilizer, emulsifier, suspending and gelling agent. It is a high calorific value food providing ~ 17 kJ g^{-1} of energy as against ~ 1 kJ g^{-1} for low calorie polysaccharides (Stephen and Charms, 1995). Starch is not utilized for food and energy source only, but also as a high sustainable and environment friendly source that can be utilized for industrial purposes. Besides it is the primary source of various sugar syrups, which provide a base to many pharmaceutical and confectionery industries.

HYDROLYSIS OF STARCH

Industrial processes for starch hydrolysis to glucose rely on inorganic acids or enzyme catalysis. Developments in starch processing have moved on from acid hydrolysis to acid-enzyme hydrolysis (AE system) to enzyme-enzyme hydrolysis (EE system). The disadvantages of acid hydrolysis include low glucose yield, formation of large amounts of salts and need to use corrosion resistant equipment. These problems encountered in the chemical conversion of starch to sugar syrups have been avoided by using enzymatic process.

Depending on the relative location of the bond under attack, as counted from the end of the chain, the products of this digestive process are dextrins, maltotriose, maltose, and glucose. Dextrins are shorter broken starch segments that form as the result of the random hydrolysis of internal glycosidic bonds. A molecule of maltotriose is formed if the third bond from the end of a starch molecule is cleaved, a molecule of maltose is formed if the point of attack is the second bond, a molecule of glucose results at the bond being cleaved is the terminal one and so on. The method of determining the degree of hydrolysis is stated as the Dextrose Equivalent (DE) value. The DE value of any syrup is the measure of the total quantity of reducing sugars, equated as D-glucose. Other terminology is the degree of polymerization i.e., DP1 (glucose), DP2 (maltose), DP3 (maltotriose) to DPn (oligo-/polysaccharide) (Bentley and Williams, 1996).

CONVENTIONAL STARCH HYDROLYSIS PROCESS

The main amylolytic enzymes used in the starch industry for the production of glucose, maltose and maltooligosaccharides are a-amylase, α-amylase, glucoamylase and pullulanase

(Hyun and Zeikus, 1985). The properties of enzymes used in the process determine the conditions under which the starch processing must operate. Glucose and maltose syrups are usually produced from starch in a two step process- liquefaction and saccharification. First, an aqueous slurry of starch (30-40% DS) is gelatinised (105°C, 5 min) and partially hydrolyzed (95°C, 2h) by highly thermostable α-amylase to about DE 5-10. The optimum pH for the reaction is 6.0-6.5 and calcium (generally 50ppm) is also needed. Then during saccharification pullulanase is added with glucoamylase (60°C, pH 4.0-4.5, 48h) to yield greater than 95-96% glucose, or with α-amylase (55°C, pH 5.0-5.5, 72h) to yield around 80-85% maltose (Fig. 1).

Pullulanase is used together with glucoamylase to improve the efficiency of starch conversion to glucose or together with α-amylase to increase the maltose level in high maltose syrups (Norman, 1982). Pullulanases are very important because they specifically increase the concentration of glucose (about 2%) or maltose (about 20-25%), reduce the reaction time (to 48 h), allow an increase in substrate concentration (to 40% DS) and allow

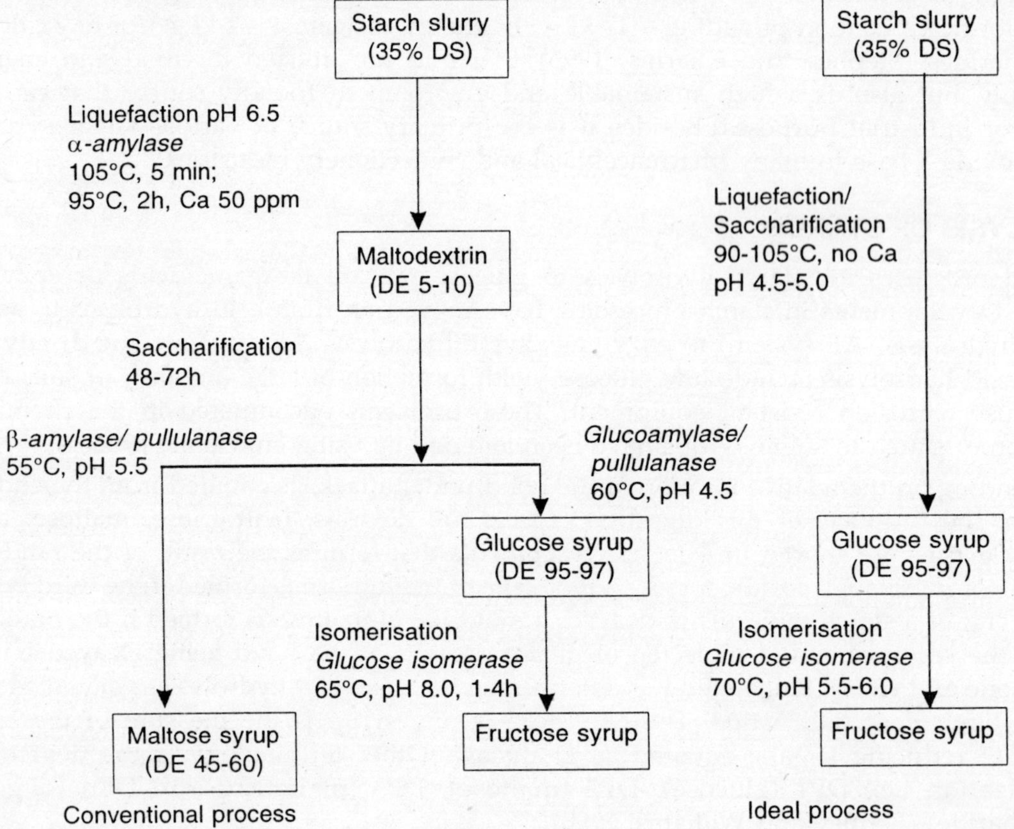

Fig. 1. Conventional and ideal starch processing

a reduction in the use of glucoamylase (upto 50%)[Saha and Zeikus, 1989]. The variation of various parameters in this process causes many handicaps in the starch industry. Due to pH variation large amounts of salts have to be removed by ion exchangers. Apart from the first step, all other steps are time consuming, leading, in most cases, to reverse reactions and lower yields. Therefore, undesirable products like branched oligosaccharides, panose, isopanose and isomaltose are formed. The improvement of the starch conversion process by finding new efficient and suitable enzymes having high thermostabilities, capable of working in the acidic to neutral range of pH and independent of requirement of metal ions for activity would, therefore, significantly lower the cost of sugar syrup production (Antranikian, 1992; Saha and Zeikus, 1989).

THE IDEAL PROCESS

Thermophilic bacteria are important sources for the production of efficient thermostable enzymes. The production of enzymes that simultaneously attack α-1,4- and α-1,6-linkages may enhance the starch saccharification process (Fig.1). For replacement of traditionally used enzymes, it is of utmost importance to find more thermostable enzymes with unique properties. Overproduction of such enzymes can be achieved by employing genetic techniques and optimization of fermentation processes (Antranikian *et al.*, 1987a,b; Vihinen and Mäntsälä, 1989). The enzymes with simultaneous α-1,4- and α-1,6-bond hydrolysing capability are a novel kind of pullulanase and have been variously called as amylase-pullulanase (Kim and Kim, 1995) and amylopullulanase (Saha *et al.*, 1989).

USE OF ENZYMES

The use of enzymes is preferred as it offers a number of advantages including improved yields and favorable economics. Microbial enzymes are of two types, viz., medical and industrial. Total market of the industrial enzymes in India alone is estimated to be Rs.1, 500 crores/annum. They are used in diverse industrial processes like detergent, textiles, leather, wine, pharmaceutical, food processing, paper, dairy and so on. Production of industrial enzymes is essentially a technology-oriented process (Ghatnekar *et al.*, 1995).

The starch-processing industry is unique within the industrial enzyme sectors, in that the use of enzymes is essential for the industry. The enzymatic hydrolysis allows greater control over amylolysis, the specificity of the reaction, and the stability of the generated products. The milder reaction conditions involve lower temperature and near neutral pH, thus reducing unwanted side reactions. Enzymatic methods are favoured because they have low energy requirements and eliminate neutralization steps (Bigelis, 1993).

STARCH HYDROLYZING ENZYMES

Many enzymes with different specificity are involved in the hydrolysis of starch. α-Amylase is an endoenzyme, which hydrolyzes internal independent α-1,4-bonds and can bypass 1,6-linkages. β-Amylase is an exoenzyme that liberates maltose by hydrolysing 1,4-linkages from the non-reducing ends. As it can not bypass 1,6-linkages, there remain β-limit dextrins after α-amylolysis. The action of glucoamylase produces glucose from starch by the cleavage of both α-1,4 and α-1,6-linkages. Isoamylase and pullulanase are debranching enzymes that hydrolyze α-1,6-linkages. They differ in their ability to hydrolyse pullulan. Only pullulanase can degrade this α-glycan (Vihinen *et al.*, 1989).

Starch hydrolyzing enzymes are among the most important enzymes that are produced on industrial scale. In addition to their application in the detergent industry they are used for the production of various sugar syrups. Alone in the USA, more than 18 billion pounds of sweeteners are produced from starch per year (Arbige *et al.*, 1989). Starch hydrolyzing enzymes accounted for nearly 15% of the global enzyme market, which was worth $1 billion in 1995.

α-amylase (1,4-α-D-Glucan-Glucanohydrolase, EC 3.2.1.1) is widely distributed in microbes and it hydrolyzes α-1,4-glycosidic linkages randomly in starch. The α-1,6-glycosidic linkages in amylopectin are not hydrolyzed by α-amylases. Its action on starch causes the formation of linear and branched oligosaccharides of varying length. Such branched oligosaccharides are called α limit dextrins. α-Amylases are also referred to as liquefying and saccharifying enzymes. Almost all of the technical α-amylases, however, needs a certain amount of calcium ions in the application, because their thermostability depends on the presence of calcium ions (Chang *et al.*, 1979).

Pullulanase is used in combination with the saccharifiying α-amylase to raise the saccharification rates and yields in the production of fructose syrups. Industrial starch saccharification processes are usually carried out at temperatures above 60°C in order to obtain higher substrate solubility and reduce microbial contamination (Hyun & Zeikus, 1985). However, most of the reported pullulanases are unstable at such temperatures. Thus, it seems expedient to identify suitable thermoactive, thermostable pullulanases for the benefit of saccharification processes.

Amylopullulanase, a thermozyme appears to have evolved in thermophilic bacteria (organisms thriving at 60-80°C). Thermozymes are thermostable enzymes that function optimally between 60 and 125°C. This is a 'hot' research topic for developing industrial enzyme sector & specialty biotechnologies. In recent years, thermozymes have attracted increasing attention owing to their biotechnological potential. This class of enzymes is capable of hydrolyzing α-1,4-linkages in addition to the branching points (α-1,6-linkages) in polysaccharides and limit dextrins. This enzyme is also capable of hydrolyzing amylose, which is composed exclusively of α-1,4-linkages (Noorvez and Satyanarayana, 1999).

The enzyme amylopullulanase was reported in the late 80's when the dual activity was considered to be the activity of α-Amylase and pullulanase. But the results from the characterization proved it to be a function of the same enzyme (Melasniemi, 1987). Saha *et al.* (1988) tentatively termed the enzyme amylopullulanase. This enzyme is a typical bacterial enzyme. Though it has been reported from some mesophilic bacteria, the major stress by researchers has been on thermophiles. This enzyme has been reported predominantly from thermophilic Archaea and eubacteria.

This stress on thermophiles had been due to the fact that starch gelatinization and saccharification necessarily occur at elevated temperatures and enzymes from thermophiles are naturally endowed with properties, which enable them to function optimally at such temperatures (Saha and Zeikus, 1989). In the last decade there had been a concerted effort to screen thermophilic bacteria for an amylopullulanase, which has the requisite properties to replace the existing battery of enzymes employed in starch hydrolysis process. Thus starch-processing industry is in need of a novel, efficient, thermostable, calcium independent amylolytic enzyme with dual activities of α amylase and pullulanase in order to significantly lower the cost of sugar syrup

THERMOPHILES

In the past twenty years, much of the research has been on enzymes from thermophiles of genera *Bacillus* and *Thermus*. These organisms are easy to maintain and grow on both large and small scale. Brock and Freeze (1969) discovered the first truly thermophilic organism, *Thermus aquaticus*. This was the organism, which later proved to be the source of Taq DNA Polymerase, the thermostable enzyme that revolutionized modern biology with the PCR technology.

Thermophiles have been isolated from diverse high temperature environments like geothermally heated volcanic regions, hotsprings and hydrothermal vents. Starch bioprocessing industry virtually depends on thermophiles for these enzymes, which are used to manufacture various sugar syrups. Important enzymes in this regard are α-amylase (*B. stearothermophilus, B. licheniformis*), α amylase, pullulanase and amylopullunase.

Many thermophilic bacteria produce enzymes that are not readily denatured at high temperature. Thermophiles have relatively high proportion of G + C content in their DNA that raise the melting point and add stability to the DNA molecule of these organisms. Several industrial processes already use thermostable enzymes, the best-known examples probably being those used in starch hydrolysis for the production of high fructose syrups.

Pullulanase was first isolated from strains of *Aerobacter aerogenes* by Bender and Wallenfels (1961). Since then it has been isolated from many mesophiles and thermophiles. Amylopullulanases are more prevalent in thermophilic anaerobes although known to be produced by some aerobic thermophiles as well as mesophiles. Among aerobes, certain *Bacillus* sp. is known to produce this enzyme. *Bacillus* strain 3183 (Shen *et al.*, 1990), *B. circulans* F-2 (Sata *et al.*, 1989; Kim *et al.*, 1990; Kim & Kim, 1995), *Bacillus* sp. TS-23 (Lin *et al.*, 1994), *Bacillus subtilis* (Takasaki, 1987) and *Bacillus* sp. DSM 405 (Brunswick *et al.*, 1999) has been reported to produce amylopullulanase.

Melasniemi (1987) described α-amylase and pullulanase activities from *Clostridium thermohydrosulfuricm,* which behaved identically at different pH and temperatures. Both these activities were stabilized by Ca^{++}. The enzyme was optimally active at 58-90°C and pH 5.6. Subsequently two forms of this enzyme were reported from C. *thermohydrosulfuricum* (Melasniemi, 1988). A similar enzyme was reported from *Bacillus* sp. 3183, which was optimally active at 75°C and pH 6.0 (Saha *et al.,* 1988). The purified enzyme cleaved α-1,6 linkages of pullulan liberating only maltotriose, but it cleaved α-1,4 and α-1,6 linkages in starch producing various saccharides. This enzyme was termed as amylopullulanase. Saha *et al.,* (1990) described an amylopullulanase from *Thermoanaerobacter,* which was optimally active at 75 °C and pH 5.0.

Sporadic efforts have been made to isolate moderately thermophilic bacteria from Indian thermal environmental samples (Sen and Satyanarayana 1993). A systematic attempt to discern the diversity of thermopiles has not, however, been made in India. The production of amylolytic enzymes such as α-amylase by moderately thermophilic *B. licheniformis* (Ramesh and Lonsane 1989,1990,1991) and *B. coagulans* (Babu and Satyanarayana 1993, 1955) has been reported. Seenayya and his co-workers have purified and characterized α-amylase and pullulanase of *Clostridium thermosulfurogenes* SV2 recently (Swamy and Seenayya 1996; Reddy *et al.* 1998). Recently, an attempt was made on the production & partial characterization of thermostable, calcium-independent α-amylase by an extreme thermophile Bacillus *thermoleovorans* (Malhotra *et al.*, 2000; Narang and Satyanarayana, 2001). We are the only group working on amylopullulanase of extremely thermophilic bacterium *Geobacillus thermoleovorans* in India.

Recently, Nazina *et al.*, (2001) proposed to create a new genus *Geobacillus* gen. nov., based on fatty acid analysis, DNA-DNA hybridization studies and 16S rRNA gene sequence analysis. This new genus includes their two isolates *Geobacillus subterraneus* gen. nov., sp. nov., *Geobacillus uzenensis* sp. nov., and the established species of thermophilic bacilli of *B. sterothermophilus, B. thermocatenulatus, B. thermoleovorans, B. kaustophilus, B. thermoglucosidasius* and *B. thermodenitrificans* have been transferred to *Geobacillus stearothermophilus, G. thermocatenulatus, G. thermoleovorans, G. kaustophilus, G. thermoglucosidasius* and *G. thermodenitrificans.*

RECOMBINANT DNA TECHNOLOGY

Recombinant DNA technology has become the main technology for the development and production of industrial enzyme products for a competitive price. Since the Dutch company Gist-Brocades introduced the a-amylase from *B. licheniformis* in 1985 and Genencor Inc. introduced a protease from *B. subtilis,* which are produced in recombinant production systems, more and more enzymes for industrial applications are produced in a homologous and heterologous expression systems with genetically modified microorganisms. The introduction of genetic modification can offer the following advantages in the production and/or quality of these enzymes:

- Higher production efficiency and thus less use of energy and raw materials and less waste,
- Availability of enzyme products which for economic, occupational or environmental reasons would otherwise not be available thus enabling new applications, and
- Technical improvement through higher specificity and purity of enzyme product.

Thermophiles are generally known to produce lower biomass. Usually very low titres of this enzyme are obtained. Since amylopullulanases are generally produced in very low titres, attempts have been made for overproduction. As mentioned above, continuous culturing has been tried, and also gene cloning is being performed. Melasniemi (1987) reported very low titres from *C. thermohydrosulfuricum.* Therefore, Melasniemi and Palheimo (1989) cloned amylopullunase gene from *Thermoanaerobium brockii* into *E. coli* and *B. subtilis. E. coli* did not export any measurable enzyme but *B. subtilis* secreted more enzyme (0.8-1.0 U/mL) than *T. brockii* (0.23 U/mL). Over expression of amylopullulanase was also reported by Lee *et al.,* (1994) when they cloned and expressed aapT gene from *Bacillus* sp. strain Xal 601 into *E. coli.* The importance of this enzyme has also boosted academic interest to carry out nucleotide sequence of amylopullulanase gene (Ramesh *et al* 1994). Recently, a gene coding for a new amylolytic enzyme from *Pseudomonas* sp. strain KFCC 10818 was cloned, and it was sequenced (Na *et al.*, 1996). Considering the impact such an enzyme would have on simplification and economization of the starch hydrolyzing process, the search is still on, and there is no report yet of its industrial applications.

During our search for thermostable and calcium-independent starch hydrolyzing enzymes, we have isolated a strain of *G. thermoleovorans* producing α-amylase, and another strain secreting amylopullulanase that cleaves both α-1,4 and α-1,6 glycosidic linkages in starch. Both these enzymes were thermostable and calcium-independent (Noorvez, 2000).

Production of amylopullulanase by *G. thermoleovorans*

The maximum amylopullulanase production of this strain has been found to be optimally at 65°C, pH 7.0 and with the incubation period of 18-20. Different physical and nutritional parameters were optimized for maximum production of amylopullulanase, which led to an increase in the production of amylase and pullulanase from 210 and 50 UL^{-1} to 2500 and 800 UL^{-1} in shake flasks. The most important parameter which led to significant increase in production were starch concentration (2%), inoculum age (10-12h) and nitrogen source. Further investigations in a 22L lab fermenter (10L medium) led to an increase in enzyme production to 5,800 and 1,900 UL^{-1} for amylase and pullulanase, respectively. The enzyme production was constitutive and independent of catabolite repression. The enzyme was purified to homogeneity by a combination of acetone precipitation, anion-exchange and gel-filtration chromatography. It was a low molecular mass amylopullulanase with an approximate molecular mass of 48 kDa and displayed both pullulanase and amylase activities as demonstrated by activity staining on starch and pullulan azure overlay gels. The enzyme was not a glycoprotein. The temperature and pH optima for both pullulanase and amylase activities were 80°C and pH 7-8, respectively. The enzyme was highly thermostable with amylase and pullulanase activities displaying half-lives of 2 and 3.5h at 100°C, respectively. The two enzyme activities demonstrated different thermostabilities, pullulanase being more stable than amylase. Experiments with mixed substrates also suggested that the enzyme belonged to the class of amylopullulanases having two different active sites for the amylase and pullulanase activities, as against the amylopullulanases having one active site responsible for both the activities.

α-amylase production of *G. thermoleovorans*

This strain produced the thermostable and calcium-independent α-amylase optimally at 70°C, with the incubation period of 12h. The α-amylase production levels in shake flasks of 250ml capacity containing 50ml medium was 14 780 UL^{-1}. In fermentor, the maximum production of α-amylase was found optimally at 60°C, pH 5.4, with the incubation period of 8h and the enzyme levels increased to 24 050 UL^{-1}. The medium components for the growth & maximum enzyme production were optimized. Starch favoured maximum α-amylase secretion as a carbon source, whereas tryptone & ammonium sulphate supported the maximum bacterial growth and α-amylase production as an organic, inorganic nitrogen sources, respectively. Yeast extract and tryptone required as essential growth factors. Partial purification of α-amylase with acetone precipitation led to 43.7% recovery with 6.2 fold purification. The α-amylase was optimally active at 100°C and pH 8.0 with $t_{1/2}$ of 3h at 100°C.

CONCLUSION

Enzymes from thermophiles are better suited for industrial processing of polysaccharides because of their increased activity and stability at high temperature. With more efficient enzyme producers, the cost of enzyme production can go down. The observations recorded in the present investigation showed some important features of the enzyme, which may be important from industrial perspective, especially its high thermostability, capability to function in a wide pH range and its independence from requirement of calcium ions for activity. Thermostable enzymes are receiving considerable applications and there are many industrial applications already. Since one of our strain, producing thermostable and calcium-independent a-amylase, further work is in progress on the use of this enzyme in starch saccharification. Most thermostable enzymes on the market have, however, been derived from mesophiles. Since amylopullulanases are known to be secreted at very low levels, further research, especially on the possibilities of cloning of a gene encoding the amylopullulanase from our strain of *G. thermoleovorans* into mesophilic 'GRAS' (generally regarded as safe) hosts will greatly increase its exploitation in starch saccharification.

REFERENCES

Antranikian, G. (1992). Microbial degradation of starch. In: *Microbial Degradation of Natural Products,* (*Ed.* G. Winkelmann), VCH, Weinheim, Germany.

Antranikian, G., Zablowski P. and Gottschalk G. (1987a). Conditions for the overproduction and excretion of thermostable a-amylase and pullulanase from *Clostridium thermohydrosulfuricum* DSM 567. *Applied Microbiology and Biotechnology* 27:75-81.

Antranikian, G., Herzberg C. and Cottschalk G. (1987). Production of thermostable a-amylase and pullulanase and a-glucosidase in continuous culture by a new Clostridium isolate. *Applied and Environmental Microbiology* 53:1668-1673.

Arbige, M. V. and Pitcher W. H. (1989). Industrial enzymology: a look towards the future. *TIBTECH* 7:330-335.

Babu, K. R. and Satyanarayana T. (1993). Extracellular calcium-inhibited alpha amylase of *Bacillus coagulans* B 49. *Enzyme Microbial Technology* 15:1066-1069.

Babu, K. R. and Satyanarayana T. (1995). a-Amylase Production by Thermophilic *Bacillus coagulans* in Solid State Fermentation. *Process Biochemistry* 30:305-309.

Bender, H. and Wallenfels K. (1961). Pullulan. II. Specific decomposition by bacterial enzyme. *Biochemistry* 334:79-95.

Bentley, I. S. and Williams E. C. (1996). Starch conversion. In: *Industrial enzymology* (*Ed.* Tony Godfrey and Stuart West), 2nd ed., Macmillan Press Ltd., London.

Bigelis, R., (1993). Carbohydrases. In: *Enzymes in Food Processing*, (*Ed.* T. Nagodawithana and G. Reed), 3rd ed., Academic Press, Inc., San Diego, California.

Brock, T. D. and Freeze H. (1969). *Thermus aquaticus* gen. N. and sp. n., a Non-sporulating Extreme Thermophile. Journal of Bacteriology 98:289-297.

Brunswick, J. M., Kelly C. T. and Fogarty W. M. (1999). The amylopullulanase of *Bacillus* sp. DSM 405. *Applied Microbiology and Biotechnology* 51:170-175.

Chang, J. P., Alter J.E. and Sternberg M. (1979). Purification and characterization of a thermostable a-Amylase from *Bacillus licheniformis. Starch/Strike* 31:86-92.

Ghatnekar, S. D., Karion M. F. and Ghatnekar G. S. (1995). Production of industrial enzymes; Lucerative venture for indian industries. In: *Biotechnology strategy for development*, BCIL, New Delhi.

Hermansson, A. M., and Svegmark K. (1996). Developments in the understanding of starch functionality. *Trends in Food Science and Technology* 7:345-353.

Hyun, H. H. and Zeikus J. G. (1985). Simultaneous and enhanced production of thermostable amylases and ethanol from starch by cocultures of *Clostridium thermosulfurogenes and Clostridium thermohydrosulfuricum. Applied and Environmental Microbiology* 499:1174-1184.

Kim, G. H., Kim D. S., Taniguchi H., and Maruyama Y. (1990). Purification of an amylase-pullulanase bifunctional enzyme by high-performance size exclusion and hydrophobic-interaction chromatography. *Journal of Chromatography* 512:131-137.

Kim, C-H. and Kim Y. S. (1995). Substrate specificity and detailed characterization of a bifunctional amylase-pullulanase enzyme from *Bacillus circulans* F-2 having two different active sites on one polypeptide. *European Journal of Biochemistry* 227: 687-693.

Lee, S. P., Morikawa, M., Takagi, M. and Imanaka T. (1994). Cloning of the *aapT* gene and characterization of its product, α-amylase-pullulanase (AapT), from thermophilic and alkaliphilic *Bacillus* sp. strain XAL601. *Applied and Environmental Microbiology* 60:3764-3773.

Lin, L. L., Tsau M. R. and Chu W. S. (1994). General characteristics of thermostable amylopullulanases and amylases from the alkalophilic *Bacillus* sp. TS-23. *Applied Microbiology and Biotechnology* 42: 51-56.

Malhotra. R., Noorwez S. M. and Satyanarayana T. (2000). Production and partial characterization of thermostable and calcium-independent α-amylase of an extreme thermophile *Bacillus thermooleovorans* NP54. *Letters in Applied Microbiology* 31: 378-384.

Melasniemi, H. (1987). Characterization of alpha-amylase and pullulanase activities of *Clostridium thermohydrosulfuricum. Biochemical Journal* 246:193-197.

Melasniemi, H., (1988). Purification and some properties of the extracellular a-amylase-pullulanase produced by *Clostridium thermohydrosulfuricum. Biochemical Journal* 250:813-818.

Melasniemi, H., and Paloheimo M. (1989). Cloning and Expression of the *Clostridium thermohydrosulfuricum* a-Amylase-pullulanase Gene in *Escherichia coli. J. Gen. Microbiol.* 135:1755-1762.

Na, H.K., Kim E. S., Lee H. B., Yoo O. J., and Jhon D. Y. (1996). Cloning and Nucleotide sequence of the α-Amylase gene from alkalophilic *Pseudomonas* sp. KFCC 10818. *Mol.Cells* 6:203-208.

Narang. S. and Satyanarayana T. (2001). Thermostable α-amylase production by an extreme thermophile *Bacillus thermooleovorans. Letters in Applied Microbiology* 32:31-35.

Nazina, T. N., Tourova, T. P., Poltaraus, A. B., Novikova, E. V., Grigoryan, A. A., Ivanova, A. E., Lysenko, A. M., Petrunyaka, V. V., Osipov, G. A., Belyaev, S. S. and Ivanov M. V. (2001). Taxonomic study of aerobic thermophilic bacilli: descriptions of *Geobacillus subterraneus* gen. Nov., sp. nov. and *Geobacillus uzenensis* sp. nov. from petroleum reservoirs and transfer of *Bacillus stearothermophilus, Bacillus thermocatenulatus, Bacillus thermoleovorans, Bacillus kaustophilus, Bacillus thermoglucosidasius* and *Bacillus thermodenitrificans* to *Geobacillus* as the new combinations *G. Stearothermophilus, G. thermocatenulatus, G. thermoleovorans, G. Kaustophilus, G. thermoglucosidasius* and *G. thermodenitrificans. International Journal of Systematic and Evolutionary Microbiology* 51:433-446.

Noorvez, S. M. (2000). Amylopullulanase of Thermophilic Bacterium *Bacillus Thermoleovorans* NP33. Ph. D Thesis, University of Delhi, India, pp. 162.

Noorvez, S. M., and Satyanarayana T. (1999). Starch hydrolysing enzymes: Pullulanases and Amylopullulanases In: *Microbial Biotechnology for Sustainable Development and Productivity*, (*Ed.* R. C. Rajak), scientific Publishers (India), Jodhpur, pp.275-278.

Norman, B.E., (1982). A novel debranching enzyme for application in the glucose syrup industry. *Starch/Stärke* 10:340-346.

Ramesh, M. V., and Lonsane B. K. (1989). Solid state fermentation for production of higher titres of thermostable alpha-amylase with two peaks for pH optima for *B. licheniformis* M 27. *Biotechnology Letters* 11:49-52.

Ramesh, M. V., and Lonsane B. K. (1990). Critical importance of moisture content of the medium in a-amylase production by *Bacillus licheniformis* M-27 in solid state fermentation system. *Appl. Microbiol. Biotechnol.* 33:501-505.

Ramesh, M. V., and Lonsane B. K. (1991). Ability of a solid state fermentation technique to significantly minimize catabolite repression of α-amylase production by *B. licheniformis* M 27. *Appl. Microbiol. Biotechnol.* 35:591-593.

Ramesh, M. V., Podkovyrov S. M. , Lowe S. E. and Zeikus J. G. (1994). Cloning and Sequencing of the *Thermoanaerobacterium saccharolyticum* B6A-RI *apu* Gene and Purification and Characterization of the Amylopullulanase from *Escherichia coli.* Applied and Environmental Microbiology 60:94-101.

Reddy, P. R. M., Swamy, M. V, and Seenayya G. (1998). Purification and characterization of thermostable a-amylase and pullulanase from high-yielding *Clostridium thermosulfurogenes* SV2. *World J. Microbiol. Biotechnol.* 14: 89-94.

Saha, B. C., and Zeikus J. G. (1989). Novel highly thermostable pullulanase from thermophiles. *TIBTECH* 7: 234-238.

Saha, B. C., Mathupala, S. P. and Zeikus J. G. (1988). Purification and characterization of a highly thermostable novel pullulanase from *Clostridium thermohydrosulfuricum. Biochemical Journal* 258: 343-348.

Saha, B. C., Shen, G. J., Srivastava, K. C., LeCureux, L. W. and Zeikus, J. G. (1989). New thermostable a-amylase-like pullulanase from thermophilic *Bacillus* sp. 3183. *Enzyme and Microbial Technology* 11:760-764.

Saha B. C., Lamed R. , Lee C. Y., Mathupala S. P. and Zeikus J. G. (1990). Characterization of an endo-acting amylopullunase from thermoanaerobacter strain B6A. *Appl. Environ. Microbiol.* 56:881-886.

Sata, H., Umeda M., Kim C. H., Taniguchi H. and Maruyama Y. (1989). Amylase-pullulanase enzyme produced by *Bacillus circulans* F-2. *Biochimica et Biophysica Acta* 991:338-394.

Sen, S. and Satyanarayana T. (1993). Optimization of alkaline protease production by thermostable *Bacillus licheniformis* S-40. *Indian J. Microbiol.* 33:43-47.

Shen, G. J., Srivastava K. C., Saha B. C. and Zeikus J. G. (1990). Physiological and enzymatic characterization of a novel pullulan-degrading thermophilic *Bacillus* strain 3183. *Applied and Environmental Microbiology* 33: 340-344.

Stephen, A.M., and Charms S. C. (1995). Introduction. In: *Food Polysaccharides and their Appplications*, (ed. A. M. Stephen), Marcel Dekker Inc., New York.

Swamy, M. V., and Seenayya G. (1996). Thermostable Pullulanase and α-Amylase Activity from *Clostridium Thermosulfurogenes* SV9-Optimization of Culture Conditions for Enzyme Production. *Proc. Biochem.* 31:157-162.

Takasaki, Y., (1987). Pullulanase-amylase complex enzyme from *Bacillus subtilis. Agricultural and Biological Chemistry* 51(2): 9-16.

Vihinen, M., and Mäntsälä P. (1989). Microbial amylolytic enzymes. *Critical Reviews in Biochemistry and Molecular Biology* 24(1-6): 329-418.

Zobel, H. F., and Stephen A. M. (1995). Starch: structure, analysis, and application. In; *Food Polysaccharides and their Applications*, (*Ed.* A. M. Stephen), Marcel Dekker Inc., New York.

Microbiology and Biotechnology for Sustainable Development (*Ed.* P.C. Jain),
CBS Publishers & Distributors, New Delhi (2004), pp. 121–140.

A-11

Biodiversity of Tropical Basidiomycetes—As Sources of Novel Secondary Metabolites

S. K. Deshmukh
Dept. of Natural Products, Quest Institute of Life Sciences
Nicholas Piramal India Limited, Post Box-17753
L. B. S. Marg, Mulund (W), Mumbai 400 080. India
E mail sdeshmukh @nicholaspiramal.co.in

Abstract

Basidiomycetes are an important bioresource of novel secondary metabolites. Such metabolites have chemical skeletons which are not observed in other fungi. In developing countries, such as India alternative systems of medicine utilize the curative properties of basidiomycetes. In this article, emphasis has been laid on anti-tumor and immunomodulating properties of the molecules detected. A majority of these are polysaccharides. This article also emphasises the Basidiomycetes diversity around Mumbai.

Keywords: Anti tumor polysaccharides, basidiomycetes, immunomodulating, secondary Metabolites

INTRODUCTION

It is estimated that some 1.5 million species of fungi are likely to exist, but only about 69,000 or so currently recorded; of these only 11,500 (17%) are represented in culture collections (Hawksworth, 1991). This estimate of fungal species is based principally on a ratio of vascular plants to fungi of about 1:6, and although six times greater than any previous estimate, it is still thought to be conservative. Among the reasons for proposing still higher figures are i) the probable underestimate of total number of vascular plants; ii) the vascular plant: fungi ratio rising with time (decadal rates of increase in number of fungi in different habitats range from about 20 to 50%) iii) plant: fungi ratio tends to reflect the more intensive mycological studies made in north temperate regions but may be higher in the tropics; and iv) no separate estimate is made for fungi associated with the enormous insect diversity. The fungal inventory will again grow when poorly explored regions and habitats are examined viz. marine ecosystem, cryptoendolithic communities, cryoconite holes on glacier and mycorrhizal and mycophyllal associates. Evidence for the richness of the fungal biota of tropical regions is also sighted in the same article.

The basidiomycetes constitute a class of fungi with an estimated number of 30,000 species whose secondary metabolites and biologically active products have scarcely been investigated, yet recent surveys reveal novel metabolites with antibiotic, antiviral, phytotoxic and cytostatic activity (Anke, 1989; Lorenzen and Anke, 1998 and Abraham, 2001).

We classify an immense variety of fungi in this category, the most advanced of all fungal classes. The true basidiomycetes consist of forms which people call mushrooms, toadstools, puffballs, and stinkhorns. Shelf fungi or bracket fungi also belong to this class, as well as the less familiar bird's-nest fungi. Mushrooms constitute a relatively large group of fungi consisting of about 4000 species and many of them are well known, being edible. The first reference of occurrence of basidiomycetes was recorded by Montagne in 1842 (Sathe, 1979). Later on Manjula (1983) complied "A revised list of Agricoid and Boletoid basidiomycetes from India and Nepal". Emphasis on distribution of this group of fungi from the Indian subcontinent was given by various workers (Sathe and Deshpande, 1979; Natrajan and Raman, 1983; Purkayastha and Chandra, 1985; Verma *et al.*, 1987; Lakhanpal, 1995; Pradeep *et al.*, 1998; Vrindra *et al.*, 1999 and Atri *et al.*, 2000). In India the work on this important group of fungi, however, is limited and about 850 species are recorded from various parts of the Indian subcontinent. As far as Mumbai is concerned very limited attempts have been made for distribution of basidiomycetes (Butler and Bisby, 1931 and Bhide *et al.*, 1987).

The present article highlights the use of tropical basidiomycetes in traditional medicine/ folk medicine, their distribution in the vicinity of Mumbai (18.55 N 72.54 E11 M altitude) for their biodiversity, and scope for obtaining novel secondary metabolites.

Basidiomycetes in traditional medicine/ folk medicine:

The invasion (migration) of the Aryans from central Asia into the Indian subcontinent took place around 1500 BC. They carried with them an intoxicating drink ***soma***. ***Soma*** was mostly used in Aryan religious rites. In the Rig Veda there are many songs on ***soma*** only subject on which there are chapters in Rigveda. According to Wasson (1969) the ***soma*** in the Rig Veda refers to *Amanita muscaria*

Inhibition of growth of influenza virus and recession of some kinds of cancer is shown by extract of Shiitake (*Lentinus edodes*). *Lentinus* contains compounds that reduce the serum cholesterol level in humans thereby lowering blood pressure. Wu Shui, a famous Chinese physician (Ming Dynasty) has written that the Lentinus is capable of curing cold, improving blood circulation, lowering blood pressure and generating stamina (Bahal, 1994).

Crude extracts of *Ganoderma tsugae* a traditional Chinese medicine, have been demonstrated to enhance splenic natural killer cell activity and serum interferon production in mice (Gan *et al.*, 1998). *Poria cocus* Wolf (Polyporaceae) is a well-known Chinese traditional medicine used for its diuretic, sedative, and tonic effects (Cueller *et al.*, 1996). Many basidiomycetes have been used for medicinal purpose in India (Vaidya and Rabba, 1993; Rai *et al.*, 1993 and Sharma, 1998).

Some of the information on the mushrooms in folk medicine in India is given in table 1.

Table 1: Medicinal uses of Basidiomycetes in India

No.	Fungus	Vernacular Name	Medicinal Properties	References
1	*Amanita muscaria*		Used as a powder or tincture for swollen glands & epilepsy. Used in highly diluted preparations for heart ailment and rheumatoid arthritis.	Bahl, 1994
2	*Amylosporus campbellii (Polyporus anthelminticus)*	Bamboo Agaric	Anthelminthic	Chopara, *et al.*, 1956
3	*Auricularia auricula*	Jew's ear	Used as poultice for inflammed eyes and as a gargle for inflammation of the throat.	Bahl, 1994
4	*Astraeus hygrometrius*	Savan Putpura	Burn care	Sharma, 1998
5	*Calvatia cyathiformis*	Dharti phool	Spore mass for wound healing and for checking pus formation	Sharma, 1998
6	*Calvatia giganta*		Used for anaesthesia	Bahl, 1994
7	*Cythus limbatus*	Nirghunti	conjunctivitis	Sharma, 1998
8	*Cythus stercoreus*	Kulhari	For curing disorder of eyes like pain, redness or conjunctivitis	Sharma, 1998
9	*Daedaleopsis flavida*	Snuff Fungus	Snuff powder to reduce bilirubin and bilivirain for jaundice	Vaidya and Rabba, 1993
10	*Fomes fomentarius*	Tinder Fungus	Cauterization of burned tissues.	Dymock *et al.*, 1890
11	*Fomes ignarius & Fomes fomentarius*		Used for rapid coagulation of blood	Bahl, 1994
12	*Inonotus obliquus*	Chaga	Anticarcinogenic properties, chronic gastritis & ulcers	Rolf and Rolf, 1925
13	*Larcifomes officinalis*	Larch - Quinine Fungus	Agarin, agaricol and agaric acid is active principle. Liver Complaints, asthma, jaundice, dysentery, stomach pain, pain in joints, cathartic, lactifuge, diuretic, expectorants, check bleeding from bites.	Nadkarni, 1954
14	*Lentinus edodes*	Shiitake mushroom	Capable of generating stamina, curing cold, improving the blood circulation and lowering blood pressure. It stimulates the immune system which acts against cancer cells. It also has antiviral activity. Lowers chlesterol content in blood.	Pegler, 1983
15	*Lycoperdon giganteum*		Used as a soft and comfortable surgical dressing	Bahal, 1994
16	Lycoperdon pusilum	Phusphus	Sporemass for controlling bleeding from cuts and also for wound heeling	Sharma, 1998

(Contd.)

No.	Fungus	Vernacular Name	Medicinal Properties	References
17	*Meripilus giganteus*		Applied in gums to prevent excessive salivation, good styptic.	Khory, 1887
18	*Microporus xanthopus*	Saja Pihiri	for curing ear pain	Sharma, 1998
19	*Phallus rubricandus*	Jhri Pihiri	For curing typhoid and for relief during labor pain.	Sharma, 1998
20	*Phellinus gilvus*		Conks used against kidney disorder	Vaidya and Rabba, 1993
21	*Phellinus linteus*		Conks growing on bhendi to purify blood in skin diseases.	Vaidya and Rabba, 1993
22	*Phellinus igniarius*	Bulgar tangali	Internally as a bitter tonic and laxative, externally as a styptic.	Nadkarni, 1954, Chopra, *et al.*, 1956
23	*Polyporus officinalis*	Agerick	Drastic purge external application to stop bleeding. Used for Chronic catarrh diseases of the breast and lung, as a remedy for night sweating in tuberculosis, for rheumatism, gout, jaundice, dropsy and intestinal worms.	Bahl, 1994
24	*Polyporus spp. on birch*	Snuff Fungus	Narcotic snuff	Barkeley, 1857
25	*Psilocybe spp.*		Halucinogenic treatment. Treatment of mental disorders	Krauseman, 1953
26	*Pycnoporus sanguineus*	Blood red mushroom	Dysentery, veneral disease, embrocation for leprous tubercies, inflamation of skin	Bahal, 1994
27	*Termitomyces microcarpus*	Bhoroan Pihiri	As a remade in case of partial paralysis, tonic for over coming weakness.	Sharma, 1998
28	*Volvariella volvacea & Flammulina velutipes*		They lower blood pressure & are active against tumor cells	Bahl, 1994

Occurence and Cultivation of Basidiomycetes:

In tropical / subtropical regions basidiomycetes occur in the monsoons generally after the first rains set in, till the end. We see these fungi growing on their natural habitat-dead, decayed or living plants, soil or dung. Cultures may be isolated either from fruiting bodies or basidiospores and maintained by subculturing, storage under mineral oil, in sterile water, and storage in liquid nitrogen. Short term storage on slants at 4°C is also possible. Lyophilization does not serve the same purpose.

Several difficulties are commonly encountered:

i) Seasonal occurrence of mushrooms and their collection in forests is difficult. They have a very short life and many are missed. To overcome these limitations, mushroom collectors have to visit the same locality time and again.

ii) Mushroom specimens, being fragile, are usually damaged while carrying them to the laboratory. In order to avoid damage during transportation, much care is required.
iii) Some of the mushrooms like those of *Coprinus, Dictyophora* etc. are deliquescent.
iv) Spores of many species e.g. from the genera *Inocybe* and *Russula* do not germinate.
v) Many mycelial cultures grow slowly on solid medium or in submerged cultures
vi) Fermentation cycles range from one week to five weeks or more.

The relatively small number of known mushrooms is because of the above constraints.

Distribution of basidiomycetes around Mumbai:

A systemic survey was done to see the distribution of basidiomycetes around Mumbai since very little work has been recorded in this region.

A field key to mushroom collection has been followed and used in describing the macro- and microcharacteristics of gill fungi (Mainse, 1944, Smith, 1949, Atkinson, 1961, Hawksworth, 1974, Pegler, 1977, Singer, 1986 and Atri and Saini, 2000) and some of the fungi were identified using various other keys.

The results of the primary survey are given in table 2. 54 species of 36 genera were recorded and further work on identification is in progress.

Table 2: Species of various wild mushrooms genera recorded from Mumbai

Sr. No.	Genus and species	Habitat
1	*Agaricus spp.*	Solitary or scattered in lawns
2	*Agaricus arvensis Schw . Fr*	Solitary or scattered in lawns
3	*Agaricus silvaticus Schaeff. Fr.*	Solitary on grassy soil
4	*Agaricus xanthodermus Genv.*	Scattered in lawns
5	*Agrocybe Spp.*	Scattered in lawns
6	*Amanita Spp.*	Growing in association of unidentified forest tree
7	*Anthracophyllum nigritum (Lev.) Kalch.*	On dead wood and logs
8	*Auricularia auricula Judiae (L.) Berk*	On dead wood and logs
9	*Auricularia polytricha (Mont.) Sacc.*	On dead wood and logs
10	*Cantharellus cibarius Fr.*	Associated with bamboo trees
11	*Cantharellus Spp*	Associated with bamboo trees
12	*Chlorophyllum molybditis (Mayer ex.Fr.) Massee*	Solitary or scattered in grassy land
13	*Clavaria Spp.*	Associated with bamboo trees
14	*Clavatia cythiformis (Bosc) Morgan*	Growing in groups on soil, grassy land and some time on the cultivated field
15	*Lepista nuda (Bull. : Fr.) Cooke*	Solitary or scattered in lawns
16	*Coprinus comatus (Fr.) Gray*	Singly to scattered on clustered in clumps on grassy land
17	*Craterrellus Spp.*	Associated with bamboo trees

(Contd.)

Sr. No.	Genus and species	Habitat
18	*Crepidotus molis (Schaelf. Fr.)Kummer*	Growing on wood
19	*Cyathus stercoreus (Schw.) de Toni.*	On manure heaps
20	*Dictyophora indusiata (Vent. : Pers.) Fischer*	Solitary or scattered in lawns
21	*Favolus Spp*	Solitary or in groups on stumps
22	*Ganoderma applanatum (Pers.) Pat.*	On trunk of trees
23	*Ganoderma lucidum (Leyss.: Fr.) Karst*	Solitary or in groups on stumps
24	*Geastrum Spp.*	Solitary or scattered on ground
25	*Hebeloma fastible (Pers. Fr.) Kummer*	Solitary or scattered on ground
26	*Hygrocybe indica Sharma & Deshpande*	Solitary or in groups on wood
27	*Hygrophorus Spp.*	Growing in association of unidentified forest tree
28	*Lactarius Spp.*	Growing in forest litter
29	*Leccinum Spp.*	Growing in forest litter
30	*Lentinus edodes (Berk.) Singer*	Growing in clusters in dead wood
31	Lentinus squarossulus Mont.	Growing in single or in clusters in dead wood
32	*Lepiota cristata (Fr.) Kummer*	Solitary or scattered in lawns and freshly manured soil
33	*Leucoagaricus badhamii (Berk & Br) Heim*	Solitary or scattered in lawns and freshly manured soil
34	*Leucocoprinus cepaestipes (Sow.ex.Fr.) Patouillard*	Growing in partial fairy rings in soil.and freshly manured soil
35	*Lycoperdon pyriforme Schaeff.*	Growing in soil along with fallen leaves
36	*Lycoperdon Spp.*	Growind in soil and grassy land
37	*Marasmius siccus Schw. Fr.*	Scattered in groups on fallen leaves
38	*Mycena aceculata*	Scattered in groups on fallen leaves
39	*Mycena janicicola(Fr.) Gillet*	Scattered in groups on fallen leaves
40	*Mycena madronicola Smith*	Scattered in groups on fallen leaves
41	*Mycena pura (Pers.: Fr.) Kummer*	Growing in soil along with fallen leaves
42	*Oudemansiella mucida (Schaeff.Fr.) Hoehnel*	Growing in soil along with fallen leaves
43	*Oudemansiella radicata (Reth .Fr.)Sing*	Growing in association of unidentified forest tree
44	*Phallus impudicus L.Fr.*	Growing in soil lawns/ grassy land
45	*Pleurotus eous (Berk) Sacc.*	Growing on dead tree in clusters.
46	*Pleurotus ostreatus (Jacq.: Fr.)Kummer*	Growing on dead tree in clusters.
47	*Pycnoporus cinnabarinus Jacq. ex. Fr.*	Growing on dead wood or logs
48	*Russula nigricans (Bull.) ex. Fr.*	Growing in association of unidentified forest tree
49	*Rhodophyllus strictus (Perk.) Sing*	Growing in soil along with fallen leaves
50	*Schizophyllum commune Fr.*	Growing onhard wood or logs
51	*Termitomyces heimii Natrajan*	On termite nests
52	*Termitomyces mamiformis Heim*	On termite nests
53	*Termitomyces microcarpus (Berk& Br.) Heim*	On termite nests
54	*Termitomyces robustus (Beeli)Heim*	On termite nests

Secondary Metabolites produced by Basidiomycetes:

Basidiomycetes produce a wide variety of secondary metabolites during their life cycle (Fig. 1). These metabolites may be excreted into the growth medium or in the fruiting bodies when existing in the wild. Table 3 indicates the nature of the biological activities of a number of interesting compounds from basidiomycetes.

Table 3: Compounds Isolated From Basidiomycetes

Producer	Compounds	Activity	Reference
1. *Aleurodiscus mirabilis*	Aleurodiscal	Antifungal antibiotic	Lauer *et al.*, 1989
2. *Cheimonophyllum candissimum*	Cheimonophyllon A-E and cheimonophyllal	Nematicidal, weak antifungal, antibacterial, cytotoxic activity	Stadler *et al.*, 1994
3. *Clitocybe cyathiformis*	Cyathiformine A-D	Antibacterial and antifungal	Arnone *et al.*, 1993
4. *Clitocybe diatreta*	Diatretol	Antibacterial	Arnone *et al.*, 1996
5. *Clitocybe inversa*	Clitocine	Insecticidal	Kubo *et al.*, 1986
6. *Crepidotus fulvotomentosus*	Strobilurin E	Antifungal and respiration inhibiting properties	Weber *et al.*, 1990
7. *Coprinus altramentarius*	Illudin C2, Illudin C3	Antimicrobial antibiotic	Lee *et al.*, 1996a
8. *Favolaschia pustulosa*	9-methoxystrobilurin E	Antifungal, antibacterial and cytotoxic	Wood et al., 1996
9. *Favolaschia* sp.	Favolon	Antifungal	Anke *et al.*, 1995
10. *Flagelloscypha pilatii*	Pilatin	Antibiotic and cytotoxic	Heim *et al.*, 1988
11. *Ganoderma tsugae*	3α-acetoxy-5α-lanosta-8,24-dien-21-oic acid ester β-D-glucoside	Cytotoxic	Gan *et al.*, 1998
12. *Ganoderma tsugae*	2β 3α 9α-trihydroxy-5α -ergosta-7,22-diene	Cytotoxic	Gan *et al.*, 1998
13. *Haploporus odorus*	Haploporic acid A		Morita *et al.* 1995
14. *Hericium ramosum* CL 24240	Erinacine E	Kappa opioid receptor binding inhibitor	Saito *et al.*, 1998
15. *Laurilla tsugicola*	Tsugicoline A-D	Inhibits germination of the water cress *Lepidium sativum*	Arnone *et al.*, 1995
16. *Lenzites betulina*	Betulinan A, Betulinan B	Lipid peroxidation inhibitor	Lee *et al.*, 1996b
17. *Mniopetalum* sp.	Mniopetals	Reverse transcriptase inhibitor, antimicrobial and cytotoxic	Kuschel *et al.*, 1994
18. *Mycena* sp. TA 87202	Mycenon	isocitrate lyase inhibitor	Hautzel *et al.*, 1990
19. *Mycena* sp.96097	Strobilurin M, Tetrachloro-pyrocatechol,	Antifungal and cytostatic, Antifungal, antibacterial and cytotoxic,	Daferner *et al.*, 1998
	Tetrachloropyrocatechol Methyl Ether	Antifungal, antibacterial and cytotoxic	
20. *Nidula candida*	Nidulal	Inducer of differentiation of human promyelocytic leukemia	Erkel *et al.*, 1996

(Contd.)

Producer	Compounds	Activity	Reference
21. *Omphalotus illudens*	Illudinic acid	Antibacterial	Dufresne *et al.*, 1997
22. *Oudemansiella radicata*	Oudemansin x	Antifungal	Anke *et al.*, 1990
23. *Phellinus* sp.	Cyclophellitol	β-glucosidase inhibitor	Atsumi *et al.*, 1990
24. *Poria cocos*	Lanostane	inhibitors of Phospholipase A2 inhibitor(group of anti-inflammatory agents)	Cuellar *et al.*, 1996
25. *Pterula* sp. 82168	Hydroxystrobilurin A, Strobilurin A, Oude-mansin A	Antifungal	Engler *et al.*, 1995
26. *Resupinatus leightonii*	Panellon	Antimicrobial, cytotoxic and phytotoxic	Sundin *et al.*, 1993
27. *Schizophyllum commune*	Schizostatin	Squalene synthase inhibitor	Tanimoto *et al.*, 1996
28. *Strobilurus tenacellus* 21602	Strobilurins	Antifungal antibiotic	Anke *et al.*, 1977
29. *Xerula melanotricha*	Dihydroxerulin, Xerulin Xerulinic acid	Cholesterol biosynthesis inhibitor	Kuhnt *et al.*, 1990

In our laboratories inhibition of the CDK4 enzyme was selected to find novel molecules from basidiomycetes as probable anticancer agents. In preliminary studies we have seen indications that some mushrooms can specifically inhibit *in vitro* the Cyclin Dependent Kinase(CDK-4) enzyme activity, thereby inhibiting the proliferation of some cancerous cell lines viz.- HeLa (cervical cancer), PC-3(prostate cancer), MCF-7(breast cancer). Interestingly the metabolites of fruiting bodies are often different from those of mycelial cultures. This may reflect the different stages of development. The compounds are a variety of polysaccharides.

Basidiomycetes as producers of Immunomodulatory and Antitumor Metabolites :

During our study we have observed compounds exhibiting immunomodulators, activity also exhibit significant anti-tumor activity and they are summarized below. It must be noted that the basidiomycetes species listed here have been reported in India (Butler and Bisby, 1931; Manjula, 1983; Sathe and Deshpande, 1979; Natrajan and Raman, 1983; Purkayastha and Chandra, 1985; Bhide *et al.*, 1987; Verma *et al.* 1987; Lakhanpal, 1995; Vindra *et al.*, 1999 and Atri *et al.*, 2000) though the identified metabolites may be referred to from elsewhere.

Agaricus blazei Murr,

A. *blazei,* known as Himematsutake in Japanese is a household remedy having many physiological activities. A β-D-glucan polysaccharide isolated from *A. blazei* exhibited immunostimulative and anti-tumor activity (Mizuno *et al.*, 1988). From the fruit body of this mushroom a protein linked (1A6) β- D-glucan was isolated. This glycoprotein exhibited anti-tumor activity (Kawagishi *et al.*, 1989). Three ergosterol derivatives (I) (II) and (III) isolated from *A. blazei* showed anti-tumor properties (Mizuno *et al.*, 1989).

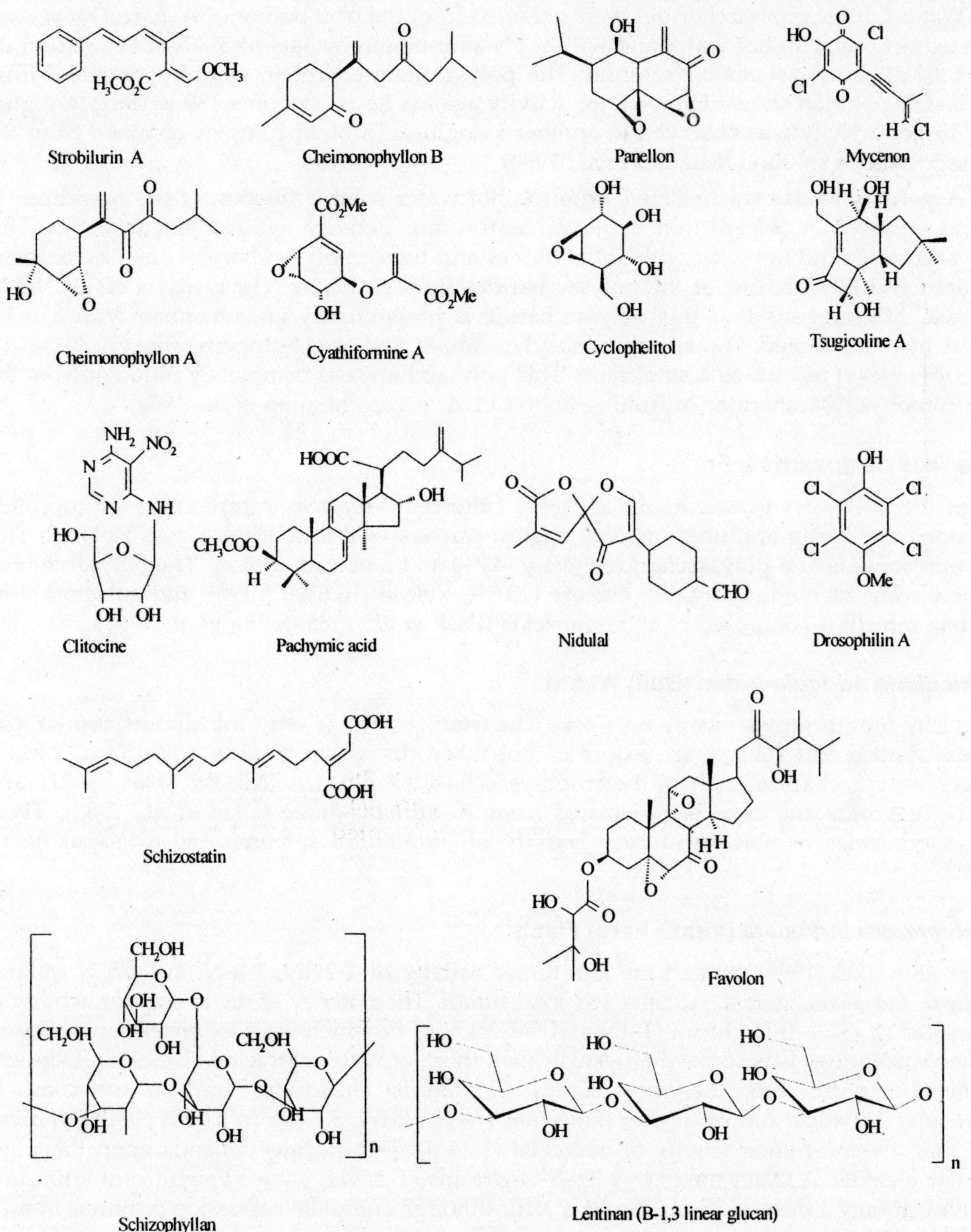

Fig. 1. Selected structures of compounds isolated from fungi belonging to Basidiomycetes

Water soluble polysaccharides were obtained from the fruit bodies of *A. blazei* by successive extractions with hot water and with i) 1% ammonium oxalate ii) 5% NaOH solution iii) 5% LiCl-dimethyl acetamide solution. The polysaccharide protein complex obtained from 5% NaOH solution showed anti-tumor activity against Rous- sarcoma 180 in mice. A higher anti-tumor activity was observed in another xyloglucan protein complex obtained from the same 5%NaOH solution (Mizuno *et al.,* 1990).

A polysaccharide was isolated from the hot water soluble fraction of the mycelium of liquid cultured *A. blazei* that exhibited anti-tumor activity against sarcoma 180. This polysaccharide did not react with antibodies of anti-tumor polysaccharides such as lentinan, gliforan and FIII-2-b, one of the polysaccharides from *A. blazei.* The analysis of 13C NMR and GC MS suggests that this polysaccharide is preliminarily glucomannan with a main chain of β-1,2 linked D-mannopyranosyl residues and *β*- D-glucopyranosyl –3-O-β-D-glucopyranosyl residue as a side chain. This polysaccharide is completely different from the anti-tumor polysaccharides of fruiting bodies of *A. blazei* (Mizuno *et al.,* 1999).

Agaricus campestris L.Fr.

From the hot water extract of the mycelial culture of *Agaricus campestris* a glycoprotein fraction , exhibiting antitumor activity against sarcoma 180 in ICR mice, was isolated. This fraction consists of a polysaccharide moiety (45%) and a protein moiety. The polysaccharide moiety contains mannose (42%), glucose (25.5%) xylose (16.6%), fucose and galactose. The protein moiety is composed of 17 aminoacids (Park *et al.,* 1986; Jeong *et al.,* 1990).

Auricularia auricula-judae (Bull) Wettst.

This jelly fungus grows mostly on wood. The fruiting body is semi-translucent, brown, cup or ear shaped and rubbery in texture except when dry when it turns quite hard. Various active polysaccharide such as heteropolysaccharides glucans (Misaki *et al.,* 1981) and acidic heteroglycans have been isolated from *A. auricula-judae* (Ukai *et al.,* 1983). These polysaccharides exhibit anti-tumor activity on implanted sarcoma 180 (Misakai *et al.,* 1981).

Dictyophora indusiata (Vent.: Pers) Fisch

Hara and Ukai (1995) studied the anti-tumor activity of T-2HN, T-4-N and T-5-N isolated from *D. indusiata* against Sarcoma 180 solid tumor. The potency of the antitumor activity of branched (1 → 3)- β-D-glucan (T-4N and T-5-N) both of which were extracted with alkaline aqueous solutions was somewhat weaker than those of water extracted (1 → 3)- β-D-glucan from other mushrooms (*Lentinus edodes, Ganoderma leucidum, Hericium erinaceus*). In particular TN-4 has a much higher molecular weight (MW: 5.5×10^5 in 0.25M NaOH) indicating that the anti-tumor activity of branched (1 → 3)- β-D-glucans depends upon their molecular weights. A O-acylated (1 → 3) -α-D-glucans (T-2-NH) showed significant antitumor activity at only a dose of 25 mg/kg/day X10, although complete regression of tumor in mice was not observed.

Flammulina velutipes (Curt. Fr.) P. Karst.

From the fruit body of *Flammulina velutipes* the β-glucan protein EA_6 was isolated. EA_6 exhibits strong antitumor activity against sarcoma 180, Lewis cancer of lung and B-16 melanoma (Ikekawa, 1995).

In addition, a new antitumor glycoprotein "Proflamin" was found in mycelia of *F. velutipes*. It is effective against allogeneic and syngeneic tumors by oral administration. Thus it is effective against solid sarcoma 180, B-16 melanoma, adenocarcinoma 775, and Gardner Lymphoma. It is also useful in combination therapy with other antitumor agents. Proflamin augments antibody formation and activates lymphocyte blastogenesis (Ikekawa *et al.*, 1985)

This edible mushroom is found in the Kashmir, Himalayas. Recently a polysaccharide, PA3 DE with an average mol. wt.5.4 x 10^6, isolated from this fungus has been shown to possess inhibitory activity against implanted Sarcoma 180 (Solid tumor) in mice (Gao *et al.*, 1989).

Ganoderma lucidum (Curt.:Fr.) P. Karst.

This polyporous fungus is an ingredient of several Chinese medicinal preprations. In China this drug is known as Lin Zhi Cao. *G. lucidum* is used in several medicinal preparations by the tribals of Madhya Pradesh in India. This fungus is rich in oxygenated lanosterol derived triterpenoids and more than 90 terpenoid compounds have been isolated from this fungus. Many of the triterpenoids isolated from this fungus are C3 epimers and C-3/C –15 positional isomers in pairs. A β-D-glucan isolated from this fungus shows immunostimulative antitumor activity (Mizuno *et. al.* 1988).

A glycoprotein fraction GL isolated from the hot watersoluble components of the basidiocarp of *G. lucidum* showed 81% inhibition of tumor growth in mice. This fraction had a mol. wt.of 47KD and analyzed for 82% polysaccharide, 8% protein and 0.9% hexosaminose. The polysaccharide moiety consisted of 63% glucose, 27% galactose, 7% mannose and 3% fucose. GL exerted the antitumor activity through immunopotentiation and not through direct cytotoxicity against the tumors. From the culture mycelium of *G. lucidum* Toth *et. al.* (1983a and b) isolated ganoderic acids Z,Y,X, W,V, and U that were cytotoxic to hepatoma cells *in vitro*.

Glucuronoglucan, xyloglucan, unannoglucan, xylomannoglucan, and other active heteroglucans and their potential complexes were extracted from *G. lucidum* for medicinal use and purified using salts, alkali, and DMSO (Mizuno *et al.*, 1984; Willard, 1990 and Wasser and Weis, 1997)

Grifola frondosa (Dick. Fr.) S.F. Gray,

Grifola frondosa commonly known as Maitake is an edible mushroom belonging to the order Aphyllophorales and the family polyporaceae and is a species of wood rotting fungus.

Active ingredient in Maitake extract is a proteoglucan, the protein with β-glucan consisting of β-1,6 main chain with β-1,3 linked glucose branches. Maitake extract exhibits antitumor effects by potentiating anti-tumor cellular functions by directly enhancing various mediators such as lymphokines and IL-1 (Nanba, 1993).

Grifolan(β-glucan), Fl-1a-β(acidic,βglucan), Flll-2c(hetro-β-glucan), xyloglucan, annoglucan, fucomannoglucan, compounds isolated from fruit bodies of *G. frondosa* have exhibited antitumor activity (Mizuno, 1997, 1998)

Heteroglucan protein, mannogalactofucan, heteroxylan , galactomannoglucan, compounds isolated from submerged cultures of *G. frondosa* have shown antitumor activity (Zhuang *et al.*, 1994 a, b)

Lentinus edodes (Berk.) Sing.

Lentinus edodes, commonly known as Shiitake has antitumor property. The antitumor properties are attributed to the polysaccharide –lentinan and emitanin. Lentinan is now used as an antitumor drug (Chihara *et al.,* 1970). Lentinan is non toxic to tumor cells, but inhibits tumor growth by stimulating the immune system (Chihara, 1978). That is, the β-D-glucan binds to lymphocyte surfaces or serum specific proteins, which activate macrophage, T-helper, NK and other effector cells. All of these increase the production of antibodies as well as interleukins (IL-1, IL-2) and interferon (IFN-γ) , which are released upon activation of effector cells (Dennert and Tucker, 1973; Hamuro *et al.,* 1976; 1978a, b and Mizuno, 1995a, b). Thus the carcinostatic effect of lentinan results due to the activation of the host's immune system.

From the extract of mycelia of *L. edodes,* α-mannan-peptide (KS-2) was isolated. KS2 was obtained by extraction of mycelium of *L. edodes* with hot water followed by precipitation with ethanol (Fujii *et. al.* 1978). KS 2 was shown to be effective on sarcoma 180 and Ehrlich's carcinoma either by i.p. or p.o. and to act via an interferon-inducing activity.

LEM, LAP from *L. edodes* mycelia and culture medium are glycoproteins containing glucose, galactose, xylose, arabinose, mannose and fructose (Iizuka *et al.*, 1990) LEM also contains various nucleic acids derivatives, vitamin B compounds, especially B1 (thiamine) B2 (riboflavin) and ergosterol (Breene, 1990). *Lentinus edodes* mycelium extract (LEM) is a preparation of the powdered mycelia extract of *L. edodes* harvested before the cap and stem grow. The precipitate obtained from a water solution of LEM by adding 4 volumes of ethanol was named LAP. LEM and LAP have both demonstrated strong antitumor activity, both orally and by injection in animals and in humans. Both of them were shown to activate the host's immune system (Mizuno, 1995 a, b). An immunoactive substance EP3 was also isolated by fractionation of LEM (Suzuki *et al.*, 1990).

Omphalotus olearius (D.C. : Fr.) Sing

Lampteromycetes japonicus (Kawamura) Sing

The above mushroom produces the cytotoxic tricyclic sesquiterpine illudin-S = (lampterol), which inhibits cancer cell growth by a unique mechanism (McMorris and Anchel 1963, 1965; Nakanishi, *et al.*, 1965; McMorris, *et al.,* 1992; Konno, 1995). It is believed that Illudin S undergoes activation by glutathione. The activated form is then capable of covalent binding to DNA. This halts DNA replication and leads to cell death. Illudin S itself is too toxic to be used as a clinical drug. A semisynthetic illudin analog 6-hydroxy-methylacyfulvene (HMAF) demonstrated a superior therapeutic profile and lower toxicity. Due to its outstanding therapeutic profile, HMAF is currently undergoing phase I human clinical trials and holds the promise of becoming a valuable new anticancer drug (Weis, 1996).

Pleurotus sajor –caju. Fr. Fr.

The above mushroom was first found by the Indian Scholar Yan Dai Ke at the foot hill of the Himalayas and then distributed to China and Australia. The protein containing polysaccharide Xyloglucan, Xylanproteins, extracted from the fruiting body of this fungus has shown antitumor activity against Sarcoma 180 tumor cells *in vivo* (Zhuang *et al.,* 1993).

Pleurotus ostereatus (Jack. :Fr.) Kumm.

Pleurotus ostereatus is an edible fungus and is cultivated in large quantities. A polysaccharide isolated from this fungus lowers the serum and liver lipids in Syrian hamsters with hyperlipoproteinemia (Bobek *et al.,* 1991).

An antitumor glucan was isolated from the neutral polysaccharide fraction from the hot water extract of this mushroom. The glucan exhibited marked antitumor activity at doses of 0.1mg /kg. It is a highly branched (1A3) β- glucan having an average structure represented by penta-saccharide segment consisting of one non –reducing terminal, one 3,6-di-O-subsituteted and 3-mono-O-substituted β-D-glucopyranosyl residues (Yoshioka *et al.,* 1985).

Schizophyllum commune Fr. Fr.

Schizophyllum commune contains schizophyllan (SPG) an active polysaccharide and shows antitumor activity against both the solid (Tabata *et al.,* 1981) and ascites forms of sarcoma 180 and also against the solid forms only of sarcoma 37, Ehrlich carcinoma, Yoshida sarcoma (Komatsu *et.al.* 1969). SPG also increases cellular immunity by restoring supressed killer-cell activity to normal levels in mice with tumors (Oka *et al.,* 1985).

SPG activates macrophages (*in vitro* and *in vivo*) which results in an augmentation of T-cell activities and increased sensitivity of cytotoxic LAK and NK to IL-2. The compound does not directly activate T cells (Shimizu *et al.,* 1992). SPG is distributed in the body in macrophagic tissues next to tumors and Kupffer cells (in bone marrow cells of mice SPG inhibited chromosomal damage caused by chemotherapeutic agents cyclophosphamide, adriamycin, and mitomycin C and by radiation). Best results against radiation damage were found when SPG was administered shortly after or at the same time as radiation, and SPG restored mitosis of bone marrow cells previously suppressed by anticancer drugs (Yang *et al.,* 1993).

Volvariella volvacea (Bull.: Fr.) Sing.

The lectin VVL, a homodimeric protein with molecular weight of 32 KDa was isolated and purified from the edible mushroom *Volvariella volvacea.* (She *et al.,* 1998) VVL is a potent mitogen as witnessed by its ability to stimulate uptake of ^{3}H thymidine by cultured murine lymphocytes at nanomolar levels. It markedly enhances transcriptional expression of interleukin–2 and interferon-γ indicating that VVL possesses a potent immunomodulatory activity. However when tumor cell lines were exposed to VVL at submicromolar levels, a remarkable inhibition of cell proliferation was observed. VVL arrests cell proliferation by blocking cell cycle progression in the G2/M phase (Liu *et al.,* 2001).

CONCLUSION

It is seen from this article that secondary metabolites of basidiomycetes are both chemically diverse and have a wide spectrum of biological activities. These activities have been explored in traditional medicine and in the new targets of molecular biology. Necessarily, this article has emphasized certain activities such as anti-tumor or immunomodulator of unusual polysaccharides (Borchers *et al.,* 1999; Ooi and Liu, 2000) Such polysaccharides are being isolated in increasing numbers and have similar structures but unique activities (Wasser and Weis, 1999).

ACKNOWLEDGEMENT

The author is thankful to Dr. Bansi Lal, President and Head-Research and Dr. T.Mukhopadhyay, Deputy Head, Research and Head of the Department, Natural Products for facilities and encouragement. Thanks are due to Dr. B.N. Ganguli, Emeritus Scientist, C. S. I. R., Govt. of India, U. D. C. T., Matunga, Mumbai for valuable suggestions and necessary help during preparation of this manuscript.

REFERENCES

Abraham,W. R. (2001). Bioactive sesquiterpenes produced by fungi : Useful for humans as well. *Current Medicinal Chemistry.* 8 : 583-606.

Anke, T. (1989). Basidiomycetes: a source for new bioactive secondary metabolites. In *Bioactive Metabolites from microorganisms.* (*Ed.* Bushell, M.E. and Grafe U.) Amesterdam: Elsevier, pp 51-66.

Anke, T., Oberwinkler, F., Steglich, W. and Schramm, G. (1977) The Strobilurins – new antifungal antibiotics from the basidiomycete *Strobilurus tenacellus* (Pers. ex. Fr.) Sing. *J. Antibiotics.* 30 : 806-810.

Anke, T., Werle, A., Bross, M. and Steglich, W. (1990) Antibiotics from basidiomycetes XXXIII, Oudemansin X, a new antifungal *E-β*-Methoxyacrylate from *Oudemansiella radicata* (Rehlan Ex Fr.) Sing. *J. Antibiotics* 43: 1010-1011.

Anke, T.,Werle, A., Zapf, S., Velten, R. and Steglich, W. (1995) Favolon, a new antifungal triterpenoid from a *Favolaschia* Species. *J. Antibiotics* 48: 725-726

Arnone, A., Capelli, S., Nasini,G., Meille, S. V., and Pava, O. V. D. (1996) Secondary mould metabolites II Structure elucidation of diatretol – A new Diketopiperzine metabolite from the fungus *Clitocybe diatreata.* Liebigs Ann. 1875-1877.

Arnone, A, Cardillo R., Nasini, G., and Pava, O.V.D. (1993) Cyathiformines A-D, new chorismate-derived metabolites from the fungus *Clitocybe cyathifomis. Tetrahedron* 49: 7251-7258.

Arnone, A., Brambilla, U., Nasini, G., and Pava, O.V.D. (1995) Isolation and structure elucidation of Tsugicolines A-D, novel protoilludane sesquiterpines from *Laurilia tsugicola. Tetrahedron.* 51: 13357-13364.

Atkinson, G. F. (1961) Mushrooms edible, poisonous etc 2nd.Hafner Publishing Co. New York.

Atri, N. S. and Saini, S.S. (2000) Collection and study of Agarics –An Introduction *Indian J. Mush.*18: 1-5.

Atri, N. S. Kaur, A. and Saini, S. S. (2000) Taxonomic studies on agarics from Punjab plains.*Indian J. Mush.*18: 6-14

Atsumi, S., Umezawa, K., Iinuma, H., Naganawa, H., Nakamura, H.,Iitaka, Y. and Takeuchi, T. (1990) Production, Isolation and Structure Determination of A Novel β- Glucosidase inhibitor, cyclophellitol, from *Phellinus* sp. *J.Antibiotics* 43: 49-53.

Bahal, N. (1994) *Handbook on Mushrooms* IIIrd Edition Oxford and IBH Publishing Co. Pvt Ltd, New Delhi, Bombay, Calcutta, pp. 157.

Berkeley, Rev.M.J. (1857). Introduction to Cryptogamic Botany. London: H.Bailliere

Bhide, V. P., Pande, A., Sathe, A. V., Rao, V. G. and Patwardhan, P. G. (1987) Fungi of Maharastra (Supp.1) M.A.C.S. Pub. pp 146.

Bobek, P., Ginter. E. Kuniak, L. Babla, J., Jurcovicova, M. and Cerven J. (1991) Effect of mushroom *Pleurotus ostereatus* and isolated fungal polysaccharides on serum and liver lipids in Syrian hamsters with hyperlipoproteinemia. Nutrition (Burhank, Calif), 7: 105-108.

Borchers, A. T., Stern, J.S., Hackman, R.M., Keen, C. L., and Gershwin, M. E. (1999) Mushrooms, tumors and immunity. Proc. Soc. Exp. Biol. Med. 221: 281-293.

Breene , W. (1990) Nutritional and medicinal value of special mushrooms. *J. Food. Prod.* 53: 883 - 894.

Butler, E. J. and Bisby, G.R. (1931) *The Fungi Of India* .Imp. Coun. Of Agric. Res. Sci. Mono. 1: XVIII pp.237, Calcutta.

Chihara, G. (1978) Antitumor and immunological properties of polyscharides from fungal origin . *Mush Sci.* 9: 797-814.

Chihara, G. Hamuro, J. Maeda, Y.Y., Arai, Y., and Fukoeka, F. (1970) Fractionation and purification of the polysaccharides with marked antitumor activity , especially lentinan from *Lentinus edodes* (Berk.) Sing (an edible mushroom). *Cancer. Res.* 30: 2776 -2781.

Chopara, R.N., Nayar, S.I. and Chopara, L.C. (1956). Glossary of Indian Medicinal Plants. ICAR Pub. New Delhi. Pp 9 and 27.

Cuellar, M. J. Giner, R. M., Recio, M. C., Just M. J., Manez, S. and Rios, J. L. (1996) Two Fungal lanostane derivative as Phospholipase A_2 Inhibitors. *J. Nat. Prod.* 59: 977 -979.

Daferner, M., Anke, T., Hellwig, V., Steglich, W. and Sterner, O. (1998) Strobilurin M, Tetrachloropyrocatechol and Tetrachloropyrocatechol methyl ether: new antibiotics from *Mycena* species. *J. Antibiotics* 51: 816-822.

Dennert, G. and Tucker, D. (1973) Antitumor polysaccharide Lentinan-a- T-cell adjuvant. J. Natl. *Cancer Res Inst.* 51: 1727- 1729.

Dufresne, C., Young, K., Pelaez, F., Val, A.G.D., Valentino, D., Graham, A., Platas, G., Bernard, A. and Zink, D. (1997) Illudinic acid, a novel Illudane sesquiterpine antibiotic. *J Nat. Prod.* 60: 188 -190.

Dymock, W. Warden, C. J.H., and Hooper, D. (1890) Pharmacographia Indica- A history of the Principal drugs of vegetable origin Part III Education Society press Byculla Bombay Pp 629-635.

Engler, M., Anke, T., Klostermeyer, D. and Steglich, W.(1995) Hydroxystrobilurin A, a new antifungal *E-β*-Methoxyacrylate from a *Pterula* species.*J.Antibiotics* 48: 884 -885.

Erkel,G., Becker, U., Anke, T. and Sterner, O. (1996) Nidulal, a novel inducer of differentiaton of Human Promyelocytic Leukemia Cells from *Nidula candida. J.Antibiotics* 49:1189-1195.

Fujii, T., Maeda, H., Suzuki, F., and Ishida, N. (1978) Isolation and characterization of a new anti-tumor polysaccharide, KS-2, extracted from culture mycelium of *Lentinus edodes*. *J. Antibiot.* 31: 1079-1090.

Gan, K. H., Fann, Y-F. , Hsu, S-H., Kou, K-W. and Lin, C-N. (1998) Mediation of the cytotoxicity of lanostanoids and steroids of *Ganoderma tsugae* through apoptosis and cell cycle. *J Nat. Prod.* 61:485-487.

Gao, P., Wu, Z., and Wang R. (1989) Isolation, purification and analysis of polysaccharides PA3DE from the fruit bodies of *Flammulina veluteps* (Curt. Fr.) Sing. *Shengwu Huaxue Yu Shen-gwa Wuli Xuebao* 21: 152-156. Chem. Abstract 112: 30286w.

Hamuro, J., Maeda, Y.Y., Fukuoka, F. and Chihara, G. (1976) Antitumor polysaccharides, Lentinan, and pachymaran as immunopotentiators. *Mushr Sci* 9: 477- 487.

Hamuro, J., Hadding, U. and Bitter –Suermann, D. (1978a) Solid phase activation of alternative pathway of complement by β-1-3 –glucans and its possible role for tumor regressing activity. *Immunology* 34: 695-705.

Hamuro, J., Wagner, H. and Rollinghoff, H. (1978b) β-(1 → 3) Glucan as a probe for T-cell specific immune adjuvants.II Enhanced *in vitro* generation of cytotoxic T Lymphocytes. Cell *Immunology*. 38:328-355.

Hara, C. and Ukai, S. (1995) Kinugasatake, *Dictyophora indusiata* Fisch: biological activities. Food. Rev. Intern. 11: 225-230.

Hautzel, R., Anke, H. and Sheldrick, W.S. (1990) Mycenon, A new metabolite from a *Mycena* species TA 87202 (Basidiomycetes) as an Inhibitor of Isocitrate Lyase. *J.Antibiotics*. 43: 1240-1244.

Hawksworth, D.L. (1974). Mycologist's Handbook , CMI Kew Surrey England.

Hawksworth, D.L. (1991) The fungal dimension of biodiversity : magnitude, significance and conservation. *Mycol. Res.* 95: 641-655.

Heim, J., Anke, T., Mocek, U., Steffan, B. and Steglich, W. (1988) Antibiotics from Basidiomycetes XXIX : Pilatin, A new antibiotically active marasmane derivative from cultures of *Flagelloscypha pilatii* Agerer. *J.Antibiotics* 41: 1752-1757.

Iizuka, C., Iizuka, H., and Ohashi, Y. (1990) Extracts of Basidiomycetes especially *Lentinus edodes* for treatment of human immunodeficiency virus (HIV). Shokin. Kogyo Co. Ltd.Eur. Pat. Appl. EP. 370673 (cl 35/84) 30 May 1990 JP Appl 88/287,316,14Nov 1988.

Ikekawa, T., Maruyama, H., Miyano, T., Okura, A., Sawasaki, Y., Naito, K. Kawamura, K. and Shiratori, K. (1985) Proflamin a new antitumor agent: preparation, physicochemcal properties and antitumor activity.Japan *J Cancer Res (Gann)* 76: 142-148.

Ikekawa, T. (1995) Enokitake *Flammulina velutipes* : Antitumor activity of extracts and polysaccharides. *Food Rev. Intern.* 11: 203-206.

Jeong, H. Lee J.W. and Lee K.H. (1990) Studies on anticomplimentary activity of Korean higher fungi. *Hanguk Kyunhakhoechi*, 18: 145-148. From CA 115:218446.

Kawagishi, H., Inagaki, R. Kamao, T, Mizuino, T., Shimura, K., Ito, H., Hagiwara, T. and Nakamura, T. (1989) Fractionation and anti tumor activity of the water –insoluble residue *of Agaricus blazei* fruiting body. *Carbohydr.Res.* 186: 267-273.

Khory, R. N. (1887) Bombay Materia Medica and their therapeutics. Pri. Raninas Union Press pp 553-555.

Komatsu, N., Okubo, S., Kimura, K., Saito, G. and Sakai, S. (1969) Host mediated antitumor action of schizophyllan , a glucan produced by *Schizophyllum commune Gann*. 60: 137-144.

Konno, K. (1995) Biologically active components of poisonous mushrooms. *Food Rev Intern* 11: 83-107.

Krauseman Van. M. J. (1953) Selected Indonesian Medicinal plants. Org. Sci.Res. *Indonesiae Bull.* 18:1- 90.

Kubo, I., Kim, M., Wood, W.F. and Naoki, H. (1986) Clitocine, A New Insecticidal Nucleoside from the mushroom *Clitocybe inversa* . *Tetrahedron Letters* 27: 4277-4280.

Kuhnt, D., Anke, T., Besl , H., Bross, M., Herrmann, R., Mocek, U., Steffan, B., and Steglich, W. (1990) Antibiotics from basidiomycetes XXXVII. New inhibitors of cholesterol biosynthesis from cultures of *Xerula melanotricha* Dorfelt. *J. Antibiotics* 43: 1413-1420.

Kuschel, A., Anke, T., Velten, R., Klostermeyer, D., Steglich, W. and Konig, B. (1994) The Mniopetals, New Inhibitors of reverse transcriptases from a *Mniopetalum* species (Basidiomycetes). *J.Antibiotics* 47: 733-739.

Lakhanpal, T. N. (1995) Mushroom flora of North West Himalayas. *In Advances In Horticulture Vol.13. Mushrooms* (*Ed.* Chandra K. L. and Sharma S. R.) MPH New Delhi India pp. 351 -373.

Lauer, U., Anke, T., Sheldrick, W.S.,Scherer, A. and Steglich, W. (1989) Antibiotics from basidiomycetes XXXI Aleurodiscal : An Antifungal Sesterterpenoid from *Aleurodiscus mirabilis.* (Berk. & Curt) Hohn. *J. Antibiotics* 42: 875-882.

Lee, I., Jeong, C-Y., Cho, S-M., Yun, B-S.,Kim, Y-S., Yu, S-H., Koshino, H. and Yoo, I-D. (1996a) Illudins C2 and C3, New Illudin C derivatives from *Coprinus atramentarius* ASI20013. *J. Antibiotics* 49: 821- 822.

Lee, I-K., Yun, B-S., Cho, S-M., Kim, W-G., Kim, J-P., Ryoo, I-J., Koshino, H. and Yoo, I-D. (1996b) Betulinans A and B, Two Benzoquinone compounds from *Lenzites betulina*. *J. Nat. Prod.* 59: 1090-1092.

Liu, W. K., Ho, J. C. K. and Ng, T. B. (2001) Suppression of cell cycle progression by fungal lectin :activation of cyclin-dependent kinase inhibitors. *Biochemical Pharmacology* 61: 33-37.

Lorenzen, K. and Anke. T. (1998) Basidiomyctes as a source for new bioactive natural products. *Current Organic Chemistry* 2:329-364.

Mainsem, B.E. (1944) Instructions to naturalists in the armed forces for botanical field work. The collection of Fungi and Lichen Publ.for Co.D, 3651 S.U. Dept of Botany, Univ. Michigan Ann. Arbor,USA.

Manjula, B. (1983). A revised list of agrigicoid and boletoid basidiomycetes from India and Nepal. *Proc. Indian. Acad. Sci.* (Plant Sci.) 92: 81-213.

McMorris, T. C. and Anchel, M. (1963). The structure of the basidiomycete metabolites illudin S and illudin M. *J. Am Chem Soc*, 85: 831.

McMorris, T. C. and Anchel, M. (1965) Fungal metabolites. The structure of the novel sesquiterpinoids illudin S and illudin M . *J. Am Chem Soc*, 87: 1954-1960.

McMorris, T. C. Michael, J. K., Wang, W., Estes, L., Montoya, M. A. and Taetle, R. (1992) Structure activity relationship of Illudin; analogs with improved therapeutic index. *J Org. Chem.* 57: 6876-6883.

Misaki, A., Kakuta, M., Sasaki, T., Tanaka, M. and Miyaji, H. (1981) Studies on interrelation of structure and antitumor effect of polysaccharides : Antitumor action of periodate –modified , branched (1→ 3)-β-D-glucan of *Auricularia auricula-judae* and other polysaccharides containing (1→ 3)- Glycosidic Kikurages). *Carbohyd. Res.* 92: 115-129

Mizuno, M., Minato, K-I, Ito H., Kawade M., Terai H., and Tsuchida H. (1999) Anti-tumor polysaccharide from the mycelium of liquid cultured *Agaricus blazei* Mill. Biochem. Mol. Biol. Int. 47: 707-714.

Mizuno, T. (1995a) Bioactive biomolecules of Mushroom: food function and medicinal effect of mushroom fungi. *Food Rev. Intern.* 11: 7-21.

Mizuno, T. (1995b) Yamabushitake, *Hericium erinaceum*: Bioactive substances and medicinal utilization. *Food Rev Intern* 11: 173-178.

Mizuno, T. (1997) "Anti-tumor Mushrooms" *Ganoderma lucidum, Grifola frondosa, Lentinus edodes and Agaricus blazei.* Gendai-shorin, Toyko 188p.

Mizuno, T. (1998.) : "Immunological special diets" *Agaricus blazei, Ganoderma lucidum, Cordyceps sinensis, Grifola frondosa, and Lentinus edodes.* Gendai-shorin, Toyko 188p.

Mizuno, T., Inagaki, R., Kanoa, T., Hagiwara, T., Nakamura , T., Ito, H., Shimura, K., Sumiya, T. and Asakura, A. (1990) Antitumor activity and some properties of water insoluble hetero-glycans from "Himematsutake"the fruiting bodies of *Agaricus blazei* Murill. Agric Biol Chem 54: 2897-2905.

Mizuno, T., Ito, H., Shimura, K., Sumitani, T., Kawagishi, H., Hagiwara, T. and Nakamura, T. (1990) Jpn. Kokai, Tokkyo, Koho, JP02,78, 630.

Mizuno, T., Kato, L., Totsuka, A., Shinkai, K. and Shimizu, M. (1984) Fractionation , stuctural features and antitumor activity of water soluble polysaccharide from "Reishi": The Fruit body of *Ganoderma lucidum* .Nippon Nogei Kagaku Kaishi. 58: 871-880.

Mizuno, T., Kawagishi H., Ito, H., and Shimura, K. (1988) Antitumor polysaccharides XII Immunostimulative antitumor effects of β-D-glucan and chitin substances isolated from some medicinal mushrooms. Shizuoka Daigaku Nogakubu Kenkyu Hokoku 29-35.CA 111 : 331186 d.

Mizuno, T., Kawagishi, H., Hagiwara, T and Nakamura, T. (1989) Ergosterol derivative and production thereof. Jpn. Kokai, Tokkyo, Koho, JP01, 246,299.

Morita, Y., Hayashi, Y., Sumi, Y., Kodaira, A., and Sibata, H. (1995) Haploporic acid A , a novel dimeric drimane sesquiterpenoid from the basidiomycete *Haploporus odorus. Biosci. Biotech. Biochem.* 59: 2008-2009.

Nanba, H., (1993) Maitake mushroom. The kind of mushrooms. Mushroom News 41: 21-25.

Nadkarni, K. M. (1954) India Materia Medica Vol 1 Edit. 3. Popular Books Depot Bombay pp 51-52 and 202.

Nakanishi, K., Ohashi, M., Toda, M., and Yamada, Y. (1965) Illudin S (lampterol). *Tetrahedron* 21: 1231-1246.

Natrajan, K. and Raman N. (1983) *South Indian Agaricales* : Today and Tomorrow ; Printers and Publishers New Delhi. P204.

Oka, T. (1985) Antitumor effects and augmentation of cellular immunity by schizophyllan and bastatin. Okayama Igakkai Zasshi 97: 527-541. From CA104:102107y.

Ooi, V.E. and Liu, F. (2000) Immunomodulation and anti-cancer activity of polysaccharide – protein complexes. Curr. Med. Chem 7: 715-729.

Park, H.J., Kim, H.W. ,Woo M. S., Shim M. J., Park W.H., Choi E. C., and Kim, B.K. (1986) Studies on constituents of the higher fungi of Korea (XLVII). Antitumor constituents of the culture mycelia of *Agaricus campastris.* Chem. Abstr. 104, 31798m.

Pegler, D. N. (1977) A preliminary agaric flora of East Africa . HMSO London. 615 pp

Pegler, D. N. (1983) The genus *Lentinus* A world monograph. *Kew Bull Addit Ser.*10:1-281.

Pradeep, C.K., Vrinda, K.B., Mathew, S. and Abraham, T. K. (1998) The genus *Volvariella* in Kerala state, India. *Mushroom Res.* 7: 53-62.

Purkayastha, R.P. and Chandra, A. (1985) *Manual of Indian Edible Mushrooms*. Jagmander Book Agency Deshbandhu Gupta Road New Delhi. p 267.

Rai, B.K., Ayachi, S.S., and Rai A. (1993) A note note on ethno-myco-medicines from central India. *The Mycologist* 7: 192-193.

Rolf, R. T. and Rolf, F. W. (1925) The romance of the Fungus world I B Lippimcott Co., Philadelphia pp 308.

Saito, T., Akoi, F., Hirai, H., Inagaki, T., Matsunaga, Y., Sakakibara, T., Sakemi, S., Suzuki, Y., Watanabe, S., Suga, O., Sujaku, T., Smogowicz, A. A., Truesdell, S.J., Wong, J.W., Nagahisa, A., Kojima, Y., and Kohjima, N. (1998) Erinacine E as a kappa opioid receptor agonist and its new analogs from a basidiomycete, *Hericium ramosum*. *J. Antibiotics* 51: 983-990.

Sathe, A.V. (1979) Agaricology in India–A review of work on Indian Agaricales. *Biovigyanam*. 5: 125-130.

Sathe, A.V. and Deshpande, S. (1979) Agaricales of Maharastra In. *Advances in Mycology and Plant pathology* (*Ed.* Chattopadhyay S.B. and Samajpati N.) pp. 82-88.

Sharma, N. (1998) Myco-myth , Mycetismus and Medicines. *Ethnobotany* 10: 16-21.

She, Q.B., Ng, T.B., and Liu, W.K. (1998) A novel lectin with potent immunomodulatory activity isolated from both fruiting bodies and cultured mycelia of the edible mushroom *Volvariella volvacea*. *Biochem Biophys Res Commun* 247: 106-111.

Shimizu, Y., Hasumi, K., and Masubuchi, K. (1992) Augmenting effect of sizofiran on the immunofunction of regional lymph nodes in cervical cancer. *Cancer*. 69:1188 -1194.

Singer, R. (1986) The Agaricales in Modern Taxonomy. 4th ed., J Cramer Germany. pp. 912.

Smith, A.H. (1949) Mushroom and their natural habitats. Hafner Press New York.

Stadler, M., Anke, H. and Sterner, O. (1994) New nematicidal and antimicrobial compounds from the basidiomycete *Cheimonophyllum candidissimum* (Berk and Curt) Sing. *J.Antibiotics*. 47:1284-1289.

Sundin, A., Anke, H., Bergquist, K-E., Mayer, A., Sheldrick, W. S., Stadler, M. and Sterner, O. (1993) The structure determination of Panellon and Panellol, two 14-Noreudesmanes Isolated from *Resupinatus leightonii*. *Tetrahedron* 49:7519-7524.

Suzuki, M. Higuchi, S., Taki, Y., Taki, S., Miwa, K., and Hamuro, J. (1990) Induction of endogenous lymphokine-activated killer activity by combined administration of Lentinan and interleukin 2 . *Int J Immunopharmacol*. 12: 613-623.

Tabata, K., Ito, W., Kojima, T., Kawabata, S. and Misaki, A. (1981) Ultrasonic degradation of schizophyllan, an antitumor polysaccharide produced by *Schizophyllum commune* Fries. *Carbohyd. Res*. 89: 121-135.

Tanimoto,T., Onodera, K., Hosoya, T., Takamatsu, Y., Kinoshita, T., Tago, K., Kogen, H.,Fujioka, T., Hamano, K. and Tsujita, Y. (1996) Schizostatin, a Novel Squalene Synthase Inhibitor Produced by the Mushroom, *Schizophyllum commune*. *J.Antibiotics* 49: 617-623.

Toth, J.O., Luu, B., Beck, J and Ourission G. (1983a) Chemistry and biochemistry of oriental drugs .Part IX . Cytotoxic Triterpines from *Ganoderma leucidum* (Polyporaceae): structures of ganoderic acids U-Z . *J. Chem. Res*.Synpo .: 299. From CA 100: 117512t.

Toth, J.O., Luu, B. and Ourission, G., (1983b) Les acides ganoderiques T a Z: Triterpenes cytotoxiques de *Ganoderma leucidum* (Polyporaceae). *Tetrahedron Lett*. 24:1081-1084.

Ukai, S. Kiho, T., Hara, C. Morita M., Gao, A. and Naomi, H.Y. (1983) Polysaccharides in FungiXIII . Antitumor activity of various polysaccharides isolated from *Dictyophora indusiata, Ganoderma japonicum ,Cordyceps cicadae, Auricularia auricula- judae* and *Auricularia* Species Chem. Pharm. Bull. (Tokyo) 31: 741-744.

Vaidya, J.C., and Rabba, A. S. (1993) Fungi in Folk medicine. *The Mycologist* 7: 131-133.

Verma, R.N. Singh, G.B. and Bilgramy, K. S. (1987) Fleshy Fungal Flora of NEH India.-I. Manipur and Meghalaya . In Indian Mushroom Science:II (*Ed.* Kaul T.N. and Kapoor B.M.) RRL CSIR Jammu Tawi 414-421.

Vrinda, K.B., Pradeep, C.K., Mathew, S. and Abraham, T. K. (1999) Agaricales from Western Ghats VII. *Mushroom Res.* 8:9-12.

Wasser, S. P. and Weis, A. L. (1997) *Medicinal Mushroom. Reishi Mushroom (Ganoderma lucidum* (Curitis:Fr.)P. Karst.) Nevo E, ed Peledfus, Haifa pp 96.

Wasser, S. P. and Weis, A. L. (1999) Therapeutic effects of sustances occuring in higher basidiomycetes mushrooms : A modern perspective. *Crit. Review in Immunology.* 19: 65-96.

Wasson, G. R. (1969) Soma -Divine mushroom of immortality XIII, Heu Court Brace and world Inc. New York pp 318.

Weber, W., Anke, T., Steffan, B. and Steglich, W. (1990) Antibiotics from Basidiomycetes XXXII Strobilurin E : A New Cytostatic and Antifungal (E)-β-Methoxyacrylate Antibiotic from *Crepidotus fulvotomentosus* Peck. *J.Antibiotics* 43: 207-212.

Weis, A. (1996) Semisynthetic drugs of fungal origin. Challenges of pre-clinical anticancer drug development. 5th Internat. Conf. On Chemical Synthesis of antibiotics and Related Microbial Products Abstracts. Debrecen, Hungarian Acad. Sci. P5.

Willard, T. (1990) Reishi Mushroom. "*Herb of spiritual potency and medical wonder.* Issaqueh Sylvan Press Vancouver BC".

Wood, K.A., Kau, D-A., Wrigley, S.K.,Beneyto, R., Renno, D. V., Ainsworth, A.M., Penn, J., Hill, D., Killacky, J. and Depledge, P. (1996) Novel β-Methoxyacrylates of the 9- Methoxystrobilurin and Oudemansin Classes Produced by the Basiodiomycete *Favolaschia pustulosa*. *J.Nat. Prod.* 59:646-649.

Yang, Z. B. Tsuchiya, Y., Arika, T. and Hosokawa, M. (1993) Inhibitory effects of sizofiran on anticancer agents or X ray induced sister chromatid exchanges and mitotic block in murine bone marrow cells. Japan. *J. Cancer Res.* 84: 538-543.

Yoshioka,Y., Tabeta, R., Saito, H., Uehera N., and Fukuoka, F. (1985) Antitumor polysaccharide from *P. ostereatus* (Fr.) Quel: isolation and structure of a beta glucan. *Carbohydr. Res.* 140: 93-100.

Zhuang , C., Mizuno, T., Shimada, A., Ito, H., Suzuki, C., Mayuzumi, Y., Okamoto, H., Ma, Y. and Li, J.(1993) Antitumor Protein-containing Polysaccharides from a Chinese mushroom Fengweigu or Houbitake, *Pleurotus sajor-caju* (Fr.) Sing *Biosci. Biotechnol. Biochem.* 57: 901-906.

Zhuang C., Mizuno, T. Ito H. Shimura K. Sumiya T. and Kawade M. (1994 a) Fractionation and anti-tumor activity of polysaccharides from *Grifola frondosa* mycelium. *Biosci Biotechnol Biochem* 58: 185-188.

Zhuang, C. Mizuno, T. Ito H. and Shimura K. (1994 b) Chemical modifications and anti-tumor activity of polysaccharides from mycelium of liquid–cultured *Grifola frondosa. Nippon Shokuhin Kogyo Gakkaishi.* 41: 733 -740.

Microbiology and Biotechnology for Sustainable Development (*Ed.* P.C. Jain),
CBS Publishers & Distributors, New Delhi (2004), pp. 141–150.

A-12

Mechanisms of Cell-Mediated Immunity in Fungal Infection

Sudhir K. Jain, P. C. Jain* and S. C. Agrawal*
Department of Applied Microbiology, College of Life Sciences
Cancer Hospital and Research Institute, Gwalior-474009, India

Abstract

Among different defense mechanisms against superficial and systemic fungal infections cell-mediated immune (CMI) response plays a pivotal role in their control and eradication. CMI triggers a cascade of events involving lymphocytes, macrophages, cytokines, peptides etc. The present review discusses cell-mediated antifungal mechanisms of host against candidiasis and cryptococcosis caused by Candida albicans and Cryptococcus neoformans, respectively. Role of phagocytes in controlling zoo-pathogenic Histoplasma capsulatum has also been discussed.

Key words: Cell-mediated immunity , *Candida albicans, Cryptococcus neoformans, Histoplasma capsulatum.*

INTRODUCTION

Effective host resistance in superficial and deep-seated fungal diseases is multifaceted. In some instances, one or more defenses may be more dominant than others. However, generally a combination of defensive measures, with an active interplay between innate and adaptive immune responses, is required for complete protection. Many species of pathogenic fungi which cause systemic infection are controlled or eradicated from the body by the hosts ability to develop a strong cell - mediated immunity (CMI). Clinical and immunological evidence also supports a role for CMI in mucocutaneous forms of some fungal infections (e.g. candidiasis), especially in patients affected by the acquired immunodeficiency syndrome (AIDS) (Klein *et al.*, 1984; Imam *et al.*, 1990; Cassone *et al.*, 1993). Overall, induction and/or expression of CMI are frequently observed to be at least transiently suppressed

* Department of Applied Microbiology and Biotechnology, Dr. Harisingh Gour University, Sagar 470003, India.

during the course of many fungal infections (Diamond and Bannett, 1973; Gray bill and Alford, 1974; Cox, 1979).

A CMI response is a complex cascade of biological events involving a number of host cells and soluble products, regulating their interaction and activation processes, such as the cytokines. When appropriately orchestrated, the CMI components enhance the elimination of fungi from tissue (Lim and Murphy, 1980; Lim *et al.*, 1980). However, when the CMI response is down regulated, there is a reduction in the clearance of fungi from tissues. The mechanisms by which activated macrophages induced by CMI kill extra cellular and intracellular pathogenic fungi are rather complicated and still controversial, especially concerning the intracellular growth inhibition and killing substances.

In this review, we provide recent evidence for the mechanisms of CMI induction and regulation as well as the nature of the growth inhibitory or killing substances against some pathogenic fungi.

T-helper (Th) cell subsets in experimental candidiasis

A major advance in immunology has been the demonstration that $CD4^+$ Th cells are composed of subsets based upon cytokines produced after stimulation, and that these distinct T-cell subsets often influence the outcome of infections (Mosmann *et al.*, 1986; Scott and kaufmann, 1991). $CD4^+$ Th1 cells produce IL-2 and IFN-γ, primary mediate CMI and are often associated with bacterial, protozoan and viral infections (Romani *et al.*, 1992; Lane *et al.*, 1993). In contrast, Th2 cells produce IL-4, IL-5 and IL-10, mediate humoral and allergic responses and are often associated with helminthes infections (Mosmann *et al.*, 1986; Scott and Kaufmann, 1991)

Bistoni and his colleagues (Romani *et al.*, 1991;Romani *et al.*, 1992; Romani *et al.*, 1992; Bistoni *et al.*, 1993) have recently reported that selective activation of either one of the $CD4^+$ Th subsets also occurs in infections with the fungus *Candida albicans* whose dissemination from the gastrointestinal tract often results in a fatal progressive disease in humans, especially in bone-marrow transplanted, neutropenic subjects (Bodey and Fainstein, 1985). Studies in mice have shown that healing and non-healing patterns of disease are detected in systemic infections with *C. albicans*. A strong correlation has been shown between disease outcome and nature of the predominant Th cell response, with healer mice developing a Th1 response and non-healer mice a predominant Th2 response. Both host genetic and yeast strain factors were found to contribute to the generation of the anti-candidal Th phenotypes. Thus, in genetically resistant mice, a protective Th1 response to virulent *C. albicans* is observed after mouse vaccination with a live vaccine strain of the yeast, PCA-2, but the same attenuated vaccine results in no protective Th2 responses in genetically susceptible DBA/2 mice (Romani *et al.*, 1993). In addition, susceptible DBA/2 mice are rendered resistant to systemic challenge when colonized intragastrically by the fungus (Bistoni *et al.*, 1993). Therefore, the immunological events occurring in the microenvironment, early in the course of the infection, could determine the subsequent outcome of infection by conditioning the dissimilar expansion of Th1 and Th2 cells.

Because Th1 and Th2 cells are defined by their secretion of distinct patterns of cytokines that mediate most of their action *in vivo*, cytokines are among the most likely candidates for the development of protective or exacerbative CD4+ cells in infection. In order to establish the pathogenetic role of cytokines in murine candidiasis, cytokines, anti-cytokine monoclonal antibodies (Mab) or cytokine antagonists were administered in vivo in healing and non-healing models of infection, obtained by injecting low-virulence PCA-2 *Candida* cells into resistant CD2F1 mice (healing infection) or into susceptible DBA/2 mice (non-healing infection). An additional model of non-healing infection was obtained by challenging CD2F1 mice with a highly virulent strain (CA-6) of *C. albicans*. Susceptibility and resistance to primary and secondary infections were evaluated by monitoring the mice for mortality, development of specific delayed-type hypersensitivity reaction (DTH) and patterns of cytokine release. The results can be summarized as follows: (i) treatment of CA-6 infected CD2F1 mice with IL-4 neutralizing M abs changed the non-healer phenotype to a healer one, in that mice survived both the infection and re-infection, developed strong DTH reactions and stopped producing IL-4 and IL-10 (Romani *et al.*, 1992); (ii) the same results were achieved by antagonizing IL-4 with soluble IL-4 receptor (Puccetti *et al.*, 1994); (iii) in DBA/2 mice injected with low-virulence *Candida* cells, a healing phenotype was obtained by neutralization of early IL-10 production, while recombinant IL-10, given exogenously, exacerbated the infection. Interestingly, neutralization of IL-10, up - regulates nitric oxide production, thus suggesting a possible link between innate resistance and adaptive immunity (iv) neutralization of endogenous IFN-γ production in CD2F1 mice injected with PCA-2 cells, while not affecting the outcome of the primary infection, rendered the mice susceptible to a secondary challenge with virulent yeast cells, accompanied by the appearance of IL-4 specific transcripts in CD4+ splenocytes (Romani *et al.*, 1992). The same results were obtained by neutralizing endogenous IL-12 (Romani *et al.*, 1994). These data indicate that cytokines can contribute to the appearance of protective and non-protective Th responses in *C. albicans* infection. In addition, the finding that Th1 and Th2 cytokines can adversely affect the anti-candidal activity of macrophages (Cenci *et al.*, 1993), points to an important role for cytokines in the control of the effecter function. Interestingly, recent data by Cassone and colleagues (1993) on CMI responses in lymphomonocyte cultures from normal human subjects have revealed a marked expression of the genes for IL-2 and IFN-y but not , or minimally so, of the genes for IL-4, IL-5 and IL-10, when the cultures were exposed to an immunodominant antigen (MP-65) target of anti-*Candida* CMI (Torosantucci *et al.*,1993; Ausiello *et al.*, 1993). Altogether these results suggest that the ability to control the emerging Th cell phenotype is critical in the induction of an appropriate immune response in fungal infections. These mechanisms are probably also operative in the natural immunosurveillance that the immune system of healthy subjects exerts against *C. albicans*.

Expression phase events of the anti-cryptococcal CMI response

Protection against *Cryptococcus neoformans* is facilitated mainly by a CMI response directed toward a mannoprotein component of the organism (Graybill *et al.*, 1974; Lim and Murphy, 1980; Lim *et al.*, 1980 Murphy *et al.*, 1983). Patients with systemic cryptococcosis typically have measurable levels of cryptococcal antigen in their serum and frequently in their spinal fluid (Gorden and Vedder, 1966). Cryptococcal antigen at levels equivalent to those found in body fluids during systemic cryptococcosis can induce a cascade of T-suppressor (Ts) cells that specifically down-regulate the CMI response as measured by DTH (Murphy and Moorhead, 1982; Murphy, 1985; Murphy and Moosley, 1985;Murphy *et al.*, 1988). The first Ts cell in the cascade, referred to as the first order Ts (Ts1) cell, can be induced by an intravenous injection of cryptococcal culture filtrate (CneF) antigen simulating the antigenaemia found in patients suffering from systemic cryptococcosis (Murphy and Moorhead, 1982). The Ts1 cells can also be induced by transferring serum from *C. neoformans* infected mice to naive mice (Murphy and Cox, 1988). The Ts1 cells suppress the induction of the DTH (Th1) cells when Ts1 cells are transferred at the time of immunization (Murphy and Moorhead, 1982;Murphy, 1985;Murphy and Moosley, 1985;Murphy *et al.*, 1988). In addition, Ts1 cells induce a second population of Ts, referred to as second-order Ts cells within 7 days of transfer of Ts1 cells into naïve mice (Murphy and Moosley, 1985;Murphy *et al.*, 1988). The Ts2 cells work in conjunction with the third order Ts (Ts3) cells that are induced by immunization to suppress the expression phase of the anti-cryptococcal DTH response (Khakpour and Murphy, 1987).

The Ts cells diminish the tissue reaction during the expression phase of the anti-cryptococcal CMI response and reduce the clearance of cryptococci from tissues, Murphy and her colleagues (Murphy and Moorhead, 1982; Murphy, 1989) got interested in determining how the Ts cells affect the cellular influxes and cytokines at the site of an anti-cryptococcal CMI reaction such as a DTH reaction. One might assume that the events occurring at the site of a DTH reaction are similar to the events at the site of the organism in an affected animal with anti-cryptococcal CMI reactivity. By understanding the cells and lymphokines at the DTH reaction site and the effects of modulators cells on those events, then it may be possible to extrapolate which parameters effect the clearance of cryptococci from tissues.

By implanting gelatin sponges into the backs of immune mice, a response was elicited in the sponges that are equivalent to a DTH reaction in the footpad of mice (Buchanan and Murphy, 1993). With the gelatin sponge model, it has been shown that mice immunized with CneF in complete Freund's adjuvant (CFA) have significantly higher numbers of leukocytes infiltrating into implanted gelatin sponges injected with CneF, than do saline-injected sponges in the same animal or CneF-injected sponges in saline CFA injected mice. The amounts of IFN-γ and, to a lesser extent, IL-5 produced in the DTH-reactive sponges of cryptococcal-sensitized mice was higher than in control sponges (Buchanan and Murphy, 1993). The sponge model was also used to study the effects of Ts1 and Ts2 cells on the cellular influx and cytokine production at the site of a DTH reaction. When Ts1 cells were given to mice at the time of immunization with CneF-CFA, the number of leukocytes infiltrating the CneF-injected sponges was not significantly different from the number of leukocytes infiltrating the CneF-injected sponges implanted in CneF-CFA immunized mice that were not given a cell transfer or in CneF-CFA immunized mice given normal lymph node cells (mock Ts1 cells). It has been noted by them that Ts1 cells did not diminish the numbers of leukocytes infiltrating into the DTH-reactive sponges, but depress the production of Th1 lymphokines (IL-2 and IFN-γ) at the DTH reaction site. In contrast, IL-5 levels were significantly increased in the DTH-reactive sponges in mice given Ts1 cells and immunized. The Th2 lymphokine, IL-4, was not detected in any of the sponges.

Injecting immunized mice with Ts2 cells intravenously at the time of challenging the sponges with CneF or saline did not alter the total numbers of leukocytes migrating into the sponges when compared to the numbers of leukocytes in sponges of immunized mice injected with mock Ts2 cells. However, Ts2 cells did significantly diminish the numbers of neutrophils, but not lymphocytes or monocytes, infiltrating into the DTH-reactive sponges. IFN-γ, IL-2 and IL-5 levels in the DTH-reactive sponges were not affected by the injection of Ts2 cells.

Their data indicate that the regulatory effects of the two different populations of anti-cryptococcal Ts cells are different. The Ts1 cells influence lymphokine production by decreasing IFN-γ and IL-2 production and by boosting production of IL-5. In contrast, the Ts2 cells do not significantly alter production of the lymphokines in the DTH-reactive sponges but cause a diminution of the influx of neutrophils. Considered together with earlier clearance studies by Murphy and her colleagues (1989), these results suggest that IFN-γ and IL-2 may be important components in protection against *C. neoformans* and down-regulation of these two lymphocytes may reduce the ability of the host to eliminate the cryptococci. Neutrophils have the potential to clear cryptococcal cells from tissues, but when the movement of neutrophils into infected tissues diminish, then clearance of the organism would be expected to be impaired. The presence of both Ts1 and Ts2 cells during infection would be expected to hamper removal of the organism, but by differing mechanisms.

Anti-*Candida* peptides produced by murine macrophages activated by IFN-□

The final effecter of CMI in protecting against infections is macrophage (MP) activated by IFN-γ released from Th1 cells (Mosmann *et al.*, 1986;Scott and Kaufmann, 1991). It has become clear from the literature that the antifungal effects of activated MP depend on the fungal target and on the kind of MP. For example, activated murine MP is fungicidal for *C. albicans* (Mosmann **et al.**, 1986; Watanabe *et al.*, 1991), but only fungi static for *Histoplasma capsulatum* (Wu-Hsieh *et al.*, 1994). In contrast, activated human MP is fungicidal for *H. capsulatum* (Brummer *et al.*, 1991). Therefore, it is evident from the above that it is difficult to generalize about antifungal mechanisms of all MP against all fungal targets.

C. albicans is known to be killed by IFN-γ activated MP (Watanabe *et al.*, 1991; Redmond *et al.*, 1993). However, the mechanisms of this intracellular killing are controversial. Many investigators have reported the role of reactive oxygen intermediates (ROI) in the candidacidal activity (Sasada **et al.**, 1987; Redmond *et al.*, 1993). On the other hand, Watanabe *et al.*, (1991) have reported that the candidacidal activity of IFN-γ activated murine peritoneal macrophages (PMP) correlated well with enhanced acidification of their phagolysosomes. They suggested that the candidacidal activity of activated MP was independent from ROI generation and was mediated by undefined proteinaceous substance(s) generated only in the strong acidic milieu of phagolysosomes by activation. Since the candidacidal substance(s) have been extracted from murine normal PMP, Kagaya *et al.*, (1994) attempted to isolate the candidacidal substance(s) from the MP cell line J774.1. The resident PMP from BALB/c mice and MP cell line, J774.1, were cultured by them with or without recombinant murine IFN-γ (100 U ml^{-1}) for 24 h, and examined for their ability to kill *C. albicans* M1012 (serotype A). PMP monolayers were infected with *C. albicans* in the presence of 10% normal fresh serum and after a 3 h incubation, the number of viable cells was determined by culture. Their results indicated that

J774.1 cells were unable to kill *C. albicans* even after stimulation with IFN-γ, although IFN-γ stimulated PMP killed 40% of the *C. albicans* inoculums. Furthermore, flow cytometry analysis of J774.1 cells containing FITC-labeled *C. albicans* cells indicated that the J774.1 cells incubated with IFN-γ for 24 h did not contain strongly acidic (pH<4) phagolysosomes (Watanabe *et al.*, 1993). Kagaya *et al.*, (1994) granule extracts obtained from normal and activated PMP and J774.1 cells by the method of Patterson-Delafield *et al.* (1980) with some modification using 0.5 M acetic acid (pH 2.6). Candidacidal activity of granule extracts dissolved in 0.01 M phosphate buffer, pH 7.0, or distilled water was assayed by colony counting after incubating with *C. albicans* for 1 h at 37°C. When granule extracts of J774.1 cells were compared with that from normal or IFN-γ activated PMP, all three granules extracts were found to be similar with respect to their candidacidal activities when they were treated with heat, trypsin, polyaspartic acid and EDTA. Their studies indicated that the granule extract of J774.1 cells had the same characteristics as those of normal PMP and activated PMP. The antimicrobial activity of the granule extract was stronger against *Staphylococcus aureus, Escherichia coli, Salmonella typhimurium* and *C. neoformans* than against *C. albicans*. However, the extract did not kill *Mycobacterium tuberculosis*. Gel filtration by Bio Gel P-2 at pH 7.0 indicated that the relative molecular mass of the effective molecules in the granule extract is approximately 1300 and 1200.

A candidacidal substance has also been obtained from acid-extracted granules of J774.1 cells. This finding strongly supports the notion that the candidacidal substance was generated only in the strong acid milieu of phagolysosomes induced by activation of PMP with IFN-γ. Candidacidal substances in neutrophils (Patterson-Delafield *et al.*, 1980) and activated alveolar macrophages (Lehrer *et al.*, 1985) were shown to be cationic proteins or peptides. On the other hand, Hiemstra *et al* (1993) have recently reported that antimicrobial proteins could be extracted from lysosomes of resident and activated murine MP and MP cell lines by acid. After purification, they resembled the members of the cationic histone family, with a molecular mass of 15.5 – 22 kDa. They killed *C. neoformans, Mycobacterium fortuitum, S. typhimurium, E. coli, Listeria monocytogenes* and *S. aureus*, whereas their activity on *C. albicans* and *M. tuberculosis* was not examined. Studies by Kagaya *et al.*, (1994) showed that: a non-cationic peptide may also play a crucial role in the candidacidal activity of activated MP; such a substance can be extracted by acidic treatment, not only from activated PMP but also from normal or a MP cell line; and an acidic milieu is induced by IFN-γ *in-vivo*.

The intracellular behavior of *H. capsulatum:* life in a phagosome

The zoo pathogenic fungus *H. capsulatum* is a facultative intracellular parasite of mononuclear phagocytes. In the tissue of an infected host, the yeasts cells of the fungus reside within MP where they survive and multiply for a time. In most human cases of histoplasmosis and in those experimental infections chosen to be sub lethal, infected individuals recover. During recovery, the intracellular replication of *H. capsulatum* is arrested and the tissues are gradually rid of the fungus (Wu-Hsieh *et al.*, 1994).

The ability of an animal sub lethally infected with *H. capsulatum* to rid itself of the fungus correlated with endogenously produced cytokines (Fleischmann *et al.*, 1990; Wu-Hsieh *et al.*, 1994). Recombinant murine interferon gamma (rMuIFN-γ) activated PMP suppress intracellular growth of the fungus. Induction of a similar suppression in murine red pulp MP requires two signals (Lane *et al.*, 1991). Growth inhibition depends on L-arginine (L-arg) metabolism. Thus, the growth inhibitory state normally induced by rMuIFN-γ and lipopolysaccharide (LPS) in resident splenic MP does not occur when the MP are cultured in the presence of N^G – monomethyl-L-arginine (N^GMMA), a competitive inhibitor of L-arginine metabolism. Resident splenic MP treated with rMuIFN-γ and LPS form nitrite (NO_2^-), an end product of L-arg metabolism. When MP are cultured in the presence of N^GMMA together with rMuIFN-γ and LPS only baseline levels of NO_2^- are detected. Spleen cells from *H. capsulatum*-infected mice produced high levels of NO_2^- in culture. The production of NO_2^- correlates with *in-vitro* inhibition of the intracellular growth of *H. capsulatum* (Lane **et al.**, 1994;Nakamura *et al.*, 1994).

The effecter molecule of arginine – dependent histoplasmostasis is thought to be nitric oxide (NO), which arises from the oxidation of the guanidino nitrogen of arginine. The anti-*Histoplasma* activity of rMuIFN-γ-treated MP of the RAW 264.7 cell line depends on the generation of NO (Nakamura *et al.*, 1994). MP of the P338D_1 cell line does not produce NO· or inhibit the intracellular growth of *H. capsulatum.* NO· is generated by the inducible enzyme nitric oxide syntheses (iNOS) formed by stimulated MP. Northern blot analysis of RAW 264.7 cells reveals the expression of iNOS mRNA after exposure to rMuIFN-γ. In contrast, rMuIFN-γ treated P388D_1 cells did not produce detectable levels of iNOS. These results suggest that the failure of P388D_1 cells to generate NO and to restrict the intracellular growth of *H. capsulatum* is due to a lack of expression of iNOS following treatment with rMuIFN-γ (Lane *et al.*, 1994). Exposure to gaseous nitrous oxide, generated from 2 mM $NaNO_2$ suspended in acid buffer and channeled across a gas-permeable but ion-impermeable membrane inhibited cells of *H. capsulatum*. But at a concentration of 1.0 M $NaNO_2$ the amount of nitrous oxide generated, killed 50% of *H. capsulatum* yeast cells in the first 24 h. Nevertheless, the survivors were able to replicate even though continuously exposed to NO. The basis for this ability is the subject of continuing investigations.

NO targets intracellular iron, a situation that further aggravates the intracellular iron depletion induced by the down-regulation of transferrin receptors induced in MP by rMuIFN-γ *H. capsulatum* requires iron for growth (Lane *et al.*, 1993). Treatment of mouse PMP with the intracellular iron chelator deferoxamine inhibits the intracellular growth of *H. capsulatum*. Exposure of MP to holotransferrin antagonized the effect of both rMuIFN-γ and deferoxamine treatment. These results suggest that iron restriction may be one of the bases of the NO· induced anti-*Histoplasma* effect of mouse MP and the iron supplementation of media can overcome the effects of NO, *In vitro*. The histoplasmostasis induced by iron-restriction resembles the stationary phase of growth induced in microbial cultures by nutrient limitation.

CONCLUSIONS

In this review, we have given examples of the complex mechanisms underlying the antifungal CMI response and its regulation in human and animal models. Central in the events, starting from antigenic recognition of fungal cells to their killing or growth inhibition, appears to be the intervention of Th1 lymphocyte subset and the consequent release of cytokines, which activate the fungicidal or fungistatic mechanisms in the macrophages. In this, a key perhaps pivotal role, is probably played by IFN-γ. A more in-depth disclosure of these mechanisms and how they are finely tuned to maximize antifungal effects certainly represents an exciting research area in the expanding field of the role of CMI in fungal infections and its possible exploitation for immunoprophylaxis or therapeutic approach to these diseases.

REFERENCES

Ausiello, C.M., Urbani, F., Gessani, S., Spagnoli, G.C., Gomez, M.J. and Cassoni, A. (1993) Cytokine gene expression in human peripheral blood mononuclear cells stimulated by mannoprotein constituents from *Candida albicans*. *Infection and Immumity, 61*: 4105-4111.

Bistoni, F., Cenci, E., Mencacci, A., Schiaffella, E., Mosci, P., Puccetti, P. and Romani, L. (1993). Mucosal and systemic T-helper cell function after intragastric colonization of adult mice with *Candida albicans*. *Journal of Infections Diseases, 168* : 1449-1457.

Bodey, G.P. and Fainstein, V. (1985). Systemic candidiasis. In Candidiasis (*Ed.* G.P. Bodey and V. Fainstein), Raven Press, New York pp. 135-168.

Brummer, E., Kurita, N., Yoshida, S., Nishimura, K. and Miyajil, M. (1991). Killing of *Histoplasma capsulatum* by gamma-interferon-activated human monocyte-derived macrophages: evidence for a superoxide anion-dependent mechanism. *Journal of Medical Microbiology, 35*: 29-39.

Buchanan, K.L. and Murphy, J.W. (1993). Characterization of cellular infiltrates and cytokine production during the expression phase of the anticryptococcal delayed-type hypersensitivity response. *Infection and Immunity, 61:* 2854-2865.

Cassone, A., Palma, C., Djeu, J.Y., Aiuti, F. and Quinti, I. (1993). Anticandidal activity and interleukin-1β and interleukin-6 production by polymorphonuclear leukocytes are preserved in subjects with AIDS. *Journal of Clinical Microbiology, 31:* 1354-1357.

Cenci, E., Romani, L., Mencacci, A., Spaccapelo, R., Schiaffella, E., Puccetti, P. and Bistoni, F. (1993). Interleukin 4 and interleukin 10 inhibit nitric oxide-dependent macrophage killing of Candida albicans. *European Journal of Immunology, 23:* 1034-1038.

Cox, R. A. (1979). Immunologic studies of patients with histoplasmosis. *American Review of Respiratory Disease, 120:* 143-149.

Diamond, R.D. and Bennett, J.E. (1973). Disseminated cryptococcosis in man: decreased lymphocyte transformation in response to *Cryptococcus neoformans*. *Journal of Infectious Diseases, 127:* 694-697.

Fleischmann, J., Wu-Hsieh, B.A. and Howard, D. H. (1990). The intracellular fate of *Histoplasma capsulatum* in human macrophages is unaffected by recombinant human interferon gamma. *Journal of Infectious Disease. 161:* 143-145.

Gordon, M.A. and Vedder, D.K. (1966). Serologic tests in diagnosis and prognosis of cryptococcosis. *Journal of the American Medical Association, 197:* 961-967.

Graybill, J.R. and Alford, R.H. (1974). Cell-mediated immunity in cryptococcosis. *Cellular Immunology, 14:* 12-21.

Hiemstra, P.S., Eisenhauer, P.B., Harwig, S.S.L., Van den Barselaar, M.T., Van Furth, R. and Lehrer, R.I. (1993). Antimicrobial proteins of murine macrophages. *Infection and immunity, 61*: 3038-3046.

Imam, N., Carpenter, C.C.J., Mayer, K.H., Fisher, A., Stein, M. and Danforth, S.B. (1990). Hierarchical pattern of mucosal *Candida* infections in HIV-seropositive women. *American Journal of Medicine, 89:* 142-146.

Kagaya, K., Fukazawa, Y., Caffone, A., Bistoni, F., Haward, D.H., Murphy, J.W., Cenci, E., Lane, T.E., Mencacci, A., Puccetti, P., Lomani, L., Spaccapelo, R., Tonnetti, L. and Wu-Hech, B.A. (1994) Host cell-fungal cell interactions. *Journal of Medical and Veterinary Mycology* 32 (1): 123-132.

Khakpour, F.R. and Murphy, J.W. (1987). Characterization of a third-order suppressor T cell (Ts3) induced by cryptococcal antigen(s). *Infection and Immunity, 55:* 1657-1662.

Klein, R.S., Harris, C.A., Smali, C.B., Moll, B., Lesser, M. and Friendland, G.H. (1984). Oral candidiasis in high risk patients as the initial manifestation of the acquired immunodeficiency syndrome. *New England Journal of Medicine, 311:* 354-358

Lane, T.E., Otero, G.C., Wu-Hsieh, B.A. and Howard, D.H. (1994). Expression of inducible nitric oxide synthase by stimulated macrophages correlates with their ant ihistoplasma activity. *Infection and Immunity, 62*: 1478-1479.

Lane, T.E., Wu-Hsieh, B.A. and Howard, D.H. (1991). Iron limitation and the gamma interferon-mediated anti histoplasma state of murine macrophages. *Infection and immunity, 59*: 2274-2278.

Lane, T.E., Wu-Hsieh, B.A. and Howard, D. H. (1993). Gamma interferon cooperates with lipopolysaccharide to activate mouse splenic macrophages to an anti-histoplasma state. *Infection and Immuniy, 61*: 1468-1473.

Lehrer, R.I., Selsted, M.E., Ganz, T. and Sherman, M.P. (1985). Multipotent antimicrobial peptides of activated macrophges. *Lymphokines, 11:* 171-186.

Lim, T.S. and Murphy, J.W. (1980). Transfer of immunity of cryptococcosis by T-enriched splenic lymphocytes from *Cryptococcus neoformans*-sensitized mice. *Infection and Immunity, 30:* 5-11.

Lim, T.S., Murphy, J.W. and Cauley, L.K. (1980). Host-etiological agent interactions in intranasally and intraperitoneally induced cryptococcosis mice. *Infection and Immunity, 29* : 633-641.

Mosmann, T.R., Cherwinski, H., Bond, M.W., Giedlin, M.A. and Coffman, R.L. (1986). Two types of murine helper T cell clone. I. Definition according to profiles of lymphokine activities and secreted proteins. *Journal of Immunology, 136*: 2348-2357.

Murphy, J.W. (1985). Effects of first-order *Cryptococcus*-specific T-suppressor cells on induction of cells responsible for delayed-type hypersensitivity. *Infection and Immunity, 48*: 439-445.

Murphy, J.W. (1989). Clearance of *Cryptococcus neoformans* from immunologically suppressed mice. *Infection and Immunity, 57:* 1946-1952.

Murphy, J.W. and Cox, R.A. (1988). Induction of antigen-specific suppression by circulating *Cryptococcus neoformans* antigen. *Clinical and Experimental Immunology, 73*: 174-180.

Murphy, J.W. and Moorhead, J.W. (1982). Regulation of Cell-mediated immunity in cryptococcosis. I. Induction of specific afferent T suppressor cells by cryptococcal antigen. *Journal of Immunology, 128:* 276-283.

Murphy, J.W. and Mosley, R.S. (1985). Regulation of cell-mediated immunity in cryptococcosis. III. Characterization of second-order T suppressor cells (Ts2). *Journal of Immunology, 134:* 577-584.

Murphy, J.W., Mosley, R.L., Cherniak, R., Reyes, G.H., Kozel, T.R. and Reiss, E.. (1988). Serological electrophoretic, and biological properties of *Cryptococcus neoformans* antigens. *Infection and Immunity, 56:* 424-431.

Murphy, J.W., Mosley, R.L. and Moorhead, J.W. (1983). Regulation of cell-mediated immunity in cryptococcosis. II. Characterization of first-order T suppressor cells (Ts1) and induction of second order suppressor cells. *Journal of Immunology, 130*: 2876-2881.

Nakamura, L.T., Wu-Hsieh, B.A. and Howard, D.H. (1994). Recombinant murine gamma interferon stimulates macrophages of the RAW cell line to inhibit intracellular growth of *Histoplasma capsulatum*. *Infection and Immunity, 62*: 680-684.

Patterson-Delafield, J., Martinez, R.J. and Lehrer, R.I. (1980). Microbicidal cationic proteins in rabbit alveolar macrophages: a potential host defense mechanism. *Infection and Immunity, 30*: 180-192.

Puccetti, P., Mencacci, A., Cenci, E., Spaccapelo, R., Mosci, P., Henssle, R.H., Romani, L. and Bistoni, F. (1994). Cure of murine candidiasis by recombinant soluble interleukin-4 receptor. *Journal of Infectious Disease, 169*: 1325-1331.

Redmond, H.P., Shou, J., Gallagher, H. J., Kelly, C.J. and Daly, J.M. (1993). Macrophage-dependent candidacidal mechanisms in the murine system. Comparison of murine Kupffer cell and peritoneal macrophage candidacidal mechanisms. *Journal of Immunology, 150:* 3427-3433.

Romani, L., Cenci.E., Mencacci, A., Spaccapelo, R., Grohmann, U., Puccetti, P. and Bistoni, F. (1992). Gamma interferon modifies $CD4^+$ subset expression in murine candidiasis. *Infection and Immunity, 60*: 4950-4952.

Romani, L., Mencacci, A., Cenci, E., Spaccapelo, R., Mosci, P., Puccetti, P. and Bistoni, F. (1993).$CD4^+$ subset expression in murine candidiasis. *Journal of Immunology, 150*: 925-931.

Romani, L., Mencacci, A., Grohmann, U., Mocci, S., Mosci, P., Puccetti, P. and Bistoni, F. (1992). Neutralizing antibody to interleukin 4 induces systemic protection and T helper type 1-associated immunity in murine candidiasis. *Journal of Experimental Medicine, 176*: 19-25.

Romani, L., Mencacci, A., Tonnetti, L., Spaccapelo, R., Cenci, E., Wolf, S., Puccetti, P. and Bistoni, F. (1994). Interleukin-12 but not interferon-g production correlates with induction of T helper type-I phenotype in murine candidiasis. *European Journal of Immunology, 24*: 909-915.

Romani, L., Mocci, S., Bietta, C., Lanfaloni, L., Puccetti, P. and Bistoni, F. (1991). Th1 and Th2 cytokine secretion patterns in murine candidiasis; association of Th1 responses with acquired resistance. *Infection and Immunity, 59*: 4647-4654.

Sasada, M., Kubo, A., Nishimura, T., Kakita, T., Moriguchi, T., Yamamoto, K. and Uchino, H. (1987). Candidacidal activity of monocyte-derived human macrophages: relationship between *Candida* killing and oxygen radical generation by human macrophages. *Journal of Leukocyte Biology, 41*: 289-294.

Scott, P. and Kaufmann, S.H. E. (1991). The role of T-cell subsets and cytokines in the regulation of infection. *Immunology Today, 12*: 346-348.

Torosantucci, A., Bromuro, C., Gomez, M.J., Ausiello, C.M., Urbani, F. and Cassone, A. (1993). Identification of a 65-kDa mannoprotein as a main target of human cell-mediated immune response to *Candida albicans*. *Journal of Infectious Diseases, 168*: 427-435.

Watanabe, K., Kagaya, K., Yamada, T. and Fukazawa, Y. (1991). Mechanism for candidacidal activity in macrophages activated by recombinant gamma interferon. *Infection and Immunity, 59:* 521-528.

Wu-Hsieh, B.A. and Howard, D.H. (1994). Histoplasmosis. In *Infectious Agents and Pathogenesis* (*Ed.* Murphy, J.W., Berdinelli, M. and Friedman, H.) Plenum Press, New York.

Microbiology and Biotechnology for Sustainable Development (*Ed.* P.C. Jain),
CBS Publishers & Distributors, New Delhi (2004), pp. 151–165.

A-13

Medical and Biological Importance of Photodynamic Action

U. S. Gupta
Department of Zoology, Dr H. S. Gour Vishwavidyalaya
Sagar (M.P.) 470003.

Abstract

In the present paper various aspects of the mechanism of photodynamic action have been discussed. The effect of photodynamic action on the microorganisms, plants, and multicellular organisms has been described. The medical and biological importance of the photodynamic action has been discussed.

Key words: Photodynamic action , Photosensitizer, microorganism.

INTRODUCTION

Photodynamic action may be defined as the dye-sensitized photoautoxidation of a biological substance. It has been with a remarkably large number of substrate, including multicellular plants and animals, single cells and cell organelles, bacteria virus and enzymes. The specific effects range from photokilling in the higher organisms to alteration of biological function at the sub cellular level (Spike, 1982).

Oscar Raab reported the first experimental study on photosensitization in biological system in 1900. Raab, a medical student found that low concentrations of certain acridines and eosin, which has no effect in the dark, led to the rapid killing of *Paramecium* on illumination. Later on many reports came and it was shown that enzymes could be inactivated and that many kinds of cells and small animals could be killed on illumination in the presence of a variety of photosensitizers.

Photosensitizers are molecules, which can absorb light to produce a chemical reaction, which would not occur in their absence. The photosensitizers may or may not be chemically changed in this process. Many compounds absorbing in the visible and near UV regions act as photodynamic sensitizers. Santamaria & Prino (1972) have listed 400 compounds which have been shown to sensitize many naturally occurring pigments, including chlorophyll and related compounds, other noniron porphyrins such as protoporphyrin IX, flavins (lumiflavin, riboflavin, FMN) and polycyclic plant pigments such as hypericin, are efficient photodynamic sensitizers. Many kinds of synthetic organic compounds also act as photosensitizers, these includes acridines (proflavin, acridine orange etc.) anthraquinones azine dyes (safranines), many ketones, thiazine dye (methylene blue, toluidine blue), thiopyronin and xanthene dye (Eosin Y, Rose Bengal etc.).

Photodynamic reaction mechanism:

The molecule which acts as photosensitizers (Sens) have the two system of electronically excited states, the singlet (1Sens) and the triplet (3Sens). On illumination the ground state sensitizer (Sens) is converted to a singlet excited state (^{1}Sens), which typically has a very short lifetime. In most efficient photodynamic sensitizers, the excited singlet undergoes conversion to another energy rich form, the triplet state (^{3}Sens). This state has a much greater chance of undergoing chemical reaction. Almost all photodynamic reactions are mediated by a triplet state.

The most effective sensitizers are therefore those which give a long-lived triplet state in high quantum yield. Many dyes (methylene blue, rose Bengal, or eosin), pigment (chlorophyll, hematoporphyrin and flavins) and aromatic hydrocarbons (rubrene & some anthracenes) are effective sensitizers. Most of these compounds absorb visible and near UV light and so that these wavelengths are effective for photosensitized oxidation.

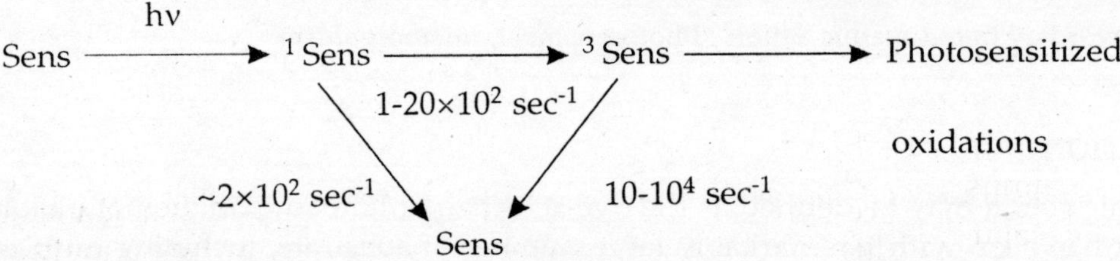

In simple photodynamic system the triplet sensitizer can react in two major ways i.e. by electron or hydrogen transfer processes (Type I or free radical reactions) or by energy transfer processes (Type II reactions). The processes depend on the chemical nature of the sensitizer and substrate and on the reaction conditions (pH, solvent, concentrations of components).

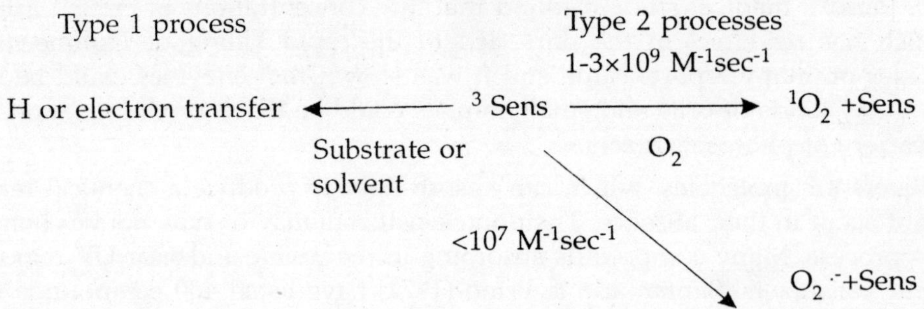

Type I (Electron transfer) Process:

Type I chemistry usually involves the production of free radical ions by interaction of the sensitizer triplet with a reducing substrate (RH or R). The product radical thus formed can react further in a variety of ways in the presence of oxygen and gives an oxidized form of the substrate and ground state sensitizer as the final products.

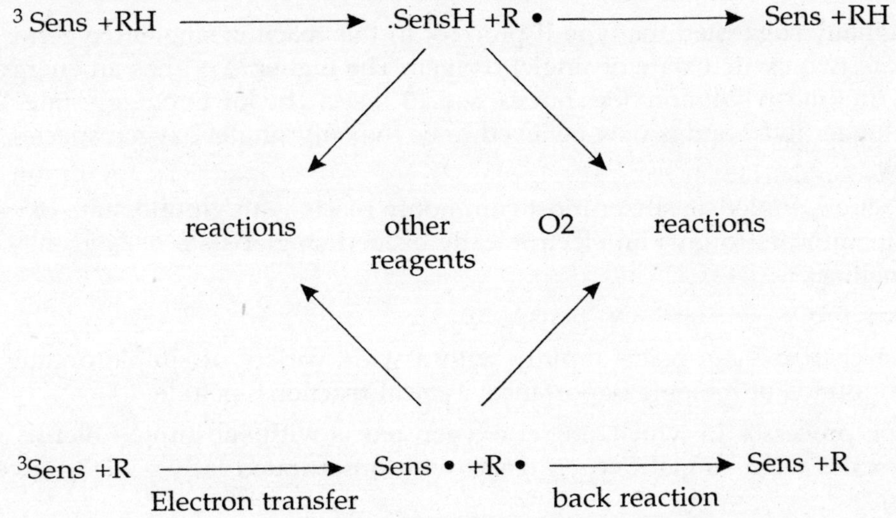

One reaction of the reduced sensitizer with oxygen is to produce O_2^- or its conjugate acid HO_2; this later can react with oxygen to give hydrogen peroxide and ground state sensitizer.

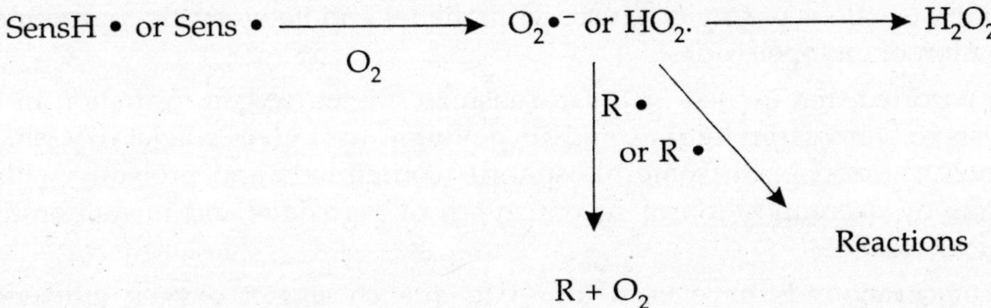

Triplet sensitizers in some cases can react with oxidants (o_x) to give a semioxidized form of the sensitizer and a reduced oxidant. Finally, triplet sensitizers can also react by transferring an electron to ground state oxygen, giving semioxidized sensitizer and oxygen superoxide.

^{3}Sens + Ox ⟶ Sens• + Ox•.- ⟶ Sens + Ox

O_2

Reactions   Reactions

An example is the reaction of the oxidized dye formed by the reaction of triplet eosin

(^3Eo) with ground- state dye; the oxidized dye then reacts with allylthiourea (ATU) regenerating Eo.

$$^3Eo + Eo \longrightarrow Eo^{\bullet +} + Eo^{\cdot -}$$
$$Eo^{\bullet +} + ATU \longrightarrow Eo + ATU\ ox$$
$$\text{Overall: } 3Eo + ATU \longrightarrow Eo^{\bullet -} + ATU\ ox$$

Kautsky originally suggested the type II process. In this reaction singlet oxygen is intermediate. These are two excited state of singlet oxygen. The higher $^1\Sigma g^+$ has an energy of 37 K cal / mole, its lifetime in solution does not exceed 10^{-11} sec. The lower energy state, 22 KCl / mole is much longer lived and is now believed to be the only singlet oxygen species which reacts in solution.

In type II reaction, triplet sensitizer most commonly reacts with ground state oxygen by an energy transfer process to give an electronically excited singlet state of oxygen $^1O_2$ and ground state sensitizer.

$$^3Sens + {}^3O_2 \longrightarrow Sens + {}^1O_2$$

The singlet excited oxygen reacts rapidly with a wide variety of simple organic compounds and compounds of biologic importance. Typical reactions include:

(a) "ene"- type processes in which singlet oxygen reacts with substituted olefins giving hydroperoxides (e.g. singlet oxygen reacts with unsaturated fatty acids to give lipid peroxides).

(b) Reaction of singlet oxygen with compounds containing heteroatoms (e.g. methionine is oxidized sulfoxide).

(c) 1-4- addition reactions of singlet oxygen with dienes and heterocyclic compounds with the formation of endoperoxides.

It has been reported that excited NO_2 can sensitize singlet oxygen formation in the gas phase. Hydrolysis of peroxyacetylnitrate, and air pollutant, also gives singlet oxygen. Singlet oxygen is formed by ozone with some phosphorus compounds and probably with many other compounds by decomposition of several types of peroxides and in numerous other nonphotochemical reactions.

A number of compounds have been found to quench singlet oxygen efficiently. For example, β- carotene inhibits Photoxidation of 2-methy-2-pentene efficiently at 10^{-4}M without itself being appreciably oxidized. Nickel complexes and polymethine dyes are also excellent quenchers for singlet oxygen. Other types of compound e.g. 1,4-diazabicyclooctane (DABCO), Azide ion, phenols, α-Tocopherol are reported as quencher of singlet oxygen.

There are two basic classes of quenching, electron transfer and energy transfer. Electron transfer quenchers and DABCO and sodium azide, these quench with rate constant on the order of 10^7 and 10^8 M^{-1} sec^{-1} respectively. The mechanism appears to be charge or electron transfer, as shown below.

$$^1O_2 + Q \longrightarrow O_2^- + Q^- \longrightarrow {}^3O_2 + Q$$

DABCO is fairly unreactive. In water, a concentration of about 5×10^{-2}M would be required to trap half the singlet oxygen present. Azide-ion is more reactive and a lower concentration is required.

The energy transfer quenchers are β- carotene and nickel complexes. These compounds quench at a rate of $1\text{-}2\times10^{10}M^{-1}sec^{-1}$ and its is likely that both react by an energy transfer process –

$$^{1}O_2 + Q \longrightarrow {}^{3}O_2 + 3\,Q \longrightarrow {}^{3}O_2 + Q$$

Cell Photosensitization Procedure

There are two types of general procedure for sensitizing cell in suspension:

(1) In the first type, the cells are incubated in the dark, with sensitizers in a suspension medium, for a sufficient time; which may be variable; usually 30 min. or longer at the physiological temperature. Then the cells are irradiated with visible light or in some cases with near-UV radiation. After irradiation the treated cells are placed for survival or tested for specific functions.

(2) In the second method excess sensitizers in the medium are removed by centrifugation or by some other means after incubation before irradiation.

Sufficient information on the cell-sensitizer interaction occurring in the incubation period is lacking. Some of the sensitizers may remain outside of the cell even after long incubation, while another group of sensitizers may only be bound to the surface of the cells. Lipid soluble sensitizers are often incorporated into the hydrophobic region of the cell membrane. Some other types of sensitizers may get in to the interior of the cell and be bound to various parts of the cell (Fig. 1).

Sensitizers and damage sites

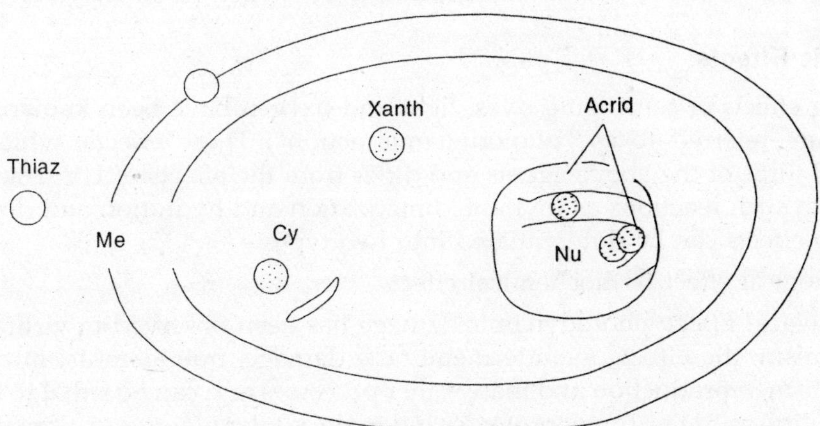

Fig 1. a schematic representation of localization of dye sensitizers and presumed sites of photodynamic damage (as proposed by Ito, 1978). Thiaz. – thiazines (O), Xanth. -xanthenes, Acrid. – acridines, Me. – membrane, Cy. – cytoplasm, Nu. – nucleus.

Thus inactivation of the cell due to photodynamic action may be classified into three modes:

1. attack from outside the cell e.g. Toluidine blue and many Thiazine dyes (Dye remains outside).
2. attack from inside e.g. Rose Bengal and Xanthenes dyes. After entering inside these dyes get inside the cell, they act on the enzymes or often cytoplasmic structures via the $^1O_2$ pathway on illumination.
3. attack from inside – In this mode DNA damage would be the major cause of inactivation. DNA binding acridine dyes belong to this category. These dyes may also be active in the production of genetic changes.

The cells can be sensitized on nutrient agar plates or in liquid nutrient medium that contains sensitizers. Immobilized sensitizers can also sensitize the cells in suspension, immobilized on plastic beads that have dimension comparable to or larger than the cells. Cells in tissue or in animal, may be sensitized topically, orally or by injection.

Irradiation by visible light or by near-UV radiation may be performed using any lamp emission covers the desired range of wavelengths with a sufficient fluence rate. Flashes and a short pulse of light have been used for particular types of experiment. A laser and in particular, a durable dye laser may find suitable application. A xenon arch lamp (e.g. 500W) with a stabilized power supply is recommended as a standard light source for quantitative work in the visible region. For a near-UV radiation source the black light lamp is a standard type.

The fluence needed to kill the sensitized cells may vary widely depending on many factors. The yeast cells are sensitized in order of 10^4 J/m^2 by acridine orange (10^{-5} M). In ordinary aerobic experiments, only stirring is required during illumination under open air however in special situation deliberate bubbling with oxygen or air may be required.

Photodynamic Effects:

The damaging effects of sensitizing dyes, light and oxygen have been known since the last century and are referred to as "photodynamic action". These effects, which require the presence of all three of the above agents and differ from the effects of UV irradiation, which typically causes such reactions as thymine dimerization and hydration and does not require oxygen. These effects can be differentiated into two types –

A. Physiological effect B. Biochemical effect

A. *Physiological Effect:* photodynamic damage has been observed in virtually all classes of organism; the effects include membrane damage, mutagenesis, interference with metabolism, reproduction and many other processes and can be lethal to the organisms such as viruses, algae, fungi, protozoa and multicellular plants and animals are affected. Dietary photosensitizers can affect grazing animals. In humans, some drug photosensitivity reactions may belong to this class. Certain porphyrins may cause genetically or liver damage, which result in the deposition of sensitizing blood porphyrins in the skin, affected individuals, receive severe skin damage or brief light exposure.

B. *Biochemical Effects:* The sites of biological lesion in the photodynamic effect have received extensive study and are well characterized, although the detailed chemistry is not well understood in most cases. Photoxidation of certain amino acids, nucleosides, lipids and certain other cell constituents appears to the cause of the lesions.

Amino acid derivatives and Peptides

Proteins, polypeptides and individual amino acids vary in susceptibility to sensitized photo oxidation; methionine, histidine, traptophan, tyrosine and cysteine are the principal amino acids affected in all cases, either with free amino acids or in peptides. No breaking of peptide or disulfide bonds occurs. Destruction of key active–site amino acids (particularly methionine and histidine) or damage leading to loss of conformational stability causes inactivation of many enzymes.

Methionine is oxidized by most sensitizing dyes to the sulfoxide with flavins, under some conditions, methanol as the product. Methionine is subject to Photoxidation at all pH , but at high pH there is evidence for H_2O_2 formation (Fig. 2).

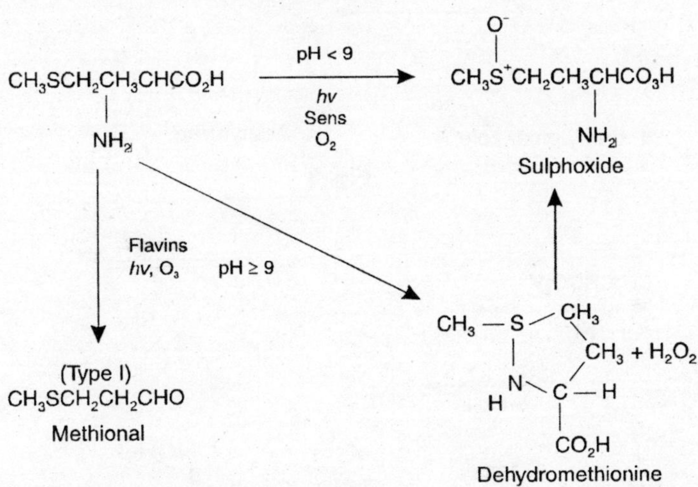

Fig. 2

Histidine (Fig. 3) gives products of cleavage of the imidazoles ring; the initial products have not been isolated but model studies on other imidazoles suggest cleavage of the examine double bond is the likely primary result followed by hydrolytic cleavage to aspartic acid. N-benzylhistidine gives compound one of the initial products whereas 4-methyl imidazole gives acetylurea.

Tryptophan: Photoxidation of tryptophan gives complex mixtures of products (Fig. 4). The isolation of N-formylkynurenine as the primary product has been reported. However, it is apparently readily converted to secondary products (Fig. 4).

Tyrosine: Tyrosine reacts by a type I mechanism in air-saturated water. Only the anionic form reacts rapidly in methylene blue sensitized oxidation. The products are not known but the reaction site in phenolic ring.

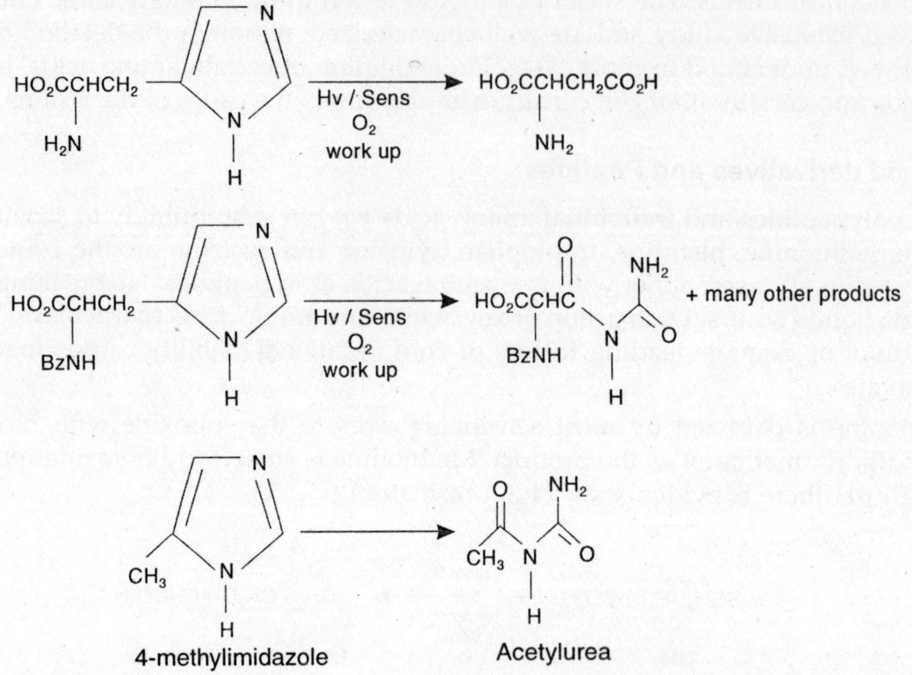

HO_2CCHCH_2 / H_2N — N, N–H
$\xrightarrow{Hv / Sens,\ O_2,\ work\ up}$
$HO_2CCHCH_2CO_2H$ / NH_2

HO_2CCHCH_2 / BzNH — N, N–H
$\xrightarrow{Hv / Sens,\ O_2,\ work\ up}$
HO_2CCHC(=O) / BzNH — NH_2, N–H, O + many other products

CH_3 — N, N–H
4-methylimidazole
$\longrightarrow$
O, NH_2, CH_3, N–H, O
Acetylurea

Fig. 3

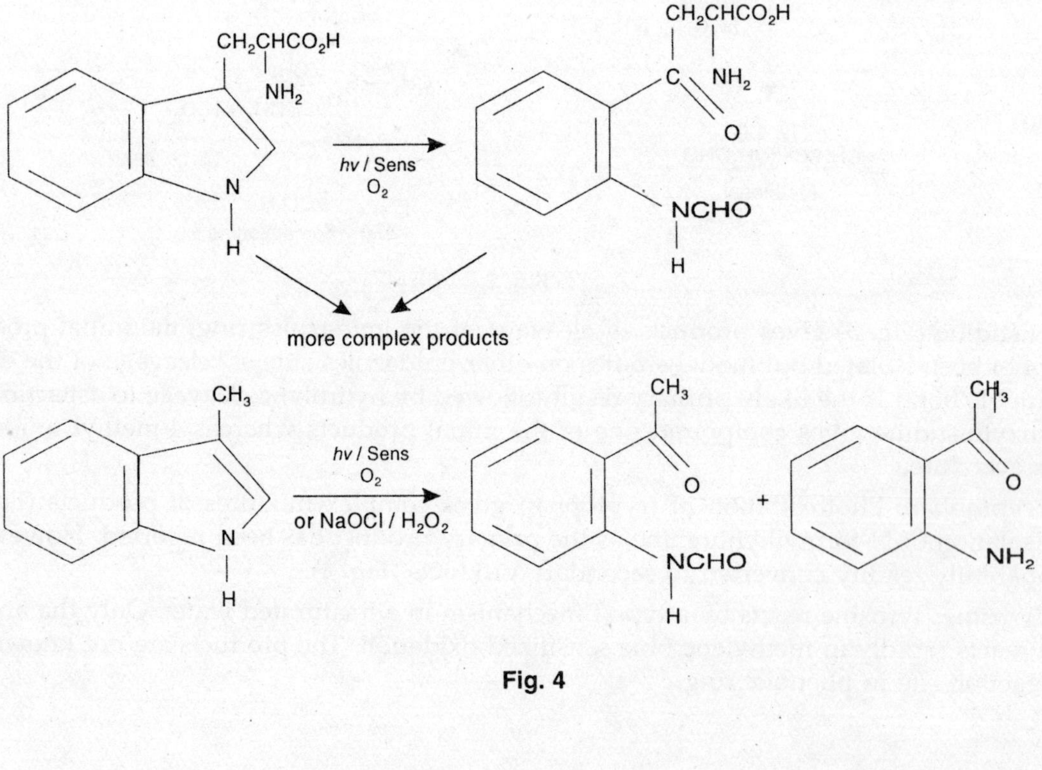

CH_2CHCO_2H / NH_2 — N–H
$\xrightarrow{hv / Sens,\ O_2}$
CH_2CHCO_2H / C(=O) / NH_2 — NCHO / H

more complex products

CH_3 — N–H
$\xrightarrow{hv / Sens,\ O_2,\ or\ NaOCl / H_2O_2}$
CH_3, O — NCHO / H + CH_3, O — NH_2

Fig. 4

Cysteine: Cystine is slowly oxidized to cysteic acid; cysteine is apparently a product under certain conditions.

Photoxidation of only a few enzymes has been studied. Nilsson and Kearns have shown that photosensitized oxygenation of yeast alcohol dehydrogenase and trypsin with methylene blue gives deactivation.

Enzyme

Singlet oxygen has been suggested to be involved in many biological processes. Examples are dioxygenases, which cleave various catechol derivatives, tryptophan pyrrolase, which gives cleavage similar to the singlet oxygen with electron- rich olefins, and lipooxygenase, which produces allulic hydroperoxides from fatty acides; prostaglandin synthetase.

Nucleic acid Derivatives

Guanine is the principal base residue destroyed in the oxidation of nucleic acid. Enamine double bonds and heterocyclic dienes are primary targets for oxidative cleavage.

Lipids

Olefins with hydrogen allylic to the double bonds are photoxidized to allylic hydroperoxide. In well-controlled laboratory studies, fatty acid derivatives and cholesterol have been shown to give photoxidation products in which the double bond is clearly shifted to the allylic position and singlet oxygen has been shown to be intermediate. Lipid oxidation is probably the cause of the membrane damage commonly reported as a result of photodynamic damage, but products are not known in most of the cases.

Polysaccharide

Sugars and cellulose materials are photoxidized fairly readily by ketonic sensitizers. This oxidation leads to acids or ketones with a decrease in molecular weight of polysaccharides, which results in tendering of textiles.

Photodynamic action at the cellular level

In the presence of light, acridines, thiazine, xanthenes and many other dyes light absorbing drugs and natural pigments or products such as furocounmarins, poly acetylenes and porphyrins act as sensitizers on many kind of biological systems.

Nuclear Damage: Nuclear damage may be induced by a sensitizer that localizes in the nucleus. Acridine derivatives usually penetrate across the cell wall and cell membrane and reach the nuclear area. By illumination with proflavine DNA & RNA synthesis were inhibited immediately in HeLa cells. Free radical scavengers reduced this photoxidative effect. Roberts (1981) has concluded that thymine and cytosine residues of DNA, in contrast to the commonly believed guanine residue, are the sites of photodamage.

Thiazine dyes like methylene blue or toluidine blue are reported to induce mutations photodynamically in bacterial cells. Neutral red is also reported to by mutagenic in *Salmonella* cells.

Cell Membrane Damage

Certain types of dye sensitizers virtually do not penetrate across cell membranes into the cytoplasmic region. This includes toluidine blue, methylene blue, xanthenes, porphyrins and acridine.

Prebble and Huda (1973) have reported that the toluidine blue (or methylene blue) sensitized the components of the respiratory chain associated with cell membrane. Photodynamic agent such as toluidine blue may cause damage in cellular DNA in E.coli (Nishida etal. 1980). Malandialdyhyde, an oxidation product of polyunsaturated fatty acids was able to induce mutation in *Salmonella* and *E. coli*.

The following observations suggest that the cell membrane damage was the primary cause of mammalian cell in activation by sensitization with porphyrin dyes.

1. Replacement of H_2O with D_2O in the cell suspension medium only enhances cell inactivation and not DNA damage.
2. Release of lysosomal enzymes occurs after most of the cells are killed.
3. Early events of photosensitization are the leakage of K^+ and membrane bound enzymes are not lysosome damage as reported earlier.
4. Significant effects on various cell-surface phenomena occurs at treatment levels that markedly reduce cell viability without affecting an intracellular events.

Naturally occurring polyactylene, and α-terthienyl sensitize human erythrocytes for photohemolysis by oxygen requiring pathway.

Photodynamic studies with multicellular organisms

Small mammals injected with a photosensitizer exhibit a characteristic pattern of responses on exposure to light, including apparent skin itching, hyperactivity and skin damage (edema, errthema, cell death and necrosis). The immediate reaction appears to be of the histamine-release type. With more sensitizer and / or light, generalized responses occur, including decreased blood pressure, intestinal hemorrhage circulatory collapse, and death.

Grazing animals often become photosensitive as a result of eating plants containing photodynamic sensitizers. Under some conditions, sheep's and goats show serious light sensitivity due to the accumulation of phylloerythrin. This is a porporphyrin produced from chlorophyll by bacterial action in the gut of the animal. Normally it is excreted in the bile; if bile discharge is interfered with, however, the sensitizers accumulates in the blood, leading to serious photodynamic injury.

Work on fish and amphibians have been reviewed by Blum(1941). Tadpoles and newts can be killed by photodynamic treatment and frog muscle has been used in studies on the photodynamic stimulation of contraction. Graham (1972) reviewed the earlier work on insect. Some of the earlier work on photosensitization of mosquito larvae suggested the use of photodynamic reactions in mosquito control. Polycyclic hydrocarbons sensitize the photodynamic killing of mosquito larvae roughly in proportion to their effectiveness as chemical carcinogens. The behavioral patterns of insects following photodynamic treatment indicate effects on the nervous system, perhaps mediated by the inactivation of acetylcholinesterase; however this mechanism has not been established.

It was demonstrated using albino mice that subcutaneous injections of photodynamic sensitizers such as hematoporphyrin promote skin-tumor formation when the animals are subsequently exposed to light.

Photodynamic Studies with Microorganisms

A number of types of photodynamic studies have been carried out with bacteria. Effects can result from photodynamic damage to nucleic acids, proteins, membrane component (lipids, proteins), to ribosomes, etc. (Table 1) Many kinds of bacteria and some mycoplasmas are killed on illumination in the presence of photodynamic sensitizers. Various metabolic activities in bacteria, including protein synthesis, respiration, glycolysis etc. can be inhibited by photodynamic treatment, some cellular enzymes are destroyed. The respiratory system in cell membranes isolated from *Sarcina lutea* is inactivated by photodynamic treatment with toluidine blue, while treatment of *Proteus mirabilis* increases the sensitivity of cell envelope to lyses. It is well known that carotenoids protect bacteria against photodynamic damage involving both endogenous and exogenous sensitizers.

Yeast and bacteria is particularly used eucaryotic microorganism. Ito (1978) has reviewed the mechanisms of photodynamic effects on yeast cells. Unicellular green plants (algae) can be killed by photodynamic treatment however, they have not been used to any great extent in photodynamic studies. Several dyes sensitize the photodynamic killing of dermatophyte fungi; under some conditions photodynamic treatment substantially reduce skin lesion formation in guinea pigs inoculated with fungi. Unicellular green plants can be killed by photodynamic treatment.

Table 1: Photodynamic action of various sensitizers on Microorganisms

Sensitizer	Organism	Photodynamic action studied
Rose Bengal (RoB)	*Saccharomyces cerevisiae*	Inactivation gene conversion
Eosine Y(EoY)	*Saccharomyces cerevisiae*	Inactivation
Rhodamine B (Rd B)	*Saccharomyces cerevisiae*	Inactivation
Thionine (TH)	*Saccharomyces cerevisiae*	Inactivation
(TP)	*Proteus mirabilis*	DNA strand break Cell envelop damage, repair
	Saccharomyces cerevisiae	Inactivation Base(uracil, adenine) uptate RNA synthesis Respiration fermentation
Methyline Blue (MB)	*Acholeplasma laidlawii*	Inactivation
	Proteus mirabilis	DNA strand break, repair
	Salmonella typhimurium	Mutation
	Sarcina lutea	Inactivation
	Saccharomyces cerevisiae	Inactivation
	Mouse L cells	Inactivation of ^{3}H thymidine
	Mouse embryo cells	incorporation
	Human erthrocytes	Hemolysis

(Contd.)

Sensitizer	Organism	Photodynamic action studied
Toluidine Blue(TB)	*Micrococcus roseus*	Inactivation
	Escherichia coli	Membrane transport
	Sarcina lutea	Membrane enzyme inactivation inactivation
	Saccharomyces cerevisiae	Membrane enzyme
	HeLa cells	inactivation
Acridines (AO)	*Eschericha coli*	Inactivation, repair
	Salmonella typhimurium	Mutation
	Saccharomyces cerevisiae	Inactivation gene conversion Miotic crossing over reverse mutation
	Mouse L cells	Inactivation of ^{3}H thymidine
	Mouse embryo cells	incorporation
Proflavin (PF)	*Saccharomyces cerevisiae*	Inactivation gene conversion
	Human fibroblast	
	HeLa cell	
Acriflavin (AF)	*Saccharomyces cerevisiae*	Inactivation gene conversion
Ethidium Bromide (TB)	*Saccharomyces cerevisiae*	Inactivation
Neutral Red	Salmonella typhimurium	Mutation
	Mouse L cells, Mouse embryo cells.	Inactivation of ^{3}H thymidine incorporation
Photoporphyrin	Human erythrocyte	Hemolysis

Medical and Biological Implications of the Photodynamic Effect

Human porphyries comprise several different syndromes, which are caused by defects in the metabolism of blood porphyrins. Some porphyrins, especially erythropoetic protoporphyria (EPP) are associated with photosensitivity; patients with the EPP disease are subject to edema and erythrema on exposure to light. This photosensitivity is caused by the deposition of photosensitizing porphyrin in the skin.

Treatment of Neonatal Jaundice

A common problem among newborn infants is jaundice; this jaundice if untreated may lead to brain damage. The cause is lake of glucuronyltransferase, which affects the conversion of the lipid–soluble yellow pigment bilirubin, to the water-soluble conjugate with glucuronic acid. The resulting excess concentration of bilirubin deposits in the skin and brain. The common treatment for neonatal jaundice is irradiation of the infant with light in the wavelength absorbed by bilirubin. Irradiation of the bleaches the bilirubin in the skin and apparently prevents brain damage.

Photodynamic carcinogenesis

It was demonstrated using albino mice, that subcutaneous injections of photodynamic sensitizers such as hematoporphyrin promote skin- tumor formation when the animals are subsequently exposed to light. These sensitizers are not themselves chemical carcinogen. This phenomenon has not been demonstrated in humans, although it has been proposed that skin cancer in older humans might involve, in part, photosensitized reactions resulting from the gradual accumulation of porphyrin phototosensitizers in the skin with age. Under proper conditions illumination with long wavelength UV radiation accelerates the development of skin tumors in mice treated with the chemical carcinogen 3, 4- benzpyrene; this compound is a good photodynamic sensitizer. Two theories of carcinogenicity involving singlet oxygen have been proposed . In the first, the "Optical Residue" theory the polynuclear hydrocarbon is bound to the cell constituent, perhaps in the photochemical step. Subsequently excitation of the bound residue produces singlet oxygen, which then produces the lesion, which directly leads to tumor growth. Alternatively it has been suggested that singlet oxygen reacts with a K region of the hydrocarbon producing a carcinogenic hydroperoxide.

Psoriasis is commonly treated by use of coal tar (which contains sensitizing hydrocarbon) and light. Ageing of skin is correlated with oxidative polymerization of elastin and particularly rapid in light exposed areas of skin, photo oxidative mechanism for this process can be visualized, but this is pure speculation. Tumor cells can be killed photodynamically. It has been reported that malignant cells take and bind hemoporphyrin to a greater extent than normal tissue; irradiation then selectivity kills the tumor cells. It is suggested that this approach may be useful in therapy of resistant tumors.

Treatment of Herpes simplex

Herpes simplex virus lesions have been effectively treated in man with neutral red followed by irradiation.

Photodynamic action and movement

The locomotion of motile organisms can be influenced or controlled by light in different ways:

1. The stationary light intensity can simply control the linear velocity of movement: photo kinesis.
2. A sudden change in light intensity can illicit a transient change in the speed and / or direction of movement: photophobic response (photophobism or phtophobotaxis)
3. The direction of light can control the direction of movement: photo taxis or photopotaxis.

Photo dynamically induced movement reactions of microorganisms such as *Spirollum volutans, Paramaecium caudatum and Navicula* species were studied by Metzner (1924). Nultsch and Hader (1984) have reported the effects of riboflavin as photosensitizers on the movement of colorless flagellate Polytomella magna. *P. magna* dose not show natural reaction to words light phototaxis,photophobic response or photo kinesis. However if riboflavin is added to the culture an avoidance response to words light field is induced. Nultsch and Kumar (1989) and Kumar and Nultsch (1983) have concluded that hydrogen peroxides is formed as photoproduct in a type I reaction which causes negative phototaxis in the colorless *Polytomella magna.*

Quenching of Singlet Oxygen

Several groups have shown that singlet oxygen can be quenched without reaction by certain compounds. The first example was a report that B- carotene quenches singlet oxygen very efficiently, essentially without reaction. Both photo chemically and none photo chemically produced singlet oxygen were quenched with the same kinetics, and carotene was kinetically shown to complete with 2-methyle-2-pentene for singlet oxygen. Nultsch and Kumar (1984) have reported that most of the $^1O_2$ quenchers such as furfurylethanol. DPDF, L- histidine and crocetin were ineffective, where as others; such as DABCO, imidazole and DMF have a slight quenching effect only at very high concentrations. In another study Gupta and Nultsch (1986) have reported that calcium chloride has some quenching property. The calcium chloride quenches the effect of riboflavin in initial stage but the long-term irradiation is lethal to the cells. When only culture is irradiated with white light (35000 lx) the formation of formazon starts decreasing after 30 minutes and up to 2 hr. very less amount of formazon is formed which clearly show that 2hr. exposure of white light is lethal to the Polytomella cells. When the Polytomella cells are irradiated in presence of calcium chloride up to forty minutes no change in the amount of formazon formation was observed but the 2hr. exposure of white light reduces the formation of formazon. However the amount was always more as compared to the 2hr. exposed Polytomella cells in presence of riboflavin, and calcium chloride or when only culture of Polytomella was irradiated. It is suggested that the white light irradiation in presence of riboflavin, damage occurs primarily due to the respiratory enzyme inactivation and calcium chloride have some quenching properties.

There are numerous medical implications of photodynamic action. Psorasis is commonly treated by use of coal tar (which contains sensitizing hydrocarbons) and light. Aging of skin is correlated with oxidative polymerization of elastin and is particularly rapid in light exposed areas of the skin. Tumor cells can be killed photodynamically. It has been reported that malignant cells take and bind hematoprhyrin to a greater extent than normal tissue irradiation then selectively kills the tumor cells (Diamond et al. (1972).

In conclusion the photodynamic reaction have applied values. They can be used in destroying pollutants in industrial wastewater; biologic contaminants such as bacteria and viruses could be destroyed. Solar UV radiation degrades many pesticides and herbicides in the environment; it may become feasible to insert photosensitizing groupings into herbicide and pesticides molecules to control their persistence in the environment. Photosensitized reactions can be used to generate chemical reagents rapidly and conveniently.

REFERENCES

Foote, C.S.(1976) Photosensitized oxidation and singlet oxygen : Consequences in biological systems: In Free radicals in Biology (*Ed.* W.A. Pryor), Academic press, U.S.A. 85 –133.

Gupta, U.S. and Nultsch, W. (1986) Effect of calcium on the viability of the colorless flagellate, *Polytomella magna* under photodynamic stress.(Unpublished, work done at Botanisches Institute, Fachbereich Biologie der Philipps- Universitat, Marburg, Germany) under cultural exchange programme.

Ito, Takashi(1983) Photodynamic agents as tools for cell biology. *In* Photochemical and Photobiological Reviews Vol.7, (*Ed.* K.C. Smith). Plenum Publishing Corporation.

Kumar, H.D. and Nultsch W. (1985) Effects of Saffron extracts and Carotenoids preparations on the photodynamically induced chemotactic response of *Polytomella magna*. Photobiochem and Photobiophy. 9,39-42.

Nultsch, W. and Kumar H.D. (1984) Effects of quenching agents on the photodynamically induced chemotactic response of the colorless flagellate *Polytomella magna*. Photochem. Photobiol. 40, 539-543.

Nultsch, W. Hader M. (1984) Light- induced chemotactic responses of the colourless flagellate *Polytomella magna*, in presence of photodynamic cells. Arch.Microbiol.139: 21-27.

Nishida, K., Wakayama, Y., Takagi, M. and Yano, K. (1980) Inactivation of *E. coli* cells by 1O2 (3) Effects on membrane DNA complex. J Radiat.Res. Abstract, 21:16.

Prebble. J. and Huda, A.S. (1973) Sensitivity of the electron transport chain of pigmented and non-pigmented *Sarcina* membranes to photodynamic action. Photochem. Photobiol. 17: 255-264.

Roberts J.E. (1981) The effects of photoxydation by proflavine on Hela cells I The molecular mechanisms. Photochem.Photobiol.33: 55-59.

Raab, O. (1900) Z. Biol. 39:524-546.

Santomariya, and Prino, G. (1972) List of photodynamic substances. In Research progress in organic, biological and medicinal chemistry Vol.3 (*Ed.* U.Gallo and L. Santamaria). North-Holland, Amsterdam, 11-35.

Spikes, J.D. (1982) Photodynamic reactions in photo medicine in The Science of Photo medicine (*Ed.* J.D. Regan and J.A. Parrish) Plenum Press, New York, 113-144.

Microbiology and Biotechnology for Sustainable Development (Ed. P.C. Jain),
CBS Publishers & Distributors, New Delhi (2004), pp. 166–184.

A-14

Use of Blue-Green Algae and *Azolla* Biofertilizers in Rice Cultivation and their Influence on Soil Properties

B. D. Kaushik
Division of Microbiology, Indian Agricultural Research Institute
New Delhi 110 012.

Abstract

Cyanobacteria play role in contributing organic carbon into the soil was demonstrated by ^{15}N studies. Though the reports indicated that under favorable conditions a good algal bloom in rice fields yields on an average about 6-8 t of fresh biomass. However in tropical rice field soils, 0.03% (672 kg ha^{-1}) increased soil organic carbon content was reported due to encouragement of native algal flora alone in a six months period. BGA are known to excrete extracellularly a number of compounds like polysaccharides, peptides, lipids etc. during their growth in soil. These compounds diffuse around soil particles, glue and hold them together in the form of microaggregates. Besides these compounds, particularly polysaccharides are made of fibers, which can also entangle clay particles and form clusters. These clusters, intern, grow and take the shape of larger soil aggregates. Inoculation with mixture of Cyanobacteria led to a 50-70 percent increased in soil aggregates in Delhi soil. Growth promoting substances from Cyanobacteria include vitamins (niacin 80-320, pentothenic acid 5-10, folic acid 0.79-1.08 and vitamin B_{12} 3.6 X 10^{-3} ng mg $^{-1}$ biomass) and indole – 3 –acetic acid and indole –3 – propionic acid or 3 –Methyl indole in addition to extracellular sugars and amino acids. BGA have the ability to mobilize bound phosphates. They have been shown to solubilise insoluble $(Ca)_3 (PO_4)_2$, $FePO_4$, $AlPO_4$ and hydrooxyapatite ($Ca_5(PO_4)_3.OH$ in soils , sediments or in pure cultures . The solubilising effect of BGA on bound PO_4^{3-} may also be used for the efficient utilization of low cost, low grade (in terms of P contents) rock-phosphate fertilizers were PO_4^{3-} remains. Quantitative estimations of nitrogen fixed by Cyanobacteria varies from region to region however on a conservative estimate Cyanobacteria provide 30-35 kg of biologically fixed N pre hectare per season to a rice crop. Algal biofertilizer is recommended only as a supplement to nitrogenous fertilizers and the supplementation effect remains perceptible even in the presence of high levels of fertilizer nitrogen. The beneficial effects of BGA application have been also shown in cotton, barley, oat, tomato, sugarcane and maize.

Beneficial effects of algalization have been observed in many countries. The work conducted at Indian Agricultural Research Institute New Delhi on rice shows that a) in areas where chemical nitrogen fertilizer is not used for various reasons, algal application as biological input provide to the rice crop the benefit of applying 20-39kg N /ha, b) where fertilizers are used, the dose can be reduced by 30 kg N/ha by algal supplementation, and c) even with high levels of nitrogen fertilizers, the yield per unit input can be increased by 10-15% through algal complementation.

Key words: Blue green algae, Cyanobacteria, nitrogen fixation, growth promoting substances, P-solubilization, organic carbon, rice yield.

INTRODUCTION

The success of rice production in the tropics and subtropics depends on an efficient and economic supply of N, an element required in the largest quantity in comparison with other essential ones. The use efficiency of N from other fertilizer sources in lowland rice is quite low, because of its loss from soil through various chemical and biochemical processes. Besides, increasing the application of nitrogenous fertilizers is neither environmental friendly nor economically viable. It has, therefore, become necessary to look for alternate renewable resources to meet at least a part of the N demand of rice crops. N_2-fixing blue-green algae (BGA) or cyanobacteria and *Azolla*, have been shown to be the most important in maintaining and improving the productivity of rice fields (Venkataraman, 1979; Kaushik, 1994a). It has been demonstrated that the N fertility of soil is sustained better under flooded conditions than under dryland conditions (Watanbe and Roger, 1984). Favourable conditions for biological N_2 fixation by such BGA is considered to be one of the reason for the relatively stable yield of rice under flooded condition. Unlike chemical N-fertilizers, BGA and *Azolla* neither contaminate the environment nor consume the photosynthates of rice plants.

A yield improvement of rice of between 5% and 25% was found when fields were inoculated with BGA even in the presence of 100-150 kg N ha^{-1} as fertilizer (Sprent and Sprent, 1990; Yanni, 1992). Since biological N_2 fixation is known to be inhibited to inorganic N, such an observation may imply that BGA confer other benefits besides adding N to the soils. BGA and *Azolla* in fact, bring about, directly or indirectly, certain changes in the physical, chemical and biological properties of the soil and soil-water interface in rice fields, which are of agronomic importance. The extracellular organic compounds liberated by the algae and the O_2 released due to photosynthesis during their active growth period, and the subsequent addition of biomass after their death, are likely to cause some important changes in the physico-biochemical properties of soil. Prevention of an algae induced pH rise, reduction in water temperature, curbing NH_3 volatilization losses and suppressing weeds under *Azolla* cover are also important effects which may cause some benefits to rice cultures.

Soil Organic Matter

The most important constituent to determine the fertility of a soil is organic carbon. Soils rich in organic carbon are productive as it helps in better nutrient utilization efficiency and checks the nutrients loss through leaching and volatilization. A continuous use of inorganic inputs mainly fertilizers without addition of organic manures like FYM, green manure or compost has led to the depletion of soil carbon reserves in soils of Punjab and Haryana states of India and the soil of these states has reached to the level of becoming unfertile. Under such situations, photosynthetic microorganisms particularly algae and cyanobacteria may play role in contributing organic carbon into the soil. As early as 1950 (De and Sulaiman, 1950) reported a build up of organic matter due to blue green algal inoculation. Later, a number of workers (Fuller and Roger, 1952; Aiyar *et al.*, 1972; Sankaran, 1971; Osmanova, 1979; Das *et al.*, 1991) supported the earlier work. However, wide variations in the reported values of organic carbon or biomass addition by BGA exists (Table 1). A well developed continuous layer of colonies of different species of BGA in rice fields yield a significant amount of biomass. Using $_{15}$N, Nekrasova and Aleksandrova (1982) confirmed that algal biomass contributed significantly to humus formation in soils despite the absence of typical lignin in them. Roger *et al.* (1987) indicated that under favourable conditions a good algal bloom in rice fields yields on an average about 6-8 t of fresh biomass. A 0.03% (672 kg ha^{-1}) increased soil organic carbon content was reported due to encouragement of native algal flora alone under laboratory conditions in a six months period (Kaushik, 1985), whereas inoculation of halotolerant cyanobacterial strains to sodic soils of Andhra Pradesh led to an addition of 5.3 – 7.6 t carbon ha^{-1} in a cropping season (Subhashini and Kaushik, 1984).

Table 1: Addition of organic carbon to soil through blue green algae (BGA).

Quantity t/ha	References
0.75	Prasad, 1949
6.70	Fuller and Roger, 1952
0.5-1.4	Gollerbach *et al.*, 1956
0.45	Rao and Burns, 1990
41.6	Reynaud and Roger, 1981
3.2-6.8	Das *et al.*, 1991

Table 2: Changes of oxidizable C and total N content of soil due to incorporation of blue green algae, *Azolla* and urea (7-35 days of incubation).

Treatments	Total N (%)	Oxidizable carbon (%)
Control	0.0770	0.644
Blue green algae	0.0840	0.674
Azolla	0.0812	0.668
Urea	0.0802	0.622

The enrichment of soils with organic matter due to incorporation or inoculation of *Azolla* is minimal (Nazeer and Prasad, 1984), although a full cover of rice with *Azolla* weighs about 10-20 t ha^{-1}. This is possibly associated with the high decomposibility of *Azolla* biomass, since it contains low amount of lignin (<5%), particularly at a young stage, when it is usually incorporated in to soils. Lales and Marte (1986) observed no significant increase in soil organic matter content inspite of five consecutive crops of rice with *Azolla* on Maahas clay soil of the Philippines. However, Singh and Singh (1987) reported a significant increase in the organic carbon content in soils due to successive *Azolla* cropping with rice. The changes in the oxidizable C and N content of soil due to incorporation of cyanobacteria and *Azolla* are given in Table 2.

Improvement in soil physical properties

At the time of puddling before transplanting rice seedlings, the soil structure is completely destroyed. The inoculation of rice fields with BGA may help to quickly regenerate and improve the soil structure (Roychoudhury *et al.*, 1979). BGA are known to excrete extracellularly a number of compound like polysaccharides, peptides, lipids etc. during their growth in soil (Misra and Kaushik, 1989 a, b; Saxena and Kaushik, 1992; Bertocchi *et al.*,1990). These compounds possibly diffuse around soil particles, glue and hold them together in the form of microaggregates. Besides these compounds, particularly polysaccharides, are made of fibers which can also entangle clay particles and form clusters. These clusters or microaggregates, in turn, grow and take the shape of macroaggregates and subsequently of larger soil aggregates. The interwoven nature of growing algal filaments may also help in binding the soil particles along with the organic C added through algal biomass. The importance of these compounds in soil-aggregate formation or soil stabilisation has been indicated by many workers (Roychoudhury *et al.*, 1979; Schulten, 1985; Rogers *et al.*, 1991; Rogers and Burns 1994). Some researchers, however, have considered polysaccharides as transient adhesives (Tisdall and Oades, 1982) and or not directly involved in the formation of aggregates, although the products of their microbial degradation like aliphatic and polyphenolic compounds are considered to be responsible for this (Haynes *et al.*, 1991). The quantity and quality of the excreted compounds also vary depending on the species of BGA, their physiological growth stages and also the associated environmental conditions (Saxena and Kaushik, 1992; Roychoudhury *et al.*, 1985). Some species give low yields of excreted compounds (e.g. *Anabaena*), while other give high yields (e.g. *Gloeotrichia, Westiellopsis*). Polysaccharides from different algal species also differ with respect to their protein, uronic acid and sugar composition (Bertocchi *et al.*, 1990) and thus in their stability in soils with respect to microbial and thermal degradation.

Kaushik and his co-workers (Kaushik and Krishna Murty, 1981; Subhashini and Kaushik, 1984; Kaushik, 1985) observed significant increases in the values of soil aggretate stability (measured as the resistance of aggregates to degradation during wetting and physical disruption) due to an increase in the polysaccharide content of soils as a result of algal inoculation (Table 3). Similarly, water-stable aggregates, which are an integral part of good (soil) aggregate formation, have also been shown to increase significantly due to algal inoculation, resulting in an improvement in the water-holding capacity and aeration status of soils (Singh, 1961; Roychoudhury *et al.*, 1979). Further, Singh (1961) reported that the mucilaginous thalli of *Aphanothece* sp. formed a compact grey substratum firmly holding the soil particles together which checked both wind and water-mediated soil erosion, particularly, in light and sandy soils subjected to heavy grazing. Such improvement in soil aggregation due to algal inoculation ultimately favoured better seedling emergence of upland crops sown after the paddy harvest (Rogers and Burns, 1994). All these results apparently suggest that the algal species, which liberate higher amounts of complex and thermostable polysaccharides, will possibly be a better choice for inoculation in rice fields for the regeneration of the soil structure. However, such algal species are known to be less efficient N_2 fixers.

Use of *Azolla* as green manure is also reported to improve soil physical properties by increasing the porosity (3.7-4.2%) and decreasing the specific gravity of soils. Long-term plots at IRRI have shown that the bulk density of the soil decreases with continued *Azolla* use (Kumarsinghe and Eskew, 1993; Ventura and Watanabe, 1993).

O_2 concentration and associated changes

BGA are aerobic photosynthetic organisms. In the medium of their growth, they release a lot of O_2 during photosynthesis through photosystem II. As a result, when they grow in rice fields they make the standing water highly oxygenated. This is an important beneficial effect in areas where rice is grown continuously throughout the year under flooded conditions in soils with relatively high organic matter contents. In these areas, continuous water-logging creating reducing conditions with redox potential values falling below 200 mV (Ponnamperuma, 1972). These conditions favour the formation and subsequent accumulation of a high amount of harmful oxidizable organic matter, a large quantity of Fe^{2+} and also S^2 which sometimes reach toxicity levels for rice plants (Aiyer *et al.*, 1971a, b). Inoculation of rice fields with BGA under such conditions may be helpful in regulating the formation of such toxic substances by maintaining the redox potential at a relatively high level. In fact, Aiyer *et al.* (1972) reported a significant reduction in the oxidizable organic matter, total S^2 and Fe^{2+} content of soils after four successive rice crops with BGA inoculation. A high O_2 tension in the soil, arising from algal photosynthesis, seems to facilitate the oxidation of these reduced components.

Table 3: Comparative effect of blue green algae and *Azolla* on soil aggregation and particle size distribution (Roychoudhury *et. al.*, 1979).

Treatments	Particle size distribution		% aggregates		% increase > 50 μ aggregates
	> 250 μ	50-250 μ	> 250 μ	50-250 μ	
Sand (>50μ)	0.5	44.5	-	-	-
Control	1.2	46.8	0.7	2.3	-
BGA	1.5	48.0	1.0	3.5	50
Azolla	1.0	47.0	0.5	2.5	-
60 kg N ha^{-1}	0.7	46.6	0.2	2.1	-
60 kg N ha^{-1}+BGA	1.6	49.0	1.1	4.5	70
60 kg N ha^{-1}+*Azolla*	0.8	47.2	0.3	2.7	-

As mentioned above, the establishment of a comparatively thick aerobic layer on the surface due to algal layer and the existence of an anaerobic, reduced layer below provide a highly favourable environment for the nitrification-denitrification process to proceed. When applied or native NH_4^+ N in soil comes into contact with this oxygenated surface layer, it is converted to NO_3^- N which on diffusion to the anaerobic layer is subjected to the process of denitrification by denitrifiers and is lost as gaseous N.

The growth of *Azolla* in rice fields also causes changes in the composition of floodwater and the soils underneath owing to variations in the light-transmission ratio (LTR) and photosynthetic activity. Krock *et al.* (1988) observed a drop in the O_2 concentration and pH to the extent of 3-8 μg g^{-1} and 1.4 units, respectively in rice-field floodwater due to *Azolla* growth. Such changes may also affect N transformation in soils. Denitrification may be reduced by the *Azolla* cover due to a thinner oxidised soil layer, a consequence of the lower O_2 concentration in floodwater and decreased oxidation of NH_4^+ to NO_3^- at lower pH values (Focht, 1979) and O_2 concentrations.

In a study conducted by Saha *et al.* (1982) comparing the availability of N through BGA, *Azolla* and urea to the rice crop observed that available N (as $NH_4^+ + NO_3 + NO_2$ - N) was gradually increased in concentration due to the decomposition of incorporated BGA and *Azolla* but a reverse trend existed with urea N. The release of N in an available form from urea to soil is more rapid than from BGA to *Azolla.* However, subsequent losses of N from the soil by nitrification and denitrification occur more quickly because of the presence of an aerobic layer overlying an anaerobic layer in flooded rice soil. The release of available N was more rapid from *Azolla* than from BGA throughout the incubation (Table 4). The greater release of *Azolla*-N compared to BGA is obviously due to its rapid decomposition in soil.

Table 4: Changes in available N in soil due to incorporation of blue green algae, *Azolla* and urea (Saha *et al.*, 1982).

Days of flooding	Treatments mg N g^{-1} soil			
	Control	Blue green algae	*Azolla*	Urea
7	5.08	13.28	17.06	23.86
14	8.46	23.59	14.85	16.33
21	7.99	23.58	21.78	15.38
28	14.10	29.79	29.70	20.12
35	10.10	33.02	29.70	13.49
LSD at 5%	Treatments mean 2.52	Days mean 2.82	Interaction 5.64	

Total N of blue green algae, 66 μg N g^{-1} soil; *Azolla*, 29μg N g^{-1} soil; urea, 25μg N g^{-1} soil.

Growth-promoting effect

The effect of BGA inocula on the yield of crops in the presence of N fertilisers has commonly been ascribed to the production of growth-promoting substances by these organisms (Brown *et al.*, 1956; Kopteva, 1970; Tupik, 1973). A large number of researchers have found better growth and germination of seeds of many crop plants after treating them with algal cultures or their extracts. The majority of them observed an enhancement in rice-seed germination, root and shoot growth, weight of rice grains and their protein content (Shukla and Gupta, 1967; Venkataraman and Neelakantan, 1967; Singh and Trehan, 1973; Jacq and Roger, 1977; Misra and Kaushik, 1989a, b); while others found similar stimulatory effects on wheat (Gupta *et al.*, 1967). Tomato (Kaushik and Venkataraman, 1979; Rodgers *et al.*, 1979) radish (Rodgers *et al.*, 1979; Vorontsova *et al.*, 1988), peas (Gupta and Gupta, 1972), banana (Ganapathi *et al.*, 1994) etc. A few negative effects on the germination of rice seeds have also been documented (Pedurand and Reynaud, 1987). Different opinions exist regarding the nature of these substances. Some have described them as hormones, i.e. gibberelin-like (Singh and Trehan, 1973) cytokinin-like (Rodgers *et al.*, 1979), auxin-like (Ahmad and Winter, 1968) or abscisic acids (Marsalek *et al.*, 1992); while others have described them either as vitamins particularly vitamin B (Grieco and Desrochers, 1978) or as amino acids (Watanable, 1951; Vorontsova *et al.*, 1988), antibiotics and toxins (Metting and Pyne, 1986). The production of these substances is however, influenced by different stress factors (Marsalek *et al.*, 1992) as well as the application of chemicals particularly Co-salts (Venkataraman and Neelankantan, 1967). Mutants of some species produce more of these substances than indigenous types (Vorontsova *et al.*, 1988). However, detailed quantitative and qualitative analyses of these substances produced by different BGA species was given by Kaushik and coworkers. They reported the different vitamins in the range of ng mg^{-1} biomass: niacin 80-320, pantothenic acid 5-10, folic acid 0.79-1.08 and vitamin B_{12} 3.6 x 10^{-3} in *Nostoc muscorum* and *Hapalosiphon fontinalis,* and stimulation in the root and shoot growth was observed with folic acid, vitamin B_{12} and pantothenic acid but not with nicotinic acid (Misra and Kaushik, 1989a). Similarly the growth hormones like indole-3-acetic acid and indole-3-propionic acid or 3-Methyl indole were identified and quantified in addition to extracellular sugars and amino acids (Misra and Kaushik, 1989b).

Transformation of soil P

BGA, like P-solubilizing bacteria, are known to have the ability to mobilize bound phosphates. They have been shown to solubilise insoluble $(Ca)_3(PO_4)_2$ (Bose *et al.*, 1971). $FePO_4$ (Wolf *et al.*, 1985), $AlPO_4$ (Dorich *et al.*, 1985) and hydroxyapatite ($Ca_5(PO_4)_3.OH$; Cameron and Julian, 1988) in soils, sediments or in pure cultures. There are mainly two hypothesis, proposed by two groups to explain how BGA solubilise such bound phosphates. One group suggested that they might synthesise a chelator (chelators?) Ca^{2+} and drive the following dissolution reaction to the right without changing the pH of the growth medium (Cameron and Julian, 1988; Roychoudhury and Kaushik, 1989):

$$Ca_{10}(OH)_2(PO_4)_6 = 10Ca^{2+} + 2OH + 6PO_4^{3+}$$

Others (Bose *et al.*, 1971) were however of the opinion that H_2CO_3 and other organic acids released by BGA during their growth could solubilise P from Ca sources following the reaction:

$$Ca_3(PO_4)_2 + 2H_2CO_3 = 2CaHPO_4 + Ca(HCO_3)_2$$

A third group (Arora, 1969; Saha and Mandal, 1979; Mandal *et al.*, 1992) believed that the above mechanisms operate simultaneously. Once solubilised, the PO_4^3 is taken up by the growing algal cells for their nutrition. After completing their growth cycle, when the cells undergo lysis the cell-bound PO_4^3 is released in the growth medium and becomes available to plants on mineralisation. Observance of an initial decrease in the available-P content in soils due to algal growth and an appreciable increase later during biomass decomposition (Saha and Mandal, 1979; Mandal *et al.*, 1992) supported this possible pathway.

Decomposition of the algal biomass also intensifies the reducing conditions of soil (Saha *et al.*, 1982) and stimulates the reduction of Fe^{3+} P to the more soluble Fe^{2+} P. This also results in the formation of various organic compounds which have chelating properties which may form chelates with Al and Fe and thus release Al- and Fe-bound forms. Inoculation with BGA may, therefore be useful in making bound P available to plants. When P in the form of water-soluble fertiliser is applied to soils, particularly lateritic ones rich in Fe and A1, it gets quickly converted to its insoluble froms, such as $FePO_4$. $AIPO_4$, $Ca_3(PO_4)_2$, $Ca_5(PO_4)_3.OH$ etc. and becomes unavailable to plants. The solubilising effects of BGA may lead to their reconversion into available forms.

The solubilising effect of BGA on bound PO_4^{3-} may also be used for the efficient utilisation of low cost, low grade (in terms of P content) rock-phsophate fertilisers where PO_4^{3-} remains bound as various forms of apatite, like hydroxyapatite, carbonapatite, choloroapatite etc. These rock phsophates are generally used in acid soils as P fertiliser. It is possible that if rock phosphate is used with BGA inoculation in acid soils, its efficacy as a source of P may be increased. In fact, Roychoudhury and Kaushik (1989) reported increased solubility of P in rock phosphate (Mussorie) due to its inoculation with BGA.

Fuller and Roger (1952) observed a greater uptake of P by plants from algal materials than from inorganic phosphates when applied in equal amounts. They concluded that: (1) P in algal material is more available to plants than inorganic phosphates over longer periods, (2) chemical fixation is not so important a factor with respect to algal material as with respect to inorganic phosphates, and (3) temporary conversion of available soil or fertilizer P into cell materials by soil algae may be a desirable process from the stand-point of long-term availability. Their proposed hypothesis was that soil algae removed available P from the sphere of chemical fixation by converting it into cell materials for by absorbing it in "luxury" amounts that might be released gradually for crop use through the process of exudation,

Table 5: Changes of available P μg g^{-1} soil due to incorporation of blue green algae, *Azolla* and urea

Days of flooding	Control	Blue green algae	*Azolla*	Urea
7	7.50	7.92	9.37	9.08
14	3.58	3.94	4.89	4.48
21	5.32	13.55	13.97	6.29
28	6.97	14.06	18.45	7.90
35	7.45	10.89	11.62	7.85
LSD at 5%	Treatment mean 1.19		Days mean 1.33	Interaction 2.66

autolysis or microbial decomposition of old algal cells. Algae also have long been known to take up P in excess of their immediate needs, which may subsequently be released in the form of dissolved organic P (Lean and Nalewajko, 1976).

Like BGA, the incorporation of *Azolla* in to rice fields also increases P availability in soils (Singh *et al.*, 1981; Saha *et al.*, 1982; Singh and Singh, 1987; Nagarajah *et al.*, 1989). This has been attributed to the decomposition of *Azolla*'s biomass, rich in organic forms of P and the subsequent release of P in the form of available P. Other possible mechanisms for increased P availability in soils on the decomposition of *Azolla* biomass may be reduction and chelation. Increased availability of P in soils on incorporation of *Azolla* ultimately increases the uptake of P by rice plants (Singh and Singh, 1987) and their P concentrations (Table 5).

Amelioration of saline and sodic soils

Saline and sodic soils constitute a large area of agricultural land in the world. Besides, a good part of prime agricultural land becomes saline every year due to poor and faulty management/irrigation practices. Sodic soils have a high pH, high exchangeable Na, measurable amounts of carbonates and undergo extensive clay dispersion (deflocculation, due to the high zeta potential of active Na^+), leading to poor hydraulic conductivity and reduced soil aeration. While saline soils contain excess amounts of soluble salts imparting high osmotic tension to plant roots for absorption of water and nutrients. Primarily, the reclamation of sodic soils requires the replacement of exchangeable Na with Ca. This is normally done by the application of suitable soil amendments, like gypsum, followed by leaching. The improvement of saline soils, on the other hand, requires leaching of excess soluble salts from the rhizosphere by good quality water. Reports of biological reclamation of these soils through the use of BGA are available (Singh, 1950; Kaushik, 1989). These methods of reclamation were possibly based on the observations of extensive growth of BGA on alkali or "*Usar*" soils of India (Singh, 1950) and on the salted "*takyr*" soils of the the USSR (Gollerbach *et al.*, 1956). These observations indicated a considerable tolerance of BGA to salinity and/or alkalinity stress. Several physiological mechanisms underlying such tolerance have now been identified. Curtailment of Na^+ influx (Subhashini and Kaushik, 1986; Apte *et al.*, 1987) and accumulation of K^+ ion (Jha *et al.*, 1987) or organic (sugar, polyols and quaternary amines etc.) osmoregulators (Blumwald *et al.*, 1983; Reed *et al.*, 1984; Kumar and Kaushik, 1994) are the important mechanisms that provide adequate protection to BGA against such salt/sodicity stress. Synthesis of salt stress specific fatty acids (Senthil *et al.*, 1993; Gautam *et al.*, 1994; Venkataraman and Kaushik, 1994) and proteins (Goel *et al.*, 1997) has been detected in several species of algae and cyanobacteria. BGA exposed to such salinity/sodicity stress may lose or have diminished nitrogenase activity possibly due to the diversion of their cellular energy towards the biosynthesis of osmoregulators (Apte *et al.*, 1987), while Jha *et al.* (1987) reported enhanced heterocyst frequency in *Westiellopsis prolifica* under salinity suggesting the increased nitrogen demand of organism to overcome the stress. In such cases, the addition of a few kilograms of N, particularly as NO_3 per hectare together with algal inoculation has been shown to be very effective in protecting them from these stresses and allowing them to establish in the stressed environment, and subsequently enhances their potential as N biofertilizer (Reddy *et al.*, 1989; Fernandes *et al.*, 1993). Once established and subsequently acclimatised to the stress, they may act in ameliorating their surrounding environment. Singh (1961) observed in laboratory experiments over a 3-year period a significant improvement in soil properties of saline-alkali soils after algal growth compared with the control covered with a black cloth. The soil pH decreased from 9.2 to 7.5 along with large increases in organic matter content (69%), total N (46%), water-holding capacity (35%), exchangeable Ca (31%) and different forms of P. A reduction in electrical conductivity, exchangeable Na and soil pH (Kaushik *et al.*, 1981; Kaushik and Subhashini, 1985) and an increase in the soluble Ca and Mg content of soils (Jain and Kaushik, 1989) have also been reported due to such algalization. The increase in soluble Ca and Mg and decrease in exchangeable Na may ultimately lower the sodium adsorption ratio – an index of alkalinity in soil – of the soils and thus alleviate the negative effects of high sodicity. In fact, Kaushik and his co-workers (Kaushik and Krishna Murthi, 1981; Subhashini and Kaushik, 1981) observed a considerable increase in the hydraulic conductivity of sodic soils due to BGA inoculation and found that it compared favourably to the use of gypsum in such soils.

A significant reduction in soil salinity (12-35%) due to repeated cultivation of *Anabaena torulosa* in soils rendered saline owing to bad farm management has also been reported (Thomas, 1977). The rice yield in saline soils is also less affected when N is given in the form of algal inocula vis-à-vis urea (Antarikanonda and Amarit, 1991). Further, such algal inocula have proved to be almost equally effective in increasing the rice yield in saline soils when compared with gypsum and/or pyrite treatments (Sharma *et al.*, 1989; Kaushik 1994b). Even when irrigated with saline water, BGA inoculation was found to be useful in minimising the deleterious effect of the increased salinity on the barley crop (Jain and Kaushik, 1989).

However, Rao and Burns (1991) opined that the then current arguments favouring BGA as a biological amendment for the reclamation of alkali soil, in particularly, were untenable. In a highly alkali soil inoculated with a mixture of seven species of BGA for 11 and 17 weeks they observed no significant changes with respect to the control in hydraulic conductivity, pH, exchangeable Na, exchangeable Ca and exchangeable Na percentage - whose changes are the essential requirements for alkali soil reclamation.

In an alkali soil almost all the problems with respect to rice cultivation are associated with the high concentration and/or activities of Na^+. If somehow its activity is checked, the whole problem is solved. BGA are quite tolerant to high alkalinity and can take up appreciable amounts of Na^+ (although disagreement exists regarding their high Na^+ absorption capacity; Apte and Thomas, 1986) (Subhashini and Kaushik, 1981; Roychoudhury *et al.*, 1985). They secrete organic acids particularly under salt stress (Singh, 1961; Sprent and Sprent, 1990) which can act on $CaCO_3$ to dissolve Ca. They also excrete a number of biologically active compounds, i.e. bioflocculants (Jha *et al.*, 1987; Levy *et al.*, 1992), which can flocculate the dispersed clay particles in alkali soils by inactivating/scavenging Na^+. All these effects of BGA may at least temporarily cause inactivation of Na^+ in alkali soils and make the soil environment favourable to the growth of plants. Successive cultivation of BGA makes the environment more favourable and after a few years it may help to produce a reasonably good yield of crops as observed by Singh (1961) for sugarcane after 3 years of reclamation with BGA. Although such biological soil amelioration is a time-consuming process, it is considered to be a sustainable approach as compared to reclamation by chemical amendments (Oikarinen, 1996). What is needed is to improve the reclamation technique with BGA by integrating its application with the use of a few hundred kilograms of gypsum per hectare (excess Ca also depresses algal growth) and selection of a suitable profusely growing and alkaline and/or saline-tolerant species of BGA *viz. Nostoc commue, Anabaena torulosa, Westiellopsis prolifica* etc. Besides, there is a good possibility of the use of genetically manipulated species of BGA tolerant of high salinity or high alkalinity for such reclamation in the near future since a few strongly alkaliphilic and saline-tolerant species have already been engineered (Apte and Haselkorn, 1990; Singh *et al.*, 1991, 1996). Detailed feasibility studies may be initiated to this end using those engineered species in order to develop a low cost and sustainable technology for the amelioration of saline/sodic soils.

Crop response

A large variety of cyanobacterial strains colonize the rice field soils and some are endowed with the capacity to fix atmospheric nitrogen. In cyanobacteria, under aerobic conditions nitrogen fixation occurs in specialized cells, called heterocysts. These structures have thick walls which allows the restricted entry of oxygen, and also lack photosystem II (Thomas, 1970). Not only heterocystous, but also non-heterocystous blue green algae are also capable of fixing nitrogen under microaerophillic conditions (Stewart *et al.*, 1979; Prasanna and Kaushik, 1994). Virtually all the dominant cyanobacteria in rice fields are nitrogen fixing, and that gives the indication how rice has been grown continuously for many centuries without the addition of fertilizer (Watanabe *et al.*, 1987). The relative contribution of BGA as a percentage of total nitrogen fixed in the paddy fields varies widely and is mainly dependent on the chemical, climatic and biotic factors. Tropical conditions ensure increased incidence of cyanobacteria in the rice fields soils and high humidity and temperature and shade provided by the crop canopy favor the luxuriant growth of cyanobacteria (Roger and Reynaud, 1979). Beneficial effects of algalization have been observed in many countries (El-Nawaway and Hamdi, 1975; Mishustin and Petrova, 1972; Kundu and Ladha, 1995). Quantitative estimations from different countries are: Philippines 18-33 kg/ha (De and Biswas, 1952; Singh 1961; Venkataraman, 1979), Senegal 0-30 kg/ha (Renaud and Roger, 1978), Mali 50-80 kg/ha (Traore *et al.*, 1978) and Japan 11-23 kg/ha (Okuda and Yamaguchi, 1955). *In situ* estimations using ARA technique have shown an addition of 18-45 Kg N ha^{-1} yr^{-1} due to activity of diazotrophic cyanobacteria (Watanabe and Cholitkul, 1979). The work conducted at Indian Agriculture Research Institute, New Delhi shows that a) in areas where chemical nitrogen fertiliser is not used for various reasons, algal application as biological input can give to the rice farmers the benefit of applying 20-30 kg N/ha, b) where fertilisers are used, the dose can be reduced by 30kg N/ha by algal supplementation, and c) even with high levels of nitrogen fertilisers, the yield per unit input can be increased by 10-15% through algal complementation. Algal biofertilizer is recommended only as a supplement to nitrogenous fertilizers and the supplementation effects remains perceptible even in the presence of high levels of fertilizer nitrogen (Venkataraman, 1978, 1979). Yoshida *et al.* (1973) reported 40-80 Kg N ha^{-1} through algal application. The water layer with extensive floating colonies of *Gloeotrichia* spp. in Moroccan rice fields has been found to show high rates of nitrogen fixing activity (44 nmoles C_2H_4 ml^{-1} hr^{-1}) (Reynault *et al.*, 1975). In long term field trials it was observed that at different levels of ammonium sulphate, algal supplementation increased the number of productive tillers as well as total grain yield (Aiyer *et al.*, 1972). Immobilized cyanobacteria also increased grain yield in paddy fields (Kannaiyan *et al.*, 1997). Even in the temperate soils, nitrogen fixation by algae is substantial. Henriksson (1971) showed annual fixation rate of 15-51 Kg N ha^{-1} yr^{-1} in an agricultural field where *Nostoc* was abundant, and 4.44 Kg N ha^{-1} yr^{-1} in a lakeside meadow containing *Nostoc, Anabaena, Cylindrospermum* and *Calothrix*. Umarova and Uromanov (1972) and Kogan and Osmanova (1972) using algae both in the presence and absence of nitrogen increased the yield of cotton in USSR. Such beneficial effects have been observed in barley, oat (Shtina, 1965), tomato (Kaushik and Venkataraman, 1979), sugarcane and maize (Singh, 1961), and also on wheat and Pea.

Using ^{15}N , Reynault *et al.* (1975) have also shown that at least some of the nitrogen fixed and liberated by *Westiellopsis prolifica* is assimilated by rice plant. Direct proof of transfer of nitrogen from the alga to the rice plant has come from ^{15}N studies (Venkataraman, 1978). Roger *et al.* (1987) suggested that attention should be given to agricultural practices that enhance the growth of endogenous strains already adapted to local environmental conditions. All that is needed is to identify and develop promising region specific stress compatible strains and place quality inoculum within easy reach of farmers. The efficiency of utilization of fixed nitrogen by rice plant is often low (Watanabe, 1984) and efforts should be made to isolate suitable strains of cyanobacteria that would provide fixed nitrogen and excrete it continuously making it available to rice plants (Boussiba, 1988). The overall conclusion is that nitrogen fixation may be an important N input in the N cycle of the rice fields and could lessen pollution problems by lowering the demand for chemical fertilizers (Quesada *et al.*, 1997). Nitrogen fixed by BGA is released either through exudation or through microbial

Table 6: Effect of different N sources and method of application (40 kg ha^{-1}) and *Azolla* on grain yield and N uptake of rice variety IR 36 (Manna and Singh, 1991).

Treatments	Wet season, 1986				Dry season 1986			
	Yield t ha^{-1}		N uptake kg ha^{-1}		Yield t ha^{-1}		N uptake kg ha^{-1}	
	- *Azolla*	+ Azolla	- *Azolla*	+ *Azolla*	- *Azolla*	+ *Azolla*	- *Azolla*	+ *Azolla*
O N	2.7	-	46	-	2.8	-	48	-
Sub-surface								
Urea	3.3	3.6	57	61	3.5	3.9	59	67
Am. Sulphate	3.6	4.0	64	69	3.7	4.3	63	72
Broadcasting								
Urea	3.0	3.3	53	57	3.3	3.6	56	61
Am. Sulphate	3.2	3.6	57	62	3.4	3.7	58	65
LSD (0.05)	0.2		2.0		0.2		2.0	

LSD, Least significant difference

decomposition after the BGA die. In paddy fields the death of algal biomass is most frequently associated with soil desiccation at the end of the cultivation cycle and algal growth has frequently resulted in a gradual build up of soil fertility with a residual effect on succeeding crop also. The pattern of distribution of total organic and mineral nitrogen studied in inoculated and uninoculated plots indicated a higher mineral nitrogen content and a low mineralisable index of N in the inoculated plots, a phenomenon very much desirable for slow release of soil reserve (Chopra and Dube, 1971).

Like blue green algae, the use of *Azolla* in rice crop has shown significant increase in crop yield. Crop response in terms of grain yield was reported to be influenced significantly by the methods of application, sources of N and the cropping season. Grain yields due to *Azolla* were higher in the dry season than the wet season. The subsurface application of ammonium sulphate recorded the highest grain yield irrespective of seasons and *Azolla* use (Table 6).

REFERENCES

Ahmad, M.R. and Winter, A. (1968). Studies on the hormonal relationship of algae in pure culture. 1. The effect of indole-3-acetic acid on the growth of blue-green and green algae. *Planta*, 78: 277-286.

Aiyer, R.S., Aboobekar, V.O., Venkataraman, G.S. and Goyal, S.K. (1971a). Effect of algalization on soil properties and yield of IR8 rice variety. *Phykos,* 10: 34-39.

Aiyer, R.S., Aboobekar, V.O. and Subramoney, N. (1971b). Effect of blue-green algae in suppressing sulphide injury to rice crop in submerged soils. *Madras Agric J.*, 58: 405-407.

Aiyer, R.S., Salahudden, S. and Venkataraman, G.S. (1972). Long term algalization field trial with high yielding varieties of rice (*Oryza sativa* L.) *Indian J Agric Sci*, 42: 380-383.

Antarikanonda, P. and Amarit, P. (1991). Influence of blue-green algae and nitrogen fertilizer on rice yield in saline soils. *Kasetsart J. Nat. Sci.*, 25: 18-25.

Apte. S.K. and Thomas, J. (1986). Membrane electrogenesis and sodium transport in filamentous nitrogen-fixing cyanobacteria. *Eur. J. Biochem.*, 154: 395-401.

Apte, S.K. and Haselkorn, R. (1990). Cloning of salinity stress-induced genes from salt tolerant nitrogen-fixing cyanobacterium *Anabaena torulosa*. *Plant Mol. Biol.*, 15: 723-733.

Apte, S.K., Reddy, B.R. and Thomas, J. (1987). Relationship between sodium influx and salt tolerance of nitrogen-fixing cyanobacteria. *Appl. Environ. Microbiol.*, 53: 1934-1939.

Arora, S.K. (1969). The role of algae on the availability of phosphorus in paddy fields. *Riso* 18: 135-138.

Bertocchi, C, Navarini, L, Cesarp, A. and Anastasio, M. (1990). Polysaccharides from cyanobacteria. *Carbohydr. Polym.,* 12: 127-153.

Blumwald, E., Mehlhorn, R.J. and Packer, L. (1983). Studies of osmoregulation in salt-adaptation of cyanobacteria with ESR spin-probe techniques. *Proc. Natl. Acad. Sci.* USA, 80: 2599-2602.

Bose, P., Nagpal, U.S., Venkataraman, G.S. and Goyal, S.K. (1971). Solubilisation of tricalcium phosphate by blue-green algae. *Curr. Sci.*, 40: 165-166.

Boussiba, S. (1988). N_2 Fixing cyanobacteria as nitrogen biofertilizer, a study with the isolate *Anabaena azollae. Symbiosis*, 6:129-138.

Brown, F., Cuthbertson, W.F.J and Fogg, G.E. (1956). Vitamin B_{12} activity of *Chlorella vulgaris* Beij and *Anabaena cylindrica* Lemm. *Nature*, 177: 188.

Cameron, H.J. and Julian, G.R. (1988). Utilisation of hydroxyapatite by cyanobacteria as their sole source of phosphate and calcium. *Plant Soil*, 109:123-124.

Chopra, T.S and Dube, J.N. (1971). Changes of N content of a rice soil inoculated with *Tolypothrix tenuis. Plant and Soil*, 35: 453-462.

Das, S.C., Mandal, B. and Mandal, L.N. (1991). Effect of growth and subsequent decomposition of blue green algae on the transformation of iron and manganese in submerged soils. *Plant Soil*, 138: 75-84.

De, P.K. and Biswas, N.R.D. (1952). Fixation of nitrogen in rice soils in the dry period. *Indian J. Agri. Sci.* 22: 375-388.

De, P.K. and Sulaiman, M. (1950). Fixation of nitrogen in rice soils by algae as influenced by crop, CO_2 and inorganic substances. *Soil Sci.*, 70:137-151.

Dorich, R.A., Nelson, D.W., Sommers, L.E. (1985). Estimating algal-available phosphorus in suspended sediments by chemical extraction. *J. Environ Qual*, 14:400-405.

El-Nawawy, A.S. and Hamdi, Y.A. (1975). In: *Nitrogen fixation by free living organisms*, WDP Stewart (ed) p 219, Camb. University Press, Cambridge.

Fernandes, T.A., Iyer, V. and Apte, S.K. (1993). Differential responses of nitrogen-fixing cyanobacteria to salinity and osmotic stresses. *Appl. Environ. Microbiol*, 59: 899-904.

Focht, D.D. (1979). Microbial kinetics of nitrogen losses in flooded soils In: *Nitrogen and rice* IRRI. Manila. pp. 119-134.

Fuller, W.H. and Roger, R.N. (1952). Utilisation of the phosphorus of algal cells as measured by the Neubauer technique. *Soil Sci*, 74: 417-429.

Ganpati, T.R., Suprasanna, P., Bapat, V.A. and Rao, P.S. (1994). Stimulatory effect of cyanobacterial extract on banana shoot tip cultures. *Trop Agric* (Trinidad), 71: 299-302.

Gautam, M., Madan, T.R. and Kaushik, B.D. (1994). Lipid profile of *Dunaliella maritima* in response to salinity stress. *Indian J Plant Physiol.*, 37: 256-258.

Goel, S., Mamta, M. and Kaushik, B.D. (1997). Nitrogen fixation and protein profile of halotolerant *Nostoc muscorum*-R strain isolated from rice fields and ARM 221 strain. *Indian J exptl Biol.*, 35: 746-750.

Gollerbach, M.M., Novichkova, L.A. and Sdubrikova, N.Y. (1956). The algae of takyrs. In: *Takyrs of western Turkmenia and routes of their agricultural conquest. Nauk. Moscow*, pp. 22-29.

Grieco, E. and Desrochers, R. (1978). Production de vitamine B_{12} parune algae belue. *Can J. Microbiol*, 24: 1562-1566.

Gupta, A.B. and Gupta, K.K. (1972). Effect of *Phormidium* extract on growth and yield of *Vigna catjang* (cowpea) T.5369. *Hydrobiologia*, 40: 127:132.

Gupta, A.B., Agarwal, V. and Kushwaha, A.S. (1967). The effect of algal growth-promoting substances on wheat. *Proc. Natl. Acad. Sci.* India, 37B: 349-355.

Haynes, R.J., Swift, R.S. and Stephen, R.C. (1991). Influence of mixed cropping rotations (pasturearable) on organic matter content, water-stable aggregation and cold porosity in a group of soils. *Soil Till Res*, 19: 77-87.

Henriksson, E. (1971). In: *Biological nitrogen fixation in natural and agricultural habitats*, TA Lie, EG Mulder (ed) p. 415, *Plant and Soil*, Special Volume.

Jacq, V. and Roger, P.A. (1977). Decrease of losses due to sulphate reducing processes in the spermosphere of rice by pre-soaking seeds in a culture of blue-green algae. *Cah ORSTOM Ser Biol*, 12: 101-108.

Jain, B.L. and Kaushik, B.D. (1989). Effect of algalization on crop response under saline irrigation. *J. Indian Soc Soil Sci.*, 37: 382-384.

Jha, M.N., Venkataraman, G.S. and Kaushik, B.D. (1987). Response of *Westiellopis prolofica* and *Anabaena* sp. to salt stress. *Mircen J. Appl. Microbiol Biotechnol*, 3: 307-317.

Kannaiyan, S., Aruna, S.J., Kumari, S.M.P. and Hall, D.O. (1997). Immobilized cyanobacteria as a biofertilizer for rice crops. *J. Appl. Phycol.*, 9, 167-174.

Kaushik, B.D. (1985). Effect of native algal flora on nutritional and physico-chemical properties of sodic soils. *Acta Bot Indica*, 13: 143-147.

Kaushik, B.D. (1989). Reclamative potential of cyanobacteria in salt-affected soils. *Phykos*, 28: 101-109.

Kaushik, B.D. (1994a). Blue green algae and sustainable agriculture. In: *Natural Resource Management for sustainable Agriculture and Environment*, (*Ed.* D.L. Deb) Angkor Publishers, New Delhi, pp. 404-416.

Kaushik, B.D. (1994b). Algalization of rice in salt-affected soils. *Ann.Agril. Res.*, 15: 105-106.

Kaushik, B.D and Venkataraman, G.S. (1979). Effect of algal inoculation on the yield and vitamin C content of two varieties of tomato. *Plant and Soil*, 52: 135-137.

Kaushik, B.D. and Krishna Murti, G.S.R. (1981). Effect of blue green algae and gypsum application on physico-chemical properties of alkali soils. *Phykos*, 20: 91-94.

Kaushik, B.D. and Subhashini, D. (1985). Amelioration of salt affected soils with blue green algae. II. Improvement in soil properties. *Proc Indian natn Sci Acad.* B 51: 386-389.

Kaushik, B.D., Krishna Murti, G.S.R. and Venkataraman, G.S. (1981). Influence of blue-green algae on saline alkali soils. *Sci. Cult.*, 47: 169-170.

Kogan, Sh. I. and Osmanova, R.S. (1972). In : *Methods of study and practical use of soil algae. Report Kirov. Agri. Inst.*, Kirov. p 195.

Kopteva, Z.H.P. (1970). Biosynthesis of thiamine, rihoflavin and vitamin B_{12} by some blue-green algae. *Mikrobiol Zh* (Kiev), 32:429-433.

Krock, T., Alkamper, J. and Watanabe, I. (1988). Effect of an *Azolla* cover on the conditions in floodwater. *J. Agron Crop. Sci.*, 161: 185-189.

Kumar, H. and Kaushik, B.D. (1994). Response of *Calothrix brevissima* to salt. *Indian J Microbiol.*, 34: 38-41.

Kumarasinghe, K.S. and Eskew, D.L. (1993). Isotopic studies of *Azolla* and nitrogen fertilisation of rice. *Kluwer*. Dordrecht. pp. 145.

Kundu, D.K and Ladha, J.K. (1995). Efficient management of soil and biologically fixed N_2 in intensively cultivated rice fields. *Soil Biology and Biochem.* (UK) 27: 431-439.

Lales, J.S. and Marte, R.S. (1986). Long term utilization of *Azolla* as organic fertilizer for low land rice. *Phil. Agric.* 69:459-464.

Lean, D.R.S. and Nalewajko, C. (1976). Phosphate exchange and organic phosphorus excretion by freshwater algae. *J. Fish Res. Bd Can.*, 33: 1312-1323.

Levy, N., Magdassi, S. and Baror, Y. (1992). Physico-chemical aspects in flocculation of bentonite suspensions by a cyanobacterial bioflocculant. *Water Res.,* 26: 249-254.

Mandal, B., Das, S.C. and Mandal, L.N. (1992). Effect of growth and subsequent decomposition of blue-green algae in the transformation of phosphorus in submerged soils. *Plant Soil*, 143: 289-297.

Manna, A.B. and Singh, P.K. (1991). Effect of nitrogen fertilizer application methods on growth and acetylene reduction activity of *Azolla pinnata* and yield of rice. *Fert Res.*, 28: 25-30.

Marsalek, B., Zahradnickova, H., Hronkova, M. (1992). Extracellular abscisic acid produced by cyanobacteria under salt stress. *J. Plant Physiol.*, 139: 506-508.

Metting, B. and Pyne, J.W. (1986). Biologically-active compounds from microalgae. *Enzyme Microbial Technol.*, 8: 386-394.

Mishustin, E.N and Petrova, A.N. (1972). In: *Methods of study and practical use of soil algae. Report of Kirov,* Agri. Inst. Kirov. P 188,

Misra, S. and Kaushik, B.D. (1989a). Growth promoting substances of cyanobacteria. I. Vitamins and their influence on rice plants. *Proc Indian natl Sci Acad.* B55: 295-300.

Misra, S. and Kaushik, B.D. (1989b). Growth promoting substances of cyanobacteria. II. Detection of amino acids, sugars and auxins. *Proc Indian natl Sci Acad.* B55: 499-504.

Nagarajah, S., Neue, H.U. and Alberto, M.C.R. (1989). Effect of *Sesbania, Azolla* and rice straw incorporation on the kinetics of NH_4^-, K, Fe, Mn, Zn and P in some flooded rice soils. *Plant Soil*, 116: 37-48.

Nazeer, M. and Prasad, N.N. (1984). Effect of *Azolla* application on rice yield and soil properties. *Phykos*, 23: 269-272.

Nekrasova, K.A. and Aleksandrove, IV. (1982). Participation of Collembola and eartworm in the transformation of algal organic matter. *Sov Soil Sci.*, 14: 31-39.

Oikarinen, M. (1996). Biological soil amelioration as the basis of sustainable agriculture and forestry. *Biol Fertil Soils*, 22: 342-344.

Okuda, A. and Yamaguchi, M. (1955). Nitrogen fixing microorganisms in paddy soils. I. Characteristics of the nitrogen fixation in paddy soils. *Soil and Plant Food*, 1: 102-104.

Osmanova, R.A. (1979). Algal biomass in the soils of the Meshed Messerian plains of south western Turkmenia. *Pochvovdeniye*, 8: 109-115.

Pedurand, P. and Reynaud, P.A. (1987). Do cyanobacteria enhance germination and growth of rice? *Plant Soil*, 101: 235-240.

Ponnamperuma, F.N. (1972). The chemistry of submerged soils. *Adv. Agron.*, 242: 90.

Prasad, S. (1949). Nitrogen recuperation by blue green algae in soils of Bihar and their growth on different types. *J. Proc. Inst. Chem India*, 21: 135-140.

Prasanna, R. and Kaushik, B.D. (1994). Physiological and molecular genetic aspects of nitrogen fixation in non-heterocystous cyanobacteria. *Indian J Exptl Biol.* 32: 248-251.

Quesada, A., Leganes, F. and Fernandezvaliente, E. (1997). Environmental factors controlling N_2 fixation in Mediterranean rice fields. *Micro. Ecol.*, 34: 39-48.

Rao, D.L.N and Burns, R.G. (1990). Use of blue Green algae and bryophyte biomass as a source of nitrogen for oilseed rape. *Biol Fertil Soils*, 10: 61-64.

Rao, D.L.N and Burns, R.G. (1991). The influence of blue-green algae on the biological amelioration of alkali soils. *Biol. Fertil. Soils*, 11: 306-312.

Reddy, B.R., Apte, S.K. and Thomas, J. (1989). Enhancement of cyanobacterial salt tolerance by combined nitrogen. *Plant Physiol.*, 89: 204-210.

Reed, R.H., Richardson, D.L., Warr, S.R.C. and Stewart, W.D.P. (1984). Carbohydrate accumulation and osmotic stress in cyanobacteria. *J. Gen Microbiol.*, 130: 1-4.

Renaud, P.A. and Roger, P.A. (1978). Nitrogen fixing algal biomass in Senegal rice fields. *Ecol. Bull.* Stockholm, 26: 148-157.

Reynaud, P.A. and Roger, P.A. (1981). Seasonal variations of algal flora and of nitrogen fixing activity in a waterloggEd sandy soils. *Rev Ecol Biol Sol*, 18: 9-27.

Reynault, J., Sasson, A., Pearson, H.W. and Stewart, W.D.P. (1975) Nitrogen fixing algae in Morocco. In: *Nitrogen fixation by free living microorganisms* (*Ed.* W.D.P. Stewart), London, Cambridge Univ. Press, pp 229-248.

Roger, P.A. and Renaud, P.A. (1979). Ecology of blue green algae in paddy soils. In: *Nitrogen and rice*, Los Banos, Philipines, Pub. IRRI, 289-309.

Roger, P.A., Grant, I.F., Reddy, P.M. and Watanabe, I. (1987). The photosynthetic aquatic biomass in wetland rice fields and its effect on nitrogen dynamics. In: *Efficiency of nitrogen fertilizers for rice*. IRRI, Manila, pp. 43-68.

Roger, P.A., Santiago-Ardales, S.P.M. and Watanabe, I. (1987) The abundance of heterocystous blue green algae in rice soils and inocula used for application in rice fields. *Biol. Fert. Soils*, 5, 98-105.

Rodgers, G.A., Bergman, B., Henriksson, E. and Udris, M. (1979). Utilisation of blue-green algae in biofertilizers. *Plant Soil*, 52: 99-107.

Rogers, S.L., Cook, K.A. and Burns, R.G. (1991). Microalgal and cyanobacterial soil inoculants and their effect on soil aggregate stability. In: Advances in soil organic matter research; the impact on agriculture and the environment. (*Ed.* W.S. Wilson) *Royal Society of Chemistry* Cambridge, pp. 175-184.

Rogers, S.L. and Burns, R.G. (1994). Changes in aggregate stability nutrient status indigenous microbial populations and seedling emergence following inoculation of soil with *Nostoc muscorum*. *Biol Fertil. Soils*, 18: 209-215.

Roychoudhury, P., Kaushik, B.D., Krishna Murty, G.S.R. and Venkataraman, G.S. (1979). Effect of blue green algae and *Azolla* application on the aggregation status of soil. *Curr Sci.*, 48: 454-455.

Roychoudhury, P., Kaushik, B.D. and Venkataraman, G.S. (1985). Response of *Tolypothrix ceylonica* to sodium stress. *Curr. Sci.*, 54: 1181-1183.

Roychoudhury, P. and Kaushik, B.D. (1989). Solubilisation of Mussorie rock phosphates by cyanobacteria. *Curr. Sci.*, 58: 569-570.

Saha, K.C. and Mandal, L.N. (1979). Effect of algal growth on the availability of P, Fe and Mn in rice soils. *Plant Soil*, 52: 139-149.

Saha, K.C., Panigrahi, B.C. and Singh, P.K. (1982). Blue-green algae or *Azolla* additions on the nitrogen and phosphorus availability and redox potential of a flooded rice soil. *Soil Biol Biochem.*, 14: 23-26.

Sankaram, A. (1971). Work done on blue green algae in relation to agriculture. Technical Bulletin No. 27. Indian Council of Agricultural Research, New Delhi.

Saxena, S. and Kaushik, B.D. (1992). Polysaccharides (biopolymers) from halotolerant cyanobacteria. *Indian J exptl Biol.*, 30: 433-434.

Schulten, J.A. (1985). Soil aggregation by cryptogams of a sand prairie. *Am J. Bot.*, 72: 1657-1661.

Senthil, C., Roychoudhury, P. and Kaushik, B.D. (1993). Lipid profile of halosensitive *Calothrix marchica bharadwajae*. *Indian J Microbiol.*, 33: 281-285.

Sharma, M.L., Bhardwaj, G.S. and Chauhan, Y.S. (1989). Study on the effect of biofertilizer, pyrite and gypsum on paddy in the salt-affected soils. *Indian J Agron.*, 34: 129:130.

Shtina, E.A. (1965). In: *The ecology and physiology of blue green algae* (VD Federov, MM Tellichenko ed.) Moscow Univ. Press.

Shukla, A.C. and Gupta, A.B. (1967). Influence of algal growth-promoting substances on growth, yield and protein contents of rice plants. *Nature*, 213: 744.

Singh, A.K., Chakravarty, D., Singh, T.P.K and Singh, H.N. (1996). Evidence for a role for L-proline as a salinity protectant in the cyanobacterium *Nostoc muscorum. Plant Cell Environ.*, 19: 490-494.

Singh, A.L. and Singh, P.K. (1987). Influence of *Azolla* management on the growth, yield of rice and soil fertility. *Plant Soil*, 102:49-54.

Singh, D.V., Tripathi, A.K. and Kumar, H.D. (1991). Isolation and characterization of salinity resistant mutant of a nitrogen-fixing cyanobacterium, *Anabaena doliolum. J. Appl. Bacteriol.*, 71: 207-210.

Singh, P.K., Panigrahi, B.C. and Satapathy, K.B. (1981). Comparative efficiency of *Azolla,* blue-green algae and other organic manures in relation to N and P availability in a flooded rice soil. *Plant soil*, 62: 35-55.

Singh, R.N. (1950). Reclamation of "usar" lands in India through blue-green algae. *Nature*, 165: 325-326.

Singh, R.N. (1961). Role of blue-green algae in nitrogen economy of Indian Agriculture. *Indian Council of Agricultural Research*, New Delhi.

Singh, V.P. and Trehan, T. (1973). Effect of extracellular products of *Aulosira fertilissima* on the growth of rice seedlings. *Plant Soil*, 38: 457-464.

Sprent, J.I. and Sprent, P. (1990). Nitrogen fixing organism – pure and applied aspects. *Chapman and Hall.* London. pp. 256.

Stewart, W.D.P, Rowell, P., Ladha, J.K. and Sampaio, M.J.A. (1979). Blue green algae (cyanobacteria) some aspects related to their role as sources of fixed nitrogen in paddy soils (WDP Stewart, JR Gallon ed.) London, Academic Press.

Subhashini, D. and Kaushik, B.D. (1981). Amelioration of sodic soils with blue-green algae. *Aust. J. Soils Res.*, 19: 361-367.

Subhashini, D. and Kaushik, B.D. (1984). Amelioration of salt affected soils with blue green algae. I. Influence of algalization on the properties of saline alkali soils. *Phykos*, 23: 273-277.

Subhashini, D. and Kaushik, B.D. (1986). Uptake of sodium and potassium by blue green algae (cyanobacteria). *Zbl fur Mikrobiol.*, 141: 177-180.

Thomas, J. (1970). Absence of the pigments of photosystem II of photosynthesis in heterocysts of biue green algae. *Nature*, 228:181-183.

Thomas, J. (1977). Biological nitrogen fixation. *Nucl India*, 15 :2-8.

Tisdall, J.M. and Oades, J.M. (1982). Organic matter and water stable aggregates in soils. *J. Soil Sci.*, 33: 141-163.

Traore, T.M., Roger, P.A., Renaud, P.A. and Sasson, A. (1978). Nitrogen fixation by blue green algae in paddy field in Malia (English summary) *Cab. ORSTOM* Ser. Biol., 13, 181-185.

Tupik, N.D. (1973). Study of the content of group B vitamins in cells of some blue-green algae in dependence on the culture age. *Ukr Bot Zh.*, 30: 636-639.

Umarova, Sh.U. and Uromanov, Z.V. (1972). In: *Methods of study and practical use of soil algae. Report Kirov.*, Agri. Inst. Kirov. P. 203.

Venkataraman, G.S. (1978). Blue green algae in rice cultivation - an evaluation. In: *Glimpses in plant research.* Vol. IV. PKK Nair (ed) p. 74-82, Vikas Publishing House Pvt. Ltd., New Delhi.

Venkataraman, G.S. (1979). Algal inoculation of rice fields. In: International Rice Research Institute. Nitrogen and Rice. Los Banos, Philippines. PP. 311-321.

Venkataraman, G.S and Neelakantan, S. (1967). Effect of cellular constituents of nitrogen fixing blue-green alga *Cylindrospermum* on root growth of rice plants. *J. Gen. Appl. Microbiol.*, 13: 53-62.

Venkataraman, S. and Kaushik, B.D. (1994). Fatty acid profile of a marine *Nostoc calcicola* under saline and non-saline conditions. *Curr Sci.*, 67: 120-122.

Ventura, W. and Watanable, I. (1993). Green manure production of *Azolla microphylla* and *Sesbania rostrata* and their long-term effects on rice yields and soil fertility. *Biol Fertil. Soils.*, 15: 241-248.

Vorontsova, G.V, Romanova, N.I., Postnova, T.I., Selyakh, I.O. and Gues, M.V. (1988). Bio-stimulating effect of cyanobacteria and ways to increase it. I. Use of nutrients – superproducers of amino acids. *Moscow Univ. Biol.Sci.Bull.*, 43: 14-19.

Watanabe, A. (1951). Production in cultural solution of some amino acids by the atmospheric nitrogen fixing blue-green algae. *Arch Biochem. Biophys.*, 34: 50.

Watanabe, I. (1984). Use of symbiotic and free living blue green algae in rice culture. *Outlook Agric.*, 13, 166-172.

Watanabe, I. and Cholitkul, W. (1979). Field studies on nitrogen fixation in paddy soils. In: *Nitrogen and Rice*, p. 223, Pub. IRRI, Los Banos, Philippines.

Watnable, I. and Roger, P.A. (1984). Nitrogen fixation in wet land rice fields. In: Subba Rao NS (ed) *Current development in biological nitrogen fixation*. Oxford IBH New Delhi, pp. 237-276.

Watanabe, I., De Datta, S.K. and Roger, P.A. (1987). Nitrogen cycling in wetland rice soils. In: *Proc. symp adv. in nitrogen cycling in agriculture ecosystems*, Brisbane, Australia. JR Wilson (ed) p.

Wolf, A.M., Baker, D.E., Pionke, H.B. and Kunichi, H.M. (1985). Soil test for estimating labile, soluble and algal available phosphorus in agricultural soils. *J. Environ. Qual.*, 14: 341-348.

Yanni, Y.G. (1992). The effect of cyanobacteria and *Azolla* on the performance of rice under different levels of fertilizer nitrogen. *World J Microbiol Biotechnol.*, 8: 132-136.

Yoshida, T., Roncal, R.A. and Bantista, E.M. (1973). Proc. 2nd. Asian Soil Conf. Indonesia.

Section B

Microbiology and Biotechnology for Sustainable Development (Ed. P.C. Jain),
CBS Publishers & Distributors, New Delhi (2004), pp. 187–194.

B-1

Survival Strategies of Lithophytic Cyanobacteria on the Temples and Monuments

S.P. Adhikary
P.G. Department of Botany, Utkal University
Bhubaneswar 751004, Orissa, India

Abstract

The biological forms occurring in the epilithic crusts/ tufts of Jagannath temple, Puri; Sun temple, Konark and seven different temples and caves of Bhubaneswar, located in the east coast of Orissa state, India were studied. Certain species of cyanobacteria were the major components of the crusts/ tufts on the exposed rock surfaces and impart blackish-brown colouration to these monuments of archaeological importance. Five species of Tolypothrix and one species each of Phormidium and Lyngbya appeared soon after wetting of the crusts/ tufts collected from different sites. These epilithic organisms possess a well- defined sheath around their cells/ trichome, grew slowly in culture and showed higher respiratory oxygen uptake rate than their corresponding rate of photosynthesis. These cyanobacterial species have been isolated into axenic culture, identified following standard monographs, assigned with a strain number and maintained in the culture collection of Utkal University.

The cyanobacterial crusts/ tufts collected even during the mid days of summer months when the temperature on the rock surfaces exceeds 60°C coupled with intense solar radiation and extreme dryness are intensely stained after treatment with 2, 3, 5-triphenyl-tetrazolium chloride (TTC) for SH group. Pre-treatment with hydrogen peroxide (1%), Urea (5 M) or even keeping in desiccated state for 4 months had no effect on TTC reduction. Even after heating the crusts in dry state to 60°C for 1 h did not abolish the ability of the corresponding cyanobacterium to reduce TTC, where as heating the crusts as well as tufts in wet state for 10 min rendered the organisms inactive. These tests indicate that the intense TTC reduction was due to the presence of high levels of SH groups in the terrestrial cyanobacterial cells, and further, the crust forming organisms were more tolerant to the adverse conditions than the cyanobacteria occurring as tufts.

Key words : Cyanobacteria, lithophytic, monuments, temple, trichome

INTRODUCTION

Cyanobacteria form characteristic coloured crusts tightly adhering the substratum or tufts/ mats of few mm thickness on the exposed rock surfaces in several regions of the globe (Hoffmann, 1989). Several lithophytic cyanobacterial communities have been reported from the ancient monuments and caves of Europe. They occur frequently in ancient Roman frescoes (Grilli Caiola *et al.*, 1987), marbles of Parthenon (Acropolis, Athens) of Greece (Anagnostidis *et al.*, 1983), Inferniglio cave of Italy (Abdelahad, 1989), cathedrals (Salmanca and Toledo) of Spain and Sweden (Ortega - Calvo *et al.*, 1993) and Roman Necropolis (Albertano *et al.*, 1994). Considerable corrosion of frescoes paintings and withering of stones under the cyanobacterial mats/crusts has been observed in many of the reports (Anagnostidis *et al.*, 1983; Grilli Caiola *et al.*, 1987; and Ortega-Calvo *et al.*, 1991, 1993). Biological weathering of rocks has also been reported previously (Krumbein and Pochon, 1964; Grant, 1982; Albertano, 1993). The cyanobacterial film on the rock surface after their spontaneous detachment showed on its reverse side the presence of grains removed from the surface, thus causing mechanical deterioration on the colonized material. Thus understanding about the lithophytic communities occurring on the exposed rock surfaces of ancient monuments and their capacity to thrive/adjust the extreme environments therein is of considerable importance.

Orissa state (22° 34' N, 87° 29' E), located in the east coast of India is a treasure trove of art and architecture. A number of gigantic temples and caves are existing specially at three locations of the state, e.g. Konark, Puri and Bhubaneswar, which were built during 6th to 13th century A.D. All these temples and caves are made up of khondalite or sandstone look blackish-brown due to occurrence of crusts or tufts of cyanobacteria imparting a characteristic blackish appearance of these magnificent temples. During mid days of summer months, the temperature on the rock surfaces goes beyond 60°C, making the environment inhospitable to any organism. Even under such extreme conditions, few cyanobacterial species survive forming crusts/ tufts. Nothing is known yet about the cyanobacterial forms occurring on the rock surfaces of these monuments and about the physiological state of these organisms in the crusts/ tufts. A detail study of the different type of crusts/ tufts occurring on different ancient temples and caves of Konark, Puri and Bhubaneswar, their cyanobacterial components and physiological state of these crusts/ tufts has been made.

Materials and methods

Sun temple, Konark (13th century A.D.), Jagannath temple, Puri (12th century A.D.), six different temples of Bhubaneswar (7th to 13th century A.D.) and the Udayagiri caves in the outskrits of Bhubaneswar (1st century B.C.) were selected as the study sites. The blackish brown crusts and/or tufts were collected from the exposed rock surface of the temples and caves, during summer season (March-May) of 1994 and 1995 using sterile needles and stored in screw capped specimen bottles. These were soaked with distilled water for 4 to 6 hours and then observed under microscope for presence of cyanobacterial forms. A pinch of the crust/ tuft, after thorough washing was transferred to BG 11 medium with or without combined nitrogen (Rippka *et al.*, 1979) and to agar plates (1% w/v, Difco nutrient agar agar in the BG 11 medium) and incubated at 25±1°C under continuous light from fluorescent tubes at an intensity of 12.5 W/m^2 up to 2 months. The organisms appeared in the agar tubes/culture flasks were studied regularly at 4 day intervals and were identified. All these organisms were isolated into unialgal culture and their morphology was studied in a Meiji TH-ML-05 trinocular research microscope. For determination of TTC reduction activity (reaction with 2, 3, Triphenyl tetrazolium chloride), the crust/ tuft was soaked with different concentrations of TTC for varied time period and observed under microscope for detection of reddish formazan crystals.

RESULTS AND DISCUSSION

Isolation, culture and identification of lithophytic cyanobacteria occurring on the temples and caves of Bhubaneswar, Puri and Konark

The survey of different microorganisms occurring on the temples and caves of Konark, Puri and Bhubaneswar of Orissa state revealed that only the cyanobacterial species form characteristic blackish-brown crusts and/or tufts on their exposed rock surfaces. Generally 3 types of crusts and/or tufts were encountered during the study: (i) crust adhering to the substratum firmly and difficult to remove (example: crust of Sun temple), (ii) blackish-brown tuft of few mm in thickness adhering to the substratum less firmly and could be removed easily (example: tuft on the monuments of Kedar-Gouri temple) and (iii) tuft forming variously coloured thick mat on the substratum loosely attached to the rock surfaces on the shaded sides of the temples and were easily removable (example: thick mat forming tuft on the rocky walls of Parasurameswar temple). Soon after wetting of all these crusts and/or tufts in distilled water or BG 11 medium, organisms belonging to the genera *Tolypothrix, Lyngbya* and *Phormidium* appeared which were clearly observed under microscope. Invariably, the crusts on the walls of Sun temple, Konark as well as Jagannath temple, Puri harboured a species of *Tolypothrix,* whereas tufts on the monuments of Kedar-Gouri temple and on the wall of Parasurameswar temple of Bhubaneswar harboured a different species of *Tolypothrix* and *Lyngbya* respectively. Several other species/strains of *Tolypothrix, Lyngbya* or *Phormidium* were also the dominant component of the crusts/tufts from various other temples and caves of Bhubaneswar. Morphological features of the organisms in the crusts/ tufts were not clearly observed under microscope. On culturing these crusts/tufts, the organisms appeared within 10-20 days. Cyanobacteria were the only components of these crusts/ tufts collected from nature during summer however, during monsoon (rainy season) many green algal members, diatoms and protozoans also occurred in these samples. These cyanobacterial forms invariably belonged to the genera *Tolypothrix, Lyngbya* or *Phormidium,* however, the species/ strains were quite different from each other, and were specific to a type of crust/ tuft and the location of the study site. Totally 5 different *Tolypothrix* species and 1 species each of *Phormidium* and *Lyngbya,* which were the dominant components on the temple walls have been isolated and identified. Based on the comparative morphological and physiological characteristics they have been assigned with strain numbers and maintained at Utkal University. The organisms were identified up to species level following Desikachary (1959) and Komárek (1993). After culturing the cyanobacterial crusts and tufts for a prolonged period, i.e. up to 60 days or more, several other cyanobacterial species appeared in the culture alongwith the dominant components of the respective crust/tuft. These associated cyanobacterial species were obtained in unialgal culture and identified.

These were invariably belonged to *Plectonema, Nostoc, Calothrix* and *Fischerella.* Details of the cyanobacterial forms which were the dominant component of the crusts/tufts from various temples and caves of Bhubaneswar, Puri and Konark and the associated minor components appeared only in culture after prolonged incubation periods have been listed in Table 1.

Table 1: Cyanobacterial forms of the epilithic crust/tuft of various temples and caves of Bhubaneswar, Puri and Konark.

Sl. No.	Collection site	Organism	Isolate number
1.	Jagannath temple, Puri	*Tolypothrix byssoidea* (+)	UU 53170
		Plectonema hansgirgi	UU 52164
2.	Sun temple, Konark	*Tolypothrix byssoidea* (+)	UU 53170
		Tolypothrix campylonemoides	UU 53171
		Nostoc ellipsosporum	UU 52184
		Lyngbya corticiocola	UU 53161
3.	Udayagiri Caves, Bhubaneswar	*Tolypothrix campylonemoides* (+)	UU 53171
		Calothrix marchica	UU 512167
4.	Parasurameswar temple, Bhubaneswar	*Lyngbya corticiocola* (+)	UU 53161
		Calothrix ghosei	UU 518169
		Fischerella muscicola	UU 512180
5.	Mukteswar temple, Bhubaneswar	*Tolypothrix scytonemoides* (+)	UU 512173
		Tolypothrix distorta (+)	UU 512176
		Calothrix scytonemicola	UU 512166
6.	Kedar-Gouri temple, Bhubaneswar	*Tolypothrix scytonemoides* (+)	UU 512173
		Tolypothrix distorta	UU 512176
		Calothrix scytonemicola	UU 512166
		Calothrix marchica	UU 512167
7.	Brahmeswar temple, Bhubaneswar	*Phormidium truncicola* (+)	UU 511160
		Tolypothrix byssoidea	UU 53170
8.	Lingaraj temple, Bhubaneswar	*Tolypothrix crassa* (+)	UU 511174
		Tolypothrix byssoidea	UU 53170
		Nostoc ellipsosporum	UU 611187
		Phormidium truncicola	UU 511160
9.	Rameswar temple, Bhubaneswar	*Tolypothrix crassa* (+)	UU 511174
		Tolypothrix campylonemoides	UU 53171

(+) Dominant component of the crust/tuft which appeared soon after wetting. *Tolypothrix byssoidea* was the minor component in the crust of Lingaraj temple and Brahmeswar temple of Bhubaneswar, which appeared in enriched cultures only.

All those crusts or tufts collected from the walls of Sun temple, Konark, Kedar-Gouri temple and Parasurameswar temple of Bhubaneswar showing characteristic blackish-brown to blackish colouration contained cyanobacterial forms with a well defined distinct sheath layer around their trichome. Interestingly, all these cyanobacterial forms, which were the dominant components survived in the tufts or crusts in vegetative state without formation of any reproductive bodies like akinetes/spores etc.

TTC reduction activity of the cyanobacterial components in the crust/tuft

To know the physiological condition of the crust/ tuft while occurring in the extreme environments, these were soaked with 2, 3, 5 Triphenyl tetrazolium chloride (TTC) solution and observed under microscope at various time intervals. The cyanobacterial component of the crust/tuft were found to maintain reducing activity in their cells even after exposure to such inhospitable environments. The cells of cyanobacteria in the crust/tuft showed reddish formazan crystals after treatment with 1% (w/v) TTC for 6 h; crystal formation in the cells was not observed upon lesser incubation periods. This shows, that the cells in the crust/ tuft became active after wetting for 6 h and, then start their reducing activity. To understand whether pre-heating of the crust/ tuft in dry or wet state has any difference in effect on the TTC reduction, 30 mg of crust from Sun temple, Konark and equal amount of tuft from Kedar-Gouri temple, Bhubaneswar was taken and incubated at 60°C in a water bath or in the incubator for up to 2 h. On pre-heating the crusts in water bath even for 10 min, TTC reduction capacity of the cells was reduced showing a negative effect of heating in wet state on the reducing activity of the cells of the cyanobacterium .But on preheating in dry state up to 1 h, TTC reduction capacity of the cells of the organism was maintained (Table 2). To the contrary, heating the tuft of Kedar-Gouri temple in dry as well as in wet state, the cells of the

Table 2: TTC reducing activity* of the crust from Sun temple, Konark and tuft from Kedar-Gouri temple, Bhubaneswar and their corresponding cyanobacteria inhabiting the crust/tuft under different treatments.

Treatment	Duration of treatment with TTC	Crust/ tuft from temple walls		Cyanobacteria from culture	
		Sun temple, Konark	Kedar-Gouri temple, Bhubaneswar	Tolypothrix byssoidea UU 53170	Tolypothrix scytonemoides UU 512173
Wet heat	10 min	-	-	-	-
	1 h	-	-	-	-
	2 h	-	-	-	-
Dry heat	10 min	+	-	+	-
	1 h	+	-	+	-
	2 h	-	-	-	-
Dessicated state	4 months	+	-	ND	ND
Hydrogen peroxide 1%	1 h	+	-	+	-
1%	2 h	+	-	+	-
1%	4 h	+	-	+	-
Urea 1M	1 h	+	-	+	+
5M	1 h	+	-	+	-
10M	1 h	-	-	-	-

* 1% (w/v) Triphenyl tetrazolium chloride (TTC) was prepared in double distilled water and used for experiment. ND; not determined.

cyanobacterium could not reduce TTC. Upon exposing the cyanobacterial filaments from culture to dry as well as wet heat, similar pattern of response of the cells to TTC was observed as per the response of the cells of the corresponding organism in the crust/ tuft. By subjecting to wet heat treatment for 10 min, the cells of *Tolypothrix byssoidea* lost their capacity to reduce TTC though the activity retained even when exposed to heating in dry state for 1 h But pre-treatment with heating at 60°C in dry and wet state, *Tolypothrix scytonemoides* UU 512173 lost its capacity to reduce TTC Further, keeping the crusts from Sun temple, Konark in a desiccator (with $CaCl_2$ and at reduced pressure) for 4 months did not show any adverse effect on their cells to reduce TTC. Cells of the same crust could maintain the TTC reducing activity even when exposed to hydrogen peroxide (1% v/v) up to 4 h. Pre treatment with urea up to 5M and then treating with TTC for 1 h also did not reduce the TTC reduction activity (Table 2). To the contrary, the cyanobacterial cells in the tufts from Kedar-Gouri temple could not form formazan crystals when treated with hydrogen peroxide or with urea (1M) for 1 h. These results showed that the cyanobacteria inhabiting in the crust of Sun temple, Konark, remained at a higher metabolically active state in comparison to the organism inhabiting in the tuft of Kedar-Gouri temple, Bhubaneswar.

Analysis of these results showed that 5 different species of *Tolypothrix* and one species each of *Lyngbya* and *Phormidium* occurred as the prominent component of the epilithic crusts and tufts on the exposed rock surface of different temples and caves of coastal regions of Orissa state, India. A species of *Tolypothrix,* i.e. *T. byssoidea* was found as the only cyanobacterial species forming characteristic crust even during summer months on the rock surface of Sun temple, Konark and Jagannath temple, Puri. It also occurred as a component of the crust/tuft in association with other species of *Tolypothrix* in certain temples of Bhubaneswar. Another species of *Tolypothrix,* i.e. *T. scytonemoides* form characteristic tuft on the rock surface of monuments in the Kedar-Gouri temple and Mukteswar temple, Bhubaneswar. Three other species of *Tolypothrix,* i.e. *Tolypothrix crassa* ,*Tolypothrix distorta* and *Tolypothrix campylonemoides* occurred in the crusts/tufts of Lingaraj temple, Rameswar temple and Udayagiri caves of Bhubaneswar. One species each of *Lyngbya corticiocola* and *Phormidium truncicola* formed characteristic blackish mat of few mm thickness on the rock surface of Parasurameswar temple and Brahmeswar temple of Bhubaneswar respectively. However, these mats harbouring *Lyngbya* species occurred in shaded places of the temples away from direct sunlight. Species of *Lyngbya* were also reported occurring on Roman frescos, Domus-aurea, Italy (Grilli Caiola *et al.,* 1987). But species of *Tolypothrix* as the dominant components of the crusts/tufts on rock surfaces of the monuments exposed to bright sunlight and/or under arid conditions in other regions of the globe has not been reported. However, there is a single report on the occurrence of *T. byssoidea* on the Pardon gate, Cathedral of Sevilla, Spain; occurrence of other *Tolypothrix* forms on the rock monuments had not been reported (Ortega Calvo *et al.,* 1991). The cyanobacterial species which form crust/ tuft in/on Roman frescos (Grilli-Caiola *et al.,* 1987), marbles of parthenon of Greece (Anagnostidis *et al.,* 1983), cave of Italy (Abdelahad, 1989), Spanish cathedrals (Ortega-Calvo *et al.,* 1993) or Roman necropolis (Albertano *et al.* 1994) were quite different from the species occurring on the temples and caves of coastal region of Orissa state, India. However, some of the cyanobacterial species belonging to genera *Plectonema, Nostoc, Calothrix, Fischerella* and also other species of *Tolypothrix* which appeared as an associated component of the dominant species in the epilithic crusts/ tufts have been found occurring in other terrestrial habitats (Budel and Wessels, 1991, Grilli Caiola *et al.*, 1987; Anagnostidis *et al.*, 1983; Johansen, 1993, Dodds *et al.*, 1995, Wessels and Budel, 1995). All those species belonging to *Tolypothrix*, *Lyngbya* or *Phormidium* which form predominant epilithic flora grew extreme slowly in comparison to the aquatic forms under the respective genus (Tripathy *et al.*, 1997).

The cyanobacterial cells in the crusts and tufts collected from the rock surface even during mid summer months could survive in the vegetative state without formation of reproductive structures like akinetes/spores. Further, even after their exposure to arid conditions and bright sunlight for several months, resumed their photosynthesis and respiration soon after wetting. This is indicative of the existing cells in the crusts/ tufts being viable after exposure to extreme environmental conditions. The organisms inhabiting the crust/ tuft did not grow within the 48 h of wetting period showing that all these cyanobacterial species survived enduring the extreme conditions on the rock surface. Hess (1962) reported that members of Scytonemataceae, Rivulariaceae and Nostocaceae were resistant to dry period of one year or longer, but not of Oscillatoriaceae family. Whitton *et al.* (1979) and Scherer *et al.* (1984) found that certain terrestrial *Nostoc* species survived in vegetative state also but not only as endospore as reported by Hess (1962). Potts *et al.* (1983) demonstrated in the desiccation resistant *Chroococcus* that internal structures of the cyanobacterium were retained without damage to the cells during dryness.

The cyanobacterial cells inhabiting the crust of Sun temple, Konark react to TTC by forming reddish formazan crystals for SH groups. This shows that the cells could maintain the reducing activity even when subjected to extreme environmental conditions. Pretreatment with up to 5M urea, 1% hydrogen peroxide or heating the crust/ tuft in dry state at 60°C up to 1 hour had no effect on TTC reduction. Keeping the crusts in desiccated state up to 4 months also did not reduce their TTC reduction activity, whereas exposing to heat by keeping in a water bath (wet state) even for 10 minutes rendered the cyanobacterial cells inactive. All these tests indicate that TTC reduction is due to presence of SH groups in lithophytic cyanobacterial cells exposed to bright sunlight. The cyanobacterial component of the tuft of Kedar-Gouri temple also reduced TTC for the SH groups. But the activity was lost after pretreatment with heat (60°C) in wet or dry state, upon exposure to H_2O_2, urea and also when kept in a desiccators for a prolonged period. This showed that cyanobacterium *T. byssoidea* inhabiting the crust of Sun temple, Konark was comparatively more tolerant to adverse conditions than that of the epilithic tuft of Kedar-Gouri temple containing *Tolypothrix scytonemoides*.

ACKNOWLEDGEMENTS

I thank the Head of the Department of Botany, Utkal University for providing laboratory facilities and to the authorities of University Grants Commission, New Delhi for financial assistance through a Research award under IXth plan.

REFERENCES

Abdelahad, N., (1989). On four *Myxosarcina* like species (cyanophyta) living in the Inferuiglio cave, Italy. *Algol . Studs*. 82:3-13.

Albertano, P., Kovacik, L. and Grilli-Caiola,M., (1994). Preliminary investigations on epilithic cyanophytes from Roman Necropolis. *Algol. Studs.* 75:71-74.

Anagnostidis,K., Economou Amilli,A. and Roussomoustakaki,M., (1983). Epilithic and chasmolithic microflora (cyanophyta/bacillariophyta) from marbles of the Parthenon (Acropolic-Athens, Greece). *Nova Hedwigia* 38: 227-277.

Budel, B. and Wessels,D.C.J., (1991). Rock inhabiting blue green algae/cyanobacteria from hot arid regions. *Algol. Studs.* 64:385-398.

Desikachary, T.V. (1959). Cyanophyta, I.C.A.R. monograph on algae, ICAR, New Delhi.p.686.

Dodds, W.K., Gudder, D.A. and Mollenhauer, D., (1995). The ecology of *Nostoc. J.Phycol.* 31:2-18.

Grant, C., (1982). Fouling of terrestrial substrates by algae and implications for control. *Biodeter.Bull.*18:57-65.

Grilli-Caiola, M., Forni, C. and Albertano, P., (1987). Characterization of algal flora growing on Roman-frescoes.*Phycologia*, 26:387-390.

Hess, U,. (1962). Uber die hydraturabhangige Entwicklung und die Austrockung stresistenz von cyanophyceen. *Arch. Microbiol.* 44:189-218.

Hoffmann, L., (1989). Algae of terrestrial habitats. *Bot.Rev.* 55: 77-105.

Johansen, J.R., (1993). Cryptogamic crusts of sub-aerial and arid lands of North America. *J. Phycol.* 29: 140-147.

Komarek,J.,(1993). Validation of the genera *Gloeocapsopsis* and *Asterocapsa* (cyanoprocaryota) with regard to species from Japan, Mexico and Himalayas. *Bull. Natl. Sci. Mus.* Tokyo Ser.B. 19: 19-37.

Krumbein, W.E. and Pochon, J., (1964). Ecologie bacterienne des pirres alterees des monuments. *Ann. Inst.Pasteur.* 107:724-732.

Ortega-Calvo, J.J., Hernandez-Marine, M. and Saiz-Jimenez, C., (1991). Biodeterioration of building materials by cyanobacteria and algae. *Int. Biodeter.* 28: 165-185.

Ortega-Calvo, J.J., Sanchez-Castillo, P.M., Hernandez-Marine, M. and Saiz-Jimenez, C., (1993). Isolation and characterization of epilithic chlorophytes and cyanobacteria from two Spanish cathedrals (Salmanca and Toledo). *Nova Hedwigia*, 57 : 239-253.

Potts, M., Ocampo-Fridmann, R., Bowman, M.A. and Tozun, B., (1983). *Chroococcus* S 24 and *Chroococcus* N 41 (cyanobacteria): morphological, biochemical and genetic characterization and effects of water stress on ultrastructure. *Arch. Microbiol.* 135: 81-90.

Rippka, R., Deruelles, J., Waterbury, J.B., Herdman, M. and Stanier, R.Y., (1979). Generic assignments, strain histories and properties of pure cultures of cyanobacteria. *J.Gen. Microbiol.* 111:1-61.

Scherer, S., Ernst, A., Chen, T.W. and Boger, P., (1984). Rewetting of drought resistant blue green algae: time course of water uptake and reappearance of respiration, photosynthesis and nitrogen fixation. *Oecologia,* 62:418-423.

Tripathy, P., Roy, A. and Adhikary, S.P., (1997). Survey of epilithic blue green algae from temples of India and Nepal. *Algol. Studs.* 87: 43-57.

Wessels, D.C.J. and Budel,B., (1995). Epilithic and cryptoendolithic cyanobacteria from Clarens sandstone Cliffs in the golden gate highlands National park, Soth Africa. *Bot. Acta*, 108: 220-226.

Whitton, B.A., Donaldson, A. and Potts, M., (1979). Nitrogen fixation by *Nostoc* colonies in terrestrial environments of Aldabra Atoll, Indian Ocean. *Phycologia,* 18: 278-287.

Microbiology and Biotechnology for Sustainable Development (Ed. P.C. Jain),
CBS Publishers & Distributors, New Delhi (2004), pp. 195–200.

B-2

Biodiversity of Acidophilic Heterotrophic Iron Oxidising Bacteria

S.R. Dave, V.V. Gajjar and D.R. Tipre
Department of Microbiology, School of Sciences
Gujarat University, Ahmedabad 380 009.

Abstract

The selected 4 samples from Malanjkhand copper mine and chemical treatment plants showed the diversity of pH, oxidation reduction potential and conductivity in the range of 3 to 6.6, 290 to 505 mV and 0.960 to 5.40 mS respectively. The MPN count of iron oxidisers in the presence of organic substrates varied between 0 to 230 per 100 ml. Sample collected from acid heap leaching site showed iron oxidation along with the dominant activity of iron reducers. Iron reducers were found to be responsible for the gradual reduction of oxidised ferrous particularly in the presence of glycerol in the medium. On the basis of time profile iron oxidation study, the samples could be arranged in the increasing order of their iron oxidation ability as, oozing water sample (MJ-5) samples from acid heap leach (MJ-6) dried samples (MJ-7) flowing water samples (MJ-3). The water samples from the different sites were having different proportion of iron oxidation. Enriched samples taken from tubes inoculated with MJ-3 for MPN study displayed iron oxidation in presence of all the three organic substrates as opposed to the rest of the samples where the iron oxidation was observed only in the presence of glucose. Addition of glucose in the medium proved to be the choice of organic material for fastest and over all iron oxidation by variety of enriched cultures. Considerable fungal growth was also observed in glucose and yeast extract containing medium inoculated with MJ-3 sample. This study resulted in growth and purification of 7 heterotrophic iron oxidisers on solid medium. Use of such isolates may prove beneficial for industrial waste treatments.

Key words: biodiversity, iron oxidising bacteria, copper mine, MPN technique

Corresponding author: *S.R. Dave.* Email:shaileshrdave@hotmail.com

INTRODUCTION

The microbial world traditionally consists of all organisms that can be seen only with a microscope i.e. the fungi, bacteria, archea, algae, protozoa and a number of newer and less known lower eukaryotes. Microbial life in extreme low pH (3) natural and man-made environment may be considerably diverse. Prokaryotic acidophiles (eubacteria and archea) have been the focus of much of the research activity in this area because of the importance of these microorganisms in biotechnology and in environmental pollution. However, obligately acidophilic eukaryotes (fungi, yeast, algae and protozoa) are also known and may form stable microbial communities with prokaryotes particularly in environment at an ambient temperature.

Interest in the biodiversity of microorganism, which inhabit extreme environments, has increased significantly over the last 25 years. Extremely acidic environments may be formed by processes, that are entirely natural. A variety of microbial activities generate net acidity. These include mainly the microbial dissimilatory oxidation of elemental sulfur, reduced sulfur compounds and ferrous iron as well as nitrification and the formation and accumulation of organic acid either during fermentation or as products of aerobic metabolism (Johnson, 1996).

Microorganisms participate in the formation, conversion and transportation of different minerals in the earth's crust. A microbial ecological surveys of various sulfidic mines and acidic environment throughout the world showed the presence of various autotrophic and heterotrophic bacteria and fungi in such environments (Modak and Natarajan, 1995).

Much work has been reported on iron and sulfur-oxidising acidophiles which are regarded as autotrophic, though the ability to assimilate organic carbon has been demonstrated with some of these (e.g. utilization of formic acid by *T. ferroxidans*) (Pronk *et al.*, 1991).

Some acidophilic heterotrophic iron oxidising microorganism requiring prefixed carbon (e.g. yeast extract) and which use iron oxidation as an energy transducing reaction have been isolated from a variety of sources (Johnson, 1995). Some prokaryotic acidophilic heterotrophic organisms have a direct role in the dissimilatory oxido-reduction of iron (Pronk and Johnson, 1992).

The contribution of heterotrophic acidophiles to the bioleaching of sulfide ores is poorly understood. They may affect mineral bioleaching indirectly by their interaction with iron-oxidising chemolithotrophs. Thus the work was carried out on biodiversity study of some acidophilic iron oxidizing bacteria with reference to influence of addition of various organic substrates in the medium.

MATERIALS AND METHODS

Various water and solid samples were obtained from Malanjkhand copper mine and chemical treatment plants.

Growth medium

The samples were inoculated in MC medium having following composition: (g/l) $(NH_4)_2SO_4$, 0.4; $MgSO_4 .7H_2O$, 0.4; $K_2HPO_4.3H_2O$, 0.056;. pH adjusted to 2-2.4 with 10% H_2SO_4 and $FeSO_4.7H_2O$,0.01%.

Non plating approach to the enumeration and identification of acidophilic heterotrophic iron oxidizing bacteria

The 3-tube most probable number (MPN) method was performed with inoculation of original sample. Aliquots like 1ml, 0.1ml and 0.01ml were used to inoculate MC medium with the addition of organic substrates like glucose (0.02 %), yeast extract (0.02%) and glycerol (1% v/v) (Johnson, 1995).

Results were checked by addition of 1% potassium thiocynate and observing the colour change from colorless to red after 21 days of incubation. Development of red colour indicated positive results (Escobar and Godoy, 1999).

Ferrous oxidation study

Enriched samples were taken from tubes inoculated with MJ-3, MJ-5, MJ-6,and MJ-7 for MPN study.

Ferrous oxidizing activity of the all the enriched environmental samples through MPN study was estimated under identical condition in 250 ml Erlenmeyer flasks containing 100 ml of the growth medium and incubation on Newtronic orbital shaker at 130-140 rpm and 32 ±2°C temperature. Test flasks were inoculated with 10% (v/v) inoculums. Ferrous iron oxidation by the microbes was estimated by titration of the residual ferrous iron using potassium dichromate solution. Growth was also ascertained by direct microscopic observation.

Solid medium was prepared with 1% washed agar, it is separately sterilized with neutral pH and mixed with growth medium (Dave, 1980).

RESULTS AND DISCUSSION

Malanjkhand open pit copper mine samples showed the presence of diversified environments in terms of pH, oxidation reduction potential and conductivity as low as 3, 290 mV and 960 μS to as high as 7.5, 505 mV and 5.40 μS respectively. Among the samples collected, except for the accumulated water sample, all other sites were showing one or other specific characteristics and they are significantly different from sample MJ-3. Sample MJ-3 was collected from the water passing through more than 100m open mine surface area. While the rest of the samples were from a closed resinity of particular sites (Table 1).

Table 1: Physicochemical characteristics of mine samples.

Sample name	Description	pH	Oxidation reduction potential (mV)	Conductivity (mS)
MJ-3	Accumulated water	6.6	290	0.960
MJ-5	Oozing water from mining site	4.9	355	2
MJ-6	Leachate from acid heap leach	3.0	505	4.3
MJ-7	Driedsample from Fe^{+3} precipitate pond	4.6	320	5.40

The most probable acidophilic iron oxidizer count was studied in the presence and absence of organic substrates in MC medium. The obtained results are given Table 2. Highest count of autotrophic iron oxidizer was observed in the sample from sample MJ-6. The microbial count of iron oxidizer in the presence of organic substrates showed significant diversity in terms of the collection sites as well as type of the organic substrates incorporated in the medium. From the MPN study, glycerol and yeast extract were found to be more preferred substrates for the growth of acidophilic iron oxidizers (Table 3).

Table 2: MPN counts per ml of various samples after 21 days.

Sample name	MPN count in various medium			
	MC	MC+Y.E.	MC+Glucose	MC+Glycerol
MJ-3	15.0	2.3	0.4	1.5
MJ-5	2.0	1.5	2.0	1.5
MJ-6	110.0	0.94	<0.3	1.5
MJ-7	2.7	2.0	<0.3	2.0

Table 3: Colonical characteristics of iron oxidisers.

Isolate Number	Isolated from sample number	Colonical characteristic on yeast extract containing medium
1	MJ-3	Round, small, isolated colony with dark orange spreaded growth.
2	MJ-3	Slightly round, bigger than previous dark orange.
3	MJ-3	Oval single colony, dark brown.
4	MJ-3	Small, uneven margin, dark orange centered.
5	MJ-6	Uneven shape, dark brown and orange colour is present surrounding the colony.
6	MJ-3	Round, small, translucent, dark brown center.
7	MJ-3	Big, uneven shape, light yellow colour surrounding the colony, uneven margin.

Samples MJ-6 and MJ-3 showed significant dominance of microbial count in the absence of organic substrates, while in case of samples MJ-5 and MJ-7, there was marginal difference in the count of iron oxidizing populations.

Due to the use of indicator, it was possible to detect the positive growth in 7 days of incubation time. Thus, this modification reduces the incubation time and helps in rapid determination of iron oxidizers.

The mixed iron oxidizing acidophilic consortia developed during MPN was studied for overall ferrous oxidizing profile and obtained results are depicted in Graph 1. The consortia developed from sample MJ-3 showed more than 10 mg/lit of iron oxidation in all the variety of the media used. Consortia developed from sample MJ-6 occupied second position in terms of overall iron oxidations. The iron oxidation activity of more than 10 mg/lit was observed only in presence of glucose in case of consortia from sample MJ-5, while sample MJ-7 showed this activity in two media.

Graph 1: Ferrous oxidation by consortia

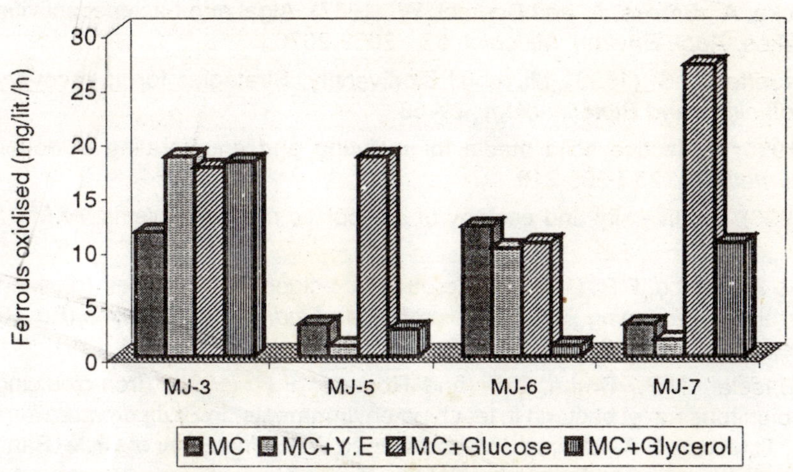

On the basis of this study the samples were arrange in the increasing order of the iron oxidation ability as MJ-5 MJ-6 MJ-7 MJ-3.

During the MPN study, acid heap leaching sample (MJ-6) showed decrease in the oxidized iron after 10 days of incubation. Similar trend was observed during the iron oxidation study in the presence of glycerol. In these flasks, there was a decrease of 2 mg ferrous but ferric was not detected. Moreover the medium of the flask showed blackening which could be due to the reduction of ferrous to ferrous sulfides and which could be due to the growth of iron reducers.

Addition of glucose in the medium proved to be the choice of organic material for fastest and overall iron oxidation by variety of enriched cultures. Considerable fungal growth was observed in glucose and yeast extract containing medium inoculated with MJ-3 and MJ-7 samples. This can be seen in Fig. 1 (Plate 1 on page 201). The study resulted in growth and purification of 7 heterotrophic iron oxidizers on solid medium (Fig. 2 in Plate 1 on page 201).

ACKNOWLEDGEMENT

We are to thankful to the Department of Biotechnology, Delhi for the project grant and for the Research Associateship to one of the authors (D.R.T.).

REFERENCES

Dave, S.R. (1980). Microbiological and bioleaching studies on metallurgical bacteria cultured from Indian sulphidic mine water. Ph.D. Thesis. The University of Mysore, Mysore, India.

Escobar, B. and Godoy, I. (1999). Determination of sulfur and iron oxidation bacteria by the most probable number (MPN) technique. In *Biohydrometallurgy and the environment towards the mining of the 21st century*. Part A (Eds. Amils, R. and Ballester, A.), IBS-99, Elsvier Publications, NewYork, pp 681-687.

Gyure, R.A., Konoka, A., Brooks, A. and Doemel, W. (1987). Algal and bacterial activities in acidic (pH 3) strip mine lakes. *Appl. Environ. Micobiol.* 53 : 2069-2076.

James, M.T. and Jeffery, I.S. (1999). Microbial Biodiversity: Strategies for its recovery. In *Manual of Industrial Microbiology and Biotechnology*, pp 56.

Johnson, D.B. (1995). Selective solid media for isolating and enumerating acidophilic bacteria. *J. Microbiological methods.* 23 : 205-218.

Johnson, D.B. (1996). Biodiversity and ecology of acidophilic microorganisms. *FEMS Microbiol. Ecol.* 27 : 307-317.

Johnson, D.B. and Francisco, F.R. (1997). Heterotrophic acidophiles and their roles in the bioleaching of sulfide minerals. In *Biomining : Theory, microbes and industrial processes* (Ed. Rawlings, D.E.)., Landes Bioscience, Austin, USA, pp 259-279.

Johnson, D.B., Bacelar, N.P., Bruhn, D.F. and Roberto, F.F. (1995). Iron-oxidising heterotrophic acidophiles : ubiquitous novel bacteria in leaching environments. In *Biohydrometallurgical porocesing I* (Eds. Vargas, T., Jerez, C.A., Weirtz, J.V. and Toledo, H.)., University of Chile, Santiago, pp 47-56.

Johnson, D.B., Said, M.F., Ghauri, M.F. and McGinness, S. (1989). Isolation of novel acidophiles and their potential use in bioleaching operations. In *Biohydromerallurgy* (Eds. Salley, J., McCready, R.G.L., and Wichlacz, P.L.)., Ottawa, Canada, pp 403-414.

Lopez, A.A.I., Marin, I. and Amils, R. (1995). Microbial ecology of an acidic river. In *Biotechnological processing II* (Eds. Vargas, T., Jerez, C.A., Wiertz, J.V. and Toledo, H.)., University of Chile, Santiago, pp 63-74.

Modak, J.M. and Natrajan, K.A. (1995). Microbial ecology of hutty gold mines with relevance to gold bioprocessing. In *Biotechnological processing II* (Eds. Vargas, T., Jerez, C.A., Wiertz, J.V. and Toledo, H.)., University of Chile, Santiago, pp 143-155.

Pronk, J.T. and Johnson, D.B. (1992). Oxidation and reduction of iron by acidophilic bacteria. *Geomicrobiol. J.*, 10 : 153-171.

Pronk, J.T., Meijer, W.M., Hazew, W., van Dijken, J.P., Bos, P. and Kuenen, J.G. (1991). Growth of *Thiobacillus ferroxidans* on formic acid. *Appl. Environ. Microbiol.* 57 : 2057-2062.

PLATE 1

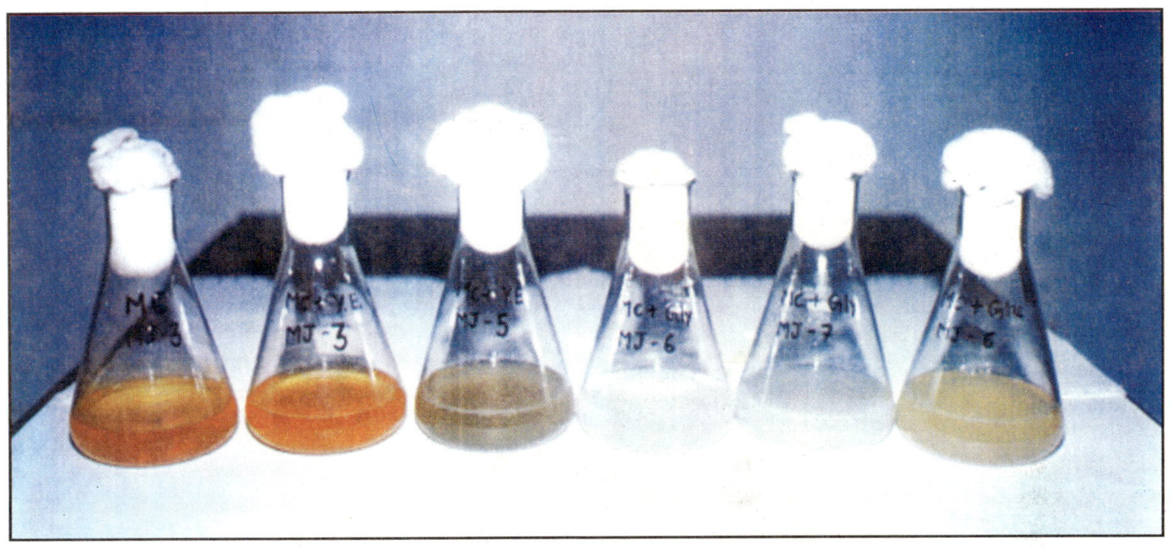

Fig. 1 : Iron oxidation along with fungal growth.

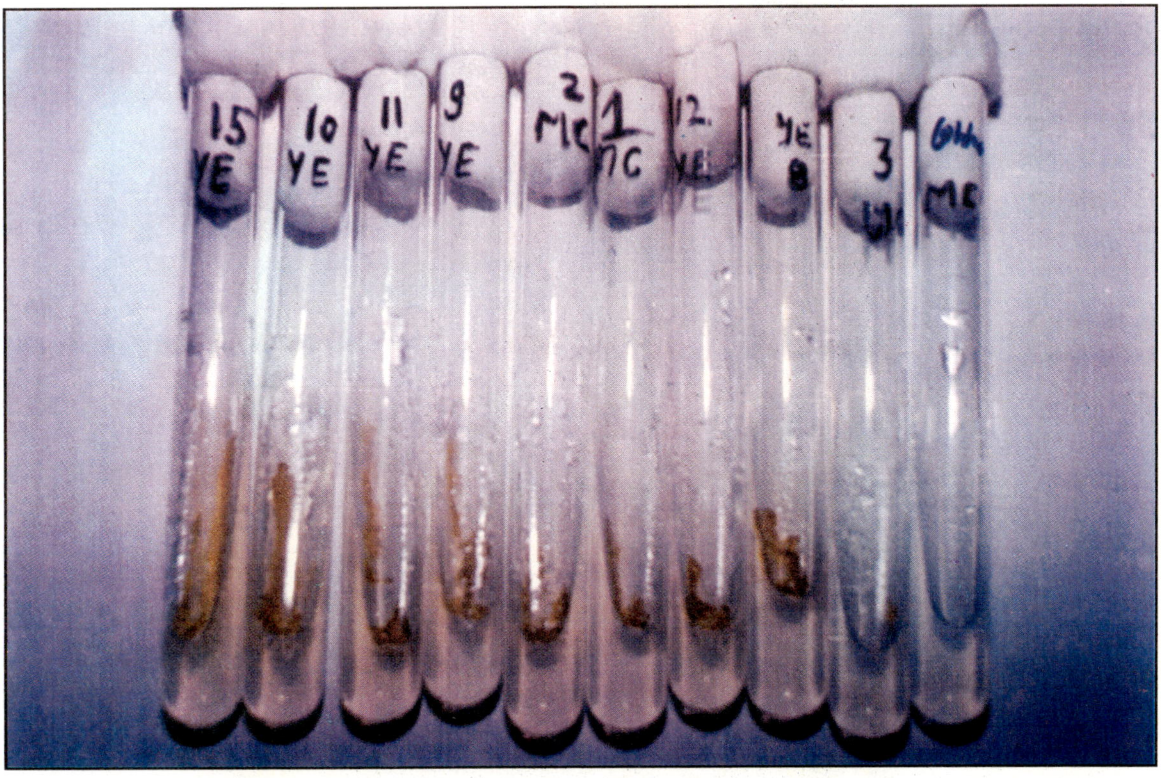

Fig. 2 : Gradation of iron oxidising growth after 72 h of incubation.

PLATE 2

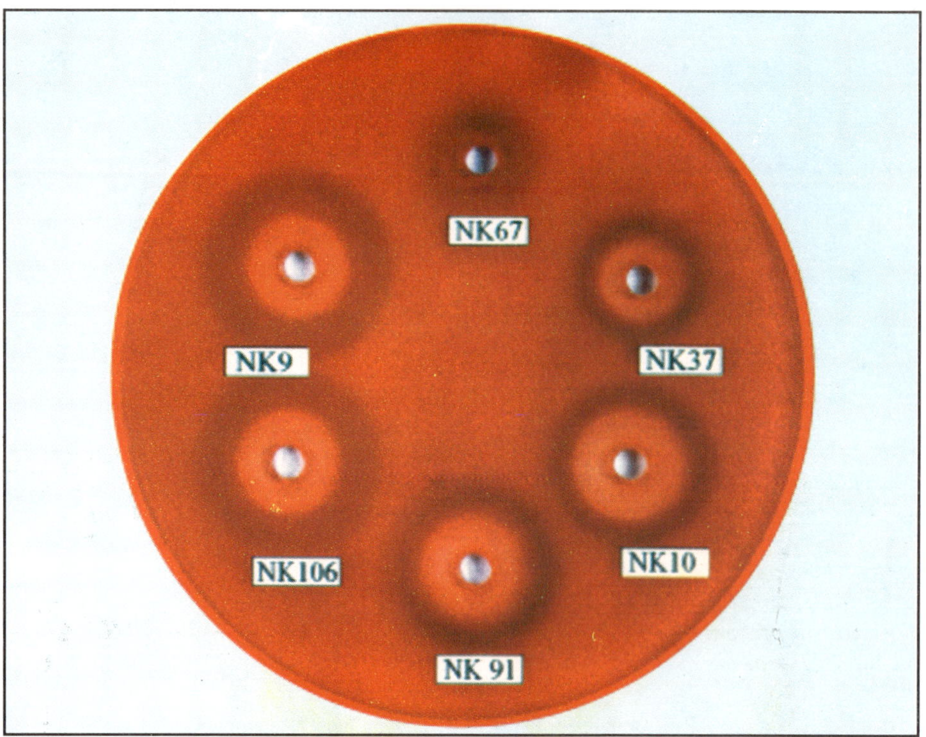

Zones of xylan hydrolysis formed by radial diffusion of crude enzyme samples on xylan agarose gel (Related text on page 296).

Microbiology and Biotechnology for Sustainable Development (Ed. P.C. Jain),
CBS Publishers & Distributors, New Delhi (2004), pp. 203–213.

B-3

Indian Thermophilic Mycoflora

R.V. Shukla and P. C. Jain*
Department of Botany, C.M.D College, Bilaspur 495001 (C.G.)

Abstract

To study thermophilic fungi occurring in Indian habitats, a total of six different habitats i.e., composts, soils, grain storages, veterinary feed, wood chip pipes and birds nest were selected. During the course of present study a total of 244 fungi were isolated. Maximum number of fungi was isolated from soil samples followed by grain storages, veterinary feed, compost, wood chip pipes and birds nest. The occurrence of thermophilic fungi in different habitats has been discussed in relation to the nature of habitat. In the present survey number of albino strains of thermophilic moulds have also been isolated.

Keywords : Thermophilic, Compost, Soil, Storages, Coalmine

INTRODUCTION

Thermophilic fungi represent a heterogeneous group of moulds consisting of a large number of morphological and physiological forms and provide information about their adaptation to high temperatures (Crisan, 1964). This group include representatives from the Zygomycetes, Ascomycetes, Basidiomycetes, and fungi Imperfecti and comprises a restricted number of species having in common, certain biochemical and ecological characteristics associated with their ability to grow at elevated temperatures, i.e., >50°C (Cooney and Emerson, 1964).

The aim of the present study, therefore, was to survey the occurrence of thermophilic fungi from different sources in India. In order to demonstrate that habitats suitable for growth of fungi at higher temperature are common, wide spread, and of long existence, Tansey and Brock (1978) reviewed the habitats in which thermophilic fungi occur and regarded geothermal heat is of major significance for the occurrence of thermophilic fungi in natural geothermal sites; including geothermal soils, hot springs and hot spring effluent channels. Evans (1971a,b) studied the distribution of thermophilic fungi in many coal spoil

* Department of Applied Microbiology and Biotechnology, Dr. H.S. Gour Vishwavidyalaya, Sagar (M.P.)

tips with high surface-soil temperatures. Maheshwari (1997) reviewed the ecology and distribution of thermophilic fungi.

The combustion heat produced by the activities of thermophilic microorganisms in self-heating of organic masses leading to combustion or self-ignition is a significant factor in creating thermal environment. Role of microorganisms, in the spontaneous heating and ignition of stored hay, have been studied by Miehe (1907) and Cooney and Emerson (1964). Gregory *et al.*, (1963) found that baled hay with an initial moisture content of 40-60% reached maximum temperatures of 60-70°C due to general increase of microorganisms. Thermophilic fungi as storage fungi supported by several descriptions (Mulinge and Apinis, 1969; Flanningan, 1969, 1972). Additional reports of thermophilic fungi in stored grain and seeds have been made by Lacey (1972); Taber and Pettit (1975), Shukla and Jain (1990). Thermophilic fungi isolated from wood chip piles, saw dust etc. participate in self heating and deterioration in wood chip piles (Tansey and Brock, 1978; Tansey, 1971; Bergman, 1974; Ofosu Asiedu and Smith, 1973; Smith, 1973; Fergus, 1969; Greaves, 1971, Singhai and Jain, 1992). Evans (1968), Craveri at al. (1966), have reported mushroom compost as a rich source of thermophilic fungi. Tansey and Brock(1973) isolated *Dactylaria gallopava* a causal agent of encephelites in chicken from geothermal habitats and from self heated coal waste piles.Thermophilic fungi of self-heated coal waste piles have been intensively studied by many workers e.g., Sumner *et al.*, (1969), Stahl (1964), Thakre and Johri (1976), Shukla and Agrawal (1987), Sastry (1996) etc.

Dravid (1940) and Geiger (1965) emphasized the solar heat radiation as main heat source producing high temperature environments in land surface. Obviously, by direct solar heating the soil surface temperature frequently rise10-20°C above the air temperature. Soil surface temperatures of 50-70°C have been recorded by Vartaza (1949). In tropical and sub tropical zones the top soil layer (at depth of 10 cm and below) are regularly warmed up to 35°C and above which is enough to enable development of sizable population of thermophiles. Apinis (1963, 1972) examined such fungi in various types of grasslands and recorded highest frequency from the litter layer, probably, because of most favorable temperature and moisture conditions. Widespread occurrence of thermophilic fungi in soils has been established (Crisan, 1964; Evans, 1968, 1971a; Udagawa *et al.*, 1973 Taber and Pettit, 1975). Besides these Ellis (1980) also reported thermophilic fungi from antartic soils.

Many thermophilic fungi are pathogens of man and other warm-blooded animals (Lacey, 1975; Cooney and Emerson, 1964; Apinis and Pugh, 1967). Birds and their nesting material also harbor thermophilic fungi and bird's assumed to be the source of heat responsible for occurrence of these.

MATERIALS AND METHODS

For the collection of samples, 6 different habitats, i.e., compost piles, soils, storage, veterinary feeds, wood chip piles and bird's nest were selected.

Soil: Samples were collected from superficial layer of soil not exceeding 1-2 inches. During survey emphasis was given to the coal mines (geothermal soil) of Madhya Pradesh and Chhattisgarh; crop fields, forests, and grasslands (alluvial soil) of northern coastal and central region of India.

Compost: Heated and self-heating habitats of India have not been investigated much where thermophilic and thermotolerant fungi are expected to be more diversified both marphologically and biochemically. In the present study samples of compost were collected from (1-2 feet deep regions) the compost piles. Composting materials such as decomposing dung, municipal waste, paddy straw, wheat straw, grasses and jute bag etc. were also collected.

Storage: Samples of cereal grains and straw were collected from deep layer of different storage. Oil seeds, cereal grains and dry fruits were collected from the storage of villagers and grain merchants.

Veterinary Feed: Samples of oil cakes, seed grains, bran, harvested green grass were collected from deep regions for the isolation.

Bird's Nest: Samples of straw and pieces of nesting materials from bird's nest were collected from various places of surveyed regions.

For the isolation of thermophilic fungi from different samples, a small amount approximately 5 gm was incubated at 45°C for 24 hours. After this treatment sample were powdered and then again incubated for 48 hrs at 45°C in to minimize the propagules of mesophilic fungi. Small amount of heat treated powdered samples was plated on Emerson's YpSs medium using direct plate method as described by Warcup (1950). The plated Petri dishes were incubated at 45°C and observed daily for any fungal growth on the medium. From the growing fungal colonies a bit of mycelium was transferred to other dishes for purification The fungi isolated were kept in petri dishes having Emerson's YpSs agar medium and grown at 20°C temperature to categorize true thermophilic fungi.

RESULT AND DISCUSSION

During the course of study a total of 244 fungi were isolated from different habitats. These isolates represent 47 species of 25 genera. Maximum number of isolates, were recorded from the soil samples, while bird's nest samples yielded only 12 isolates. *Absidia corymbifera, Aspergillus fumigatus, A.flavus, A. nidulans, Chaetomium thermophile, Humicola lanuginosa, Rhizomucor miehei, R.pusillus, Scytalidium thermophilum* were recorded from almost all the habitats (Table 1).

The soil samples collected from north, central and coastal regions of the country representing the alluvial soil yielded good numbers of fungi. The details of distribution of thermophilic fungi in soils of different places are presented in Table-2. The maximum number of thermophilic fungi were recorded from coal mines of Korba. The coal mines area of Korba representig the geothermal soil where the soil surface and atmospheric temperature recorded usually higher. Some points it was recorded more than 100°C due to self ignition of fuel rocks *Aspergillus fumigatus, A.nidulans, C. thermophile,* and *S. thermophilum* have been isolated from soil of most of the places. A total of 8 species of *Thielavia* have been recorded during present survey. Out of these, six were recorded from soil samples. Geothermal soils and alluvial soils of north region also yielded a good number of fungi (Table 2). In order to confirm thermophilic nature of isolated fungi they were also grown at 20°C on Emerson's YpSs medium for seven days. Apinis (1963) has also reported high number of thermophilic fungi in the soils rich in organic matter. Evans (1972) explained the role of organic matter, soil water content and the high temperature particularly for the growth of obligate thermophilic fungi. Qualitatively, a number of unique albino strains of *A. fumigatus, A. nidulans, C. thermophile, H.lanuginosa, Penicillium citrinum* mutant *alba, S. thermophilum* strain 1, *S.thermophilum* strain 2 were isolated from coal mines of Korba (Shukla, 1992), which

Table 1: Occurrence of thermophilic fungi in different habitats.

Organisms	Bird's nest	Compost	Soil	Storages	Veterinary feeds	Wood chip piles
Absidia corymbifera	1	2	3	4	5	1
Absidia sp.	–	–	–	1	–	–
Acremonium alabamense	–	–	–	1	–	–
Acremonium thermophilum	–	–	1	–	–	–
Aspergillus candidus	–	–	1	1	1	–
A. fumigatus	3	4	5	5	5	5
A. fumigatus, albino strain 1	–	–	1	–	–	–
A. flavus	1	1	1	3	3	1
A. nidulans	1	3	5	3	2	3
A. nidulans, albino strain 1	–	–	1	–	–	–
A. terreus	–	2	3	1	1	1
Achaetomium sp.	–	–	1	–	–	–
Coprinus sp.	–	1	–	–	–	–
Chaetomium thermophile	1	3	5	2	4	2
C. thermophile, albino strain 1	–	–	1	–	–	–
Chaetomium sp.	–	–	–	1	–	–
Cladosporium oxysporum	–	1	3	–	1	2
Myceliophthora fergusii	–	1	–	–	–	–
Corynascus sepedonium	–	–	2	–	–	–
Emericella nidulance	1	3	5	3	2	3
Humicola lanuginosa	1	5	4	5	3	3
H. lanuginosa, albino strain 1	–	–	1	–	–	–
H. stellata	–	–	–	1	–	–
Malbranchea sulfurea	–	–	1	–	–	–
Myceliophthora thermophila	–	2	1	–	1	1
Paecilomyces variotii	–	–	2	–	1	1
Penicillum citrinum mutant *Alba* mutant Nov.	–	–	1	–	–	–
P. dupontii	–	2	1	2	1	–
Phoma sorghina	–	–	–	–	–	1
Rhizomucor miehei	1	3	3	3	5	1
R. pusillus	1	1	2	2	3	1
Rhizopus rhizopodiformis	–	1	2	4	3	1
Scytaladium thermophilum	1	3	5	4	3	1
S. thermophilum, albino strain 1	–	–	1	–	–	–
S. thermophilum, albino strain 2	–	–	1	–	–	–
Chrysosporium sp.	–	–	1	–	–	–
Thermoascus aurantiacus	–	–	2	–	–	–
Thielavia basicola strain 1	–	–	1	–	–	–
T. basicola strain 2	–	–	1	–	–	–

(Contd.)

Organisms	Bird's nest	Compost	Soil	Storages	Veterinary feeds	Wood chip piles
T. fragilis	–	–	2	–	–	–
T. octospora	–	–	1	–	–	–
T. terricola	–	1	2	–	–	–
T. terristris	–	–	–	1	–	–
T. variospora	–	–	1	–	–	–
T. novoguineensis	–	1	–	–	–	–
Thielavia sp.	–	–	1	–	–	–
Total number of isolates	12	40	75	47	44	28

may be because of extremes of soil temperatures and the presence of high concentration of sulphur. The study on cultural characteristics of individual isolates of *Monascus* sp. at various temperatures (Keshari *et al.*, 1971) suggested that at a temperature above optimum or above 40°C, pigment production is considerably reduced. Sastry (1996) studied extracellular and intracellular enzyme profiles of black and albino strains of *S. thermophilum* at 45°C and 55°C temperatures in relation to their thermostability.

Table 2: Distribution of thermophilic fungi in some soil types.

Organisms	Coal mine soil		Alluvial soil		
	Chhindwara	Korba	R1	R2	R3
Absidia corymbifera	+	+	–	–	+
Acremonium thermophilum	–	–	+	–	–
Aspergillus candidus	–	+	–	–	–
A. flavus	–	+	–	–	–
A. fumigatus	+	+	+	+	+
A. fumigatus, albino strain 1	–	+	–	–	–
A. nidulans	+	+	+	+	+
A. nidulans, albino strain 1	–	+	–	–	–
A. terreus	+	+	+	–	–
Achaetomium sp.	–	–	+	–	–
Chaetomium thermophile	+	+	+	+	+
C. thermophile, albino strain 1	–	+	–	–	–
Corynascus sepedonium	–	+	+	–	–
Emericella nidulans	+	+	+	+	+
Humicola lanuginosa	+	+	+	–	+
H. lanuginosa, albino strain 1	–	+	–	–	–
Malbranchea sulfurea	–	+	–	–	–
Myceliopthora thermophila	–	+	–	–	–
Paecilomyces variotii	+	+	–	–	–
Penicillum citrinum mutant *alba* mutant Nov.	–	+	–	–	–

(Contd.)

Organisms	Coal mine soil		Alluvial soil		
	Chhindwara	Korba	R1	R2	R3
P. dupontii	–	+	–	–	–
Rhizomucor miehei	+	+	–	+	–
R. pusillus	–	+	–	+	–
Rhizopus rhizopodiformis	–	+	+	–	–
Chrysosporium sp.	–	–	+	–	–
S. thermophilum	+	+	+	–	–
S. thermophilum, albino strain 1	–	+	–	–	–
S. thermophilum, albino strain 2	–	+	–	–	–
Scytalidium sp.	–	+	–	–	–
Thermoascus aurantiacus	+	+	–	–	–
Thielavia basicola strain 1	–	+	–	–	–
T. basicola strain 2	+	–	–	–	–
T. fragilis	–	–	+	+	–
T. octospora	–	–	+	–	–
T. terricola	–	+	+	–	–
T. variospora	–	+	–	–	–
Thielavia sp.	–	+	–	–	–

R1: Soil from U.P. & Himalayan regions; R2: Soil from M.P. & Maharashtra; R3: Soil from coastal regions of Mumbai & Goa.

A total of 19 different species of thermophilic fungi have been recorded from different compost samples (Table 3). Maximum number of species, have been recorded from decomposing cattle shed sweepings mixed with the animal feeds and straw in the compost piles.

Table 3: Distribution of thermophilic fungi in compost / municipal waste.

Organisms	Dung	Straw	Municipal waste
Absidia corymbifera	–	+	–
Aspergillus fumigatus	+	+	+
A. flavus	–	+	–
A. nidulans	+	+	+
A. terreus	–	+	+
Coprinus sp.	–	–	+
Chaetomium thermophile	+	+	+
Humicola lanuginosa	+	+	+
Myceliophthora fergusii	–	–	+ jute
M. thermophila	–	+	+
Penicillum dupontii	–	+	+
Rhizomucor miehei	+	+	+
R. pusillus	–	+	–
Rhizopus rhizopodiformis	–	+	+
Scytalidium thermophilum	+	+	+
Sclerotium sp.	–	–	+ jute
Thielavia novoguineensis	+	–	–
T. terricola	–	+	–

The decomposing cow dung of compost piles and sun heated dung upala yielded most of the true thermophilic fungi. *Myceliophthora fergusii* an anamorph of *Corynascus sepedonium* and *Sclerotium* sp. were recorded from decomposed jute fiber (Sigler *et al.*, 1997). Kane and Mullins (1973) showed that samples from the surface layer of municipal compost system did contain more propagules of thermophiles than those taken at a depth of 2 ft. and stated that low pH and anaerobic conditions are unfavourable for growth of thermophilic fungi.

Thermophilic fungi are regarded as storage fungi because they damage grains or plant products when they are stored. Although, they are present while in the field but they do not damage the grains prior to storage (Tansay and Brock, 1978; Jain, 1999). In all 20 fungal species collected from different storage of cereals, oil cakes, animal fodder, dry fruits and tobacco. *Acremonium alabamense, Cladosporium oxysporum, Thielavia terrestris* are the important fungi obtained during the study (Table 4). Taber and Pettit (1975) isolated thermophlic fungi from various storages of pea nuts. Apinis and Eggins (1966) isolated lipolytic thermophilic fungi from oil palm kernels. A number of thermophilic fungi reported pathogenic to human and warm-blooded animals (Lacey, 1975, Scholer, 1974). Among these *A. corymbifera, A.fumigatus, R. pusillus* are recorded from most of the samples while a pathogenic species *H. stellata* has also been recorded from one sample.

Table 4: Distribution of thermophilic fungi in storages.

Organisms	Food grains	Oil seeds spices	Dry fruits	Animal fodder (straw)	Tobacco
Absidia corymbifera	+	+	+	+	–
Absidia sp.	–	–	+	–	–
Acremonium albamense	–	–	+	–	–
Aspergillus candidus	+	–	–	–	–
A. flavus	+	–	+	+	–
A. fumigatus	+	+	+	+	+
A. nidulans	+	–	–	+	+
A. terreus	–	–	–	+	–
Chaetomium thermophile	+	–	–	+	–
Chaetomium sp.	–	–	–	+	–
Cladosporium oxysporum	–	–	+	–	–
Emericella nidulans	+	–	–	+	+
Humicola lanuginosa	+	+	+	+	+
H. stellata	–	–	–	+	–
Penicillum dupontii	+	–	+	–	–
Rhizomucor miehei	+	+	+	–	–
R. pusillus	+	–	–	+	–
Rhizopus rhizopodiformis	+	+	+	+	–
Scytalidium thermophilum	+	+	+	+	–
Thielavia terrestris	–	–	+	–	–

Samples of three categories of animal feeds have been collected which on isolation yielded 16 species of thermophilic fungi (Table 5). The bran samples of unidentified nature collected from the various stores yielded maximum number of fungi. From the freshly harvested crop fodder and grasses occasionally stored for animal feed, only 11 thermophilic species could be collected. The same number of fungi, have been recorded from the veterinary oil cakes (khali) of different base (mustard, linum etc).

Table 5: Distribution of thermophilic fungi in samples of veterinary feeds.

Organisms	Bran & seeds	Crop fodders & grasses	Oil cakes
Absidia corymbifera	+	+	+
Aspergillus candidus	+	–	–
A. flavus	+	+	+
A. fumigatus	+	+	+
A. nidulans	+	–	+
A. terreus	+	–	–
Chaetomium thermophile	+	+	+
Humicola lanuginosa	+	+	+
Myceliophthora thermophila	–	+	–
Paecilomyces variotii	+	–	–
Penicillum dupontii	+	–	–
Rhizomucor miehei	+	+	+
R. pusillus	+	+	+
Rhizopus rhizopodiformis	+	+	+
Scytalidium thermophilum	+	+	+
Total number of fungal species	14	10	10

In the present investigation nesting material of different birds yielded only 12 thermophilic species. Among these, *Aspergillus fumigatus* has been found most frequent in the bird nest samples. In all 28 isolates belonging to 17 different species have recorded from the samples of wood chips. *Phoma sorghina* and two basidiomycetes forms have been collected from wood chip piles. Flannigan and Sagoo(1977) isolated a number of thermophilic fungi from wood chips and other cellulosic materials and concluded that both hemicelluloses and cellulose in bark of wood chips were used as substrates by the commonest thermophilic fungi like *A.fumigatus* and *C.thermophile*.

Microorganisms, during the millennia of their evolution have become adapted to occupy a wide series of temperature niches. In this context, thermophiles, which occur frequently in the habitats where temperature remains most of the time higher, adapted themselves to wide array of ecological niches like compost, soil, storage, bird's nest etc. Thermophilic fungi inhabiting in different environmental conditions in different habitats may show a great variation in their temperature requirement for their optimum growth. Whether different fungal species and their isolates inhabiting different habitats possessing same temperature growth relations is a subject of active interest and enquiry. Cochrane (1958), Johri *et al.*, (1999) suggested that subtropical strains of a particular fungus, may have higher optimum growth temperatures than strains from temperate regions and hence geographical isolates of the same species may differ in their temperature-growth relationships needs further investigation.

The results of the present investigation also indicate occurrence of many albino strains of thermophilic moulds in Indian habitats and hence many more surveys are required to find out such mutants, which can be used as tools to understand the physiology of thermophilic moulds and nature of heat sock proteins.

REFERENCES

Apinis, A.E. (1963) Occurrence of thermophlilous microfungi in certain Alluvial soils near Nottingham. Nova Hedwigia, 5:57-58

Apinis, A E. and Pugh, G. J. F. (1967) Thermophilic fungi of bird's nest. Mycopathol. Mycol. Appl., 33: 1-9

Apinis, A.E. (1972) Thermophilous fungi certain grasslands. Mycopathol. Mycol. Appl., 48: 63-74

Bergman, O. (1974) Thermal degradation and spontaneous ignition in outdoor chip storage. Res.Note r91, 36pp. Institution for Virkeslara, Skogshogskolan, Stockholm.

Cochrane, V. W. (1958) Physilogy of fungi. New York: J. Wiley.

Cooney, D. G., Emerson, R. (1964) Thermophilic fungi: An account of their biology, activities and classification, pp.188. San Francisco: W. H. Freeman and Company.

Craveri, R., Guicciardi, A. and Pacini, N. (1966) Distributin of thermophilic actinomycetes in compost for mushroom production. Annal.Microbiol, 16:111-113

Crisan, E. V. (1964) Isolation and culture of thermophilic fungi. Contri. Boyece Thompson Inst., 22:291-302

Crisan, E.V. (1973) Current concept of thermophilism and thermophilic fungi. Mycologia, 1117- 1198.

Dravid, R. K. (1940) Studies on soil temperatures in relation to other factors controlling the disposalof solar radiation. Indian Jour. Agric. Sci. 10 (3): 352-387

Ellis, D.H. (1980) Ultra structure of thermophilc fungi. 1. Ascocarp morphology of Thermoascus aurantiacus. Trans. Brit. Mycol. Soc., 76:457-466

Evans, H. C. (1968) British records. Trans. Br. Mycol. Soc., 51:587-588

Evans, H.C. (1971a) Thermophilous fungi of coal spoil tips. 1 Taxonomy. Trans Brit. Mycol. Soc., 57: 241-254.

Evans H. C. (1971b) Thermophilous fungi of coal spoil tips.11 Occurrence, distribution and temperature relationships. Trans. Brit. Mycol. Soc., 57:255-266

Evans H. C. (1972) Thermophilous fungi isolated from the air. Trans. Br. Mycol. Soc. 59: 516-519.

Fergus, C. L.(1964) Thermophilic and thermotolerant molds and actinomycetes of mushroom compost during peak heating. Mycologia (N.Y.), 56:267-284

Fergus, C. L. (1969) The cellulolytic activity of thermophilic fungi and actinomycetes. Mycologia, 61:426-431

Flanningan, B. (1969) Microflora of dried barley grain. Tran. Brit. Mycol. Soc., 53: 371-379

Flanningan, B. (1972) In 'Bio deterioration of materials' (Eds. A. H. Walters and E. H. Hueck-Van der Plas), Vol. 2, 35-41. Wiley, New York.

Flanningan, B. (1974) Distribution of seed-born microorganisms in nacked barley and wheat before harvest. Trans. Brit. Mycol.Soc., 62: 51-58.

Flanningan, B. and Sagoo, G. S. (1977) Degradation of wood by Aspergillus fumigatus isolated from self heated wood chips. Mycologia 69: 514-523.

Geiger, R. (1965) The Climate Near the Ground. 4th ed. Harvard University Press.

Greaves, H. (1971) Biodeterioration of tropical hard wood chips in outdoor storage. TAPPI, 54:1128-1133

Gregory, P.H., lacey,M. E.Festenstein, G. N. and Skinner, F.A. (1963) Microbial and biochemical changes during the moulding of hay. J. Gen. Microbiol., 33: 147-174.

Hedger, J.N. (1975) The biology of thermophilic fungi in Indonesia. In Biodegradation and Humification (ed. G. Kilbertus, O. Reisinger, A. Moury &Cancela de Fonseca) pp.59-65 Edition Pierron

Jain, P. C.(1999) Spoilage of stored products. In Thermophilic Moulds in Biotechnology (*Ed.* B.N. Johri, T. Satyanarayana and J. Olson). Kluwer academic publishers, Drodrecht, Netherlands. pp. 289-316

Johri, B.N., T. Satyanarayana and J.Olsen (1999) Thermophilic Moulds in Biotechnology, Kluwer academic publishers, Drodrecht, Netherlands. p. 342.

Kane, B.E. and Mullins, J.T. (1973) Thermophilic fungi in a municipal waste compost system. Mycologia 65: 1087-1100.

Keshari, L. Manandhar and Apinis, A.E. (1971) Temperature relation in Monascus, Trans. Br. Mycol. Soc. 57: (3) 465-472.

Kushner, D. J. (1978) Microbial Life in Extreme Environments. Academic Press, New York, p. 465.

Kuthubutheen, A. J. (1982) Thermophilic fungi from Malasia, Trans. Bri. Mycol. Soc. 79 (3) 146-150.

Lacey, J. (1972) The microbiology of grain stored underground in Iron Age type pits. J.Stored Prod. Res., 82: 151-154.

Lacey, J. (1975) Potential hazards to animals and man from microorganisms in fodder and grains. Trans. Brit. Mycol. Soc. 65: 171-184.

Maheshwari, R. (1997) The ecology of thermophilic fungi, In: Tropical Mycology (*Ed.* K.K. Janardhanan, C. Rajendran, K. Natarajan and D. L. Hawksworth) Oxford & IBH publishers, Delhi, pp. 277-289.

Mehrotra, B. S. and Monica Basu. (1980) Taxonomic studies of thermophilic fungi from India 1. Nova Hedwigia , 32:1-8

Miehe, H. (1907) 'Die Selbesterhitzung des Heus Sinebiologische Studie' Gustav Fischer, Jena.

Mulinge, S. K. and Apinis, A. E. (1969) Occurrencs of thermophilous fungi in stored barley grain. Ann, Appl. Biol., 65: 277-284.

Ofosu-Asiedu, A, and Smith, R. S. 1973.Some factors affecting wood degradation by thermophilic and thermotolerant fungi. Mycologia, 65: 87-98.

Sastry, M. S. R. (1996) Morhological and biochemical studies on thermophilic fungi of Korba, Madhya Pradesh. Ph. D. Thesis G. D. University Bilaspur (India)

Scholer, H.J. (1974) In Aspergillosis and Farmer's Lungs in man and animals. (*Ed.* R. de Haller and F. Suter),. Hans Huber Publisers, Bern, Stuttgart, Vienna. pp. 35-40.

Sigler, L. Aneja, K. R., Kumar, R., Maheshwari, R., Shukla, R. V. (1997) New records from India and redescription of *Corynascus thermophilus* and its anamorph *Myceliophthora fergusii*, M*ycotaxon* 68: 185-192.

Singhai Sharmeela and Jain, P.C. (1992) Thermophilious fungi form decomsing organic matter: compost and saw dust. Geobios New Reports. 11: 41-44.

Shukla, A.K. and Jain P.C. (1990) Thermophilous mould flora: A major deteriogenic factor for wheat grain. In. Shetty, H.S. and Prakash, M.S. (ed) Proc. Nat. Seminar on Adv. Seed Sc. and Tech. 14-16 Dec.1989. Mysore Printing and Publishing House, Mysore, India. pp. 356-357.

Shukla, R. V. (1985) Morphological and biochemical studies of some thermophilic fungi Ph. D. Thesis Dr. H. S. Gour Vishwavidyalaya Saugar (India).

Shukla, R. V. (1992) Albinism at higher temperature in fungi / lower plants. JBS Halden Centinary Congress on Evolution, Bionature 8-9.

Smith, R. S. (1973) Colonization and degradation of outside stored softwood chips by fungi .Res. note no. R83, 16PP. Dept. For. Prod., R. Coll, For Stockholm.

Stahl, R. W. (1964) Survey of burning coal-mine rfuse banks. U.S. Bur. Mines Inform. Circ.8209, 39pp.

Sumner, J. L., Morgan, E. D. and Evans, H. C. (1969). The effect of growth temperature on fatty acid composition of fungi in the order Mucorales. Can. J. Microbiol., 15: 515-520.

Taber, R. A. Pettit, R. E. (1975) Occurrence of thermophilic microoganisms in peanuts and peanut soil.Mycologia, 67: 157-161.

Tansey, M. R. (1971) Isolation of thermophilic fungi from self- heated, industrial wood chip piles. Mycolgia, 63:537-547.

Tansey, M. R. and Brock, T.D. (1978) Microbial life at high Temperatures: Ecological aspects. In. Microbial Life in Extreme Environments (*Ed.* D.J. Kushner). Academic Press, New York pp. 159-216.

Thakre, R. P. and Johri, B. N. (1976) Occurrence of thermophilic fungi in coal-mine soils of Madhya Pradesh. Curr. Sci., 45: 271-273.

Udagawa, S., Furuya, K. and Horie, Y. (1973) Notes on some ascomycetous micro fungi from soil. Bull. Natl. Sci. Mus. (Tokyo), 16: 503-520.

Vartaja, O. (1949) High surface soil temperatures. Oikos 1: 6-28

Warcup, J. H. (1950) The soil-plate method for isolation of fungi from soil. Nature, London, 166: 117-118.

Microbiology and Biotechnology for Sustainable Development (Ed. P.C. Jain),
CBS Publishers & Distributors, New Delhi (2004), pp. 214–224.

B-4

Soil Microbial Diversity with Reference to Utilization Patterns of Carbon and Nitrogen Sources

N.A. Haque, H.P. Soni and S.R. Dave
Department of Microbiology, School of Sciences
Gujarat University, Ahmedabad 380 009.

Abstract

Microorganisms play a crucial role for maintaining the fertility and productivity of soils. Understanding the functional abilities of microorganisms may help to improve agricultural practices. The role of diversity of microorganism, and the relationship between microbial diversity and function is largely unknown. Therefore the use of microbial functioning for examination of changes in biological diversity needs to be exploited for the benefit of soil quality within agroecosystem. Substrate utilisation patterns based on sole carbon source utilisation can characterise bacterial communities. Viable organisms will respond to the substrate that they can metabolise providing an overall community fingerprint. In present study 7 different amino acids as sole nitrogen source and 15 different carbon substrates were used for quick and inexpensive assessment of functional diversity of microbial communities of agricultural fields with different management practices. Shannon-Wiener diversity index (H'), Richness and Evenness indices were calculated for all the soils. Diversity index varied from 0 to 2.68. Richness index varied from 0 to 4.87 and evenness ranged from 0 to 0.95. Agricultural fields where there was crop rotation throughout the year or where vegetables were cultivated along with other crop round the year showed high diversity and richness as compared to the fields where only seasonal crops were grown. Barren and some non-organic soils failed to utilise any substrate out of the 22 substrates used, indicating degraded soil health. Among the varieties of substrates, organic acids were preferably used. Principal component analysis and detailed statistical analysis will be discussed.

Key words: functional diversity, soil microbial community, Shannon-Weiner diversity index, agroecoystems

---

Corresponding author: *S.R. Dave.* Email:*shaileshrdave@hotmail.com*

INTRODUCTION

The activities of the soil microbiota are indispensable to the long-term sustainability of agricultural systems. This is because individual species and consortia of soil microorganisms have key roles in the many functional processes that maintain such systems. However, despite the importance of these functional processes in agricultural systems, very little is known about the biodiversity of soil microbial communities that support them. This is partly due to (1) the fact that in many intensive agricultural systems, some of the functional processes carried out by the microbial communities are overridden by the use of agrochemicals and (2) the technical difficulties involved in sampling and quantifying the diversity of soil microorganisms (Pankhurst *et al.*, 1996). An alternative approach is to examine components of biodiversity for which there exists a reasonable chance of detecting patterns that are biologically meaningful. One such alternative is functional diversity (Zak *et al.*, 1994).

Functional diversity can be examined in various ways viz. physiology, enzyme activities, stress response of the community etc. (Kennedy and Smith, 1995). One of the methods is based on substrate richness i.e. the number of different substrate that are utilised by a microbial community in a defined habitat. Substrate utilisation profiles of multiple sole sources by mixed microbial communities can be rapidly obtained through direct inoculation of environmental samples (e.g. water and soil suspensions) into microtitre plates containing various substrates as a sole source and a redox indicator dye (Garland and Mills, 1991). Utilisation of different sole sources is quantified by measuring the reduction of the dye to coloured compound in respiring cells. The obtained patterns of substrate utilisation or community level physiological profiles (CLPP) can consistently discriminate spatial and temporal gradients within microbial communities (Winding, 1994; Garland *et al.*, 1997).

Substrate utilisation measures of diversity provide the basis for grouping soils with respect to microbial community similarity and differences (Kennedy and Lewin, 1997). The presence or absence of response to a particular substrate in a community level assay reflects the presence or absence of individuals in community capable of utilising the substrate (Haack *et. al.*, 1995). Individual communities can be separated through Principal Component Analysis (PCA) of the specific combination of substrates that the communities utilise (Zak *et al.*, 1994; Garland, 1996a).

The usefulness of substrate utilisation is dependent on its ability to consistently characterise microbial communities based on sole substrate utilisation and to elucidate changes in community response due to some perturbation (Garland, 1996b). Substrate utilisation assays have also been successfully used in assessing differences due to some natural and anthropogenic factors (Garland, 1996a; Garland, 1996b).

Microbial diversity indices can function as bio indicators of stability of a community. They can also be used to describe the ecological dynamics and impact of stress on community (Kennedy and Smith, 1995). For example, decrease in Shannon diversity index was seen with severe disturbances such as tillage, overgrazing and pollutants (Kennedy and Lewin, 1997).

Our objective was to characterise soil community structural differences with respect to the type of soil and management practices through analysis of utilisation patterns of seven different sole nitrogen sources and fifteen different sole carbon sources on whole soil samples.

By analysing various measures of diversity, attempt was made to understand the functional microbial diversity on the bases of applied soil management practices and soil types.

MATERIALS AND METHODS

Soil sampling

Top layer soil (0-15 cm) was collected randomly from 19 different sites from Tharad and Vav Taluka, which are semi-arid regions in Banaskantha district, Gujarat, India. Two samples were collected from Ahmedabad, Gujarat for reference point of view. The samples were collected in July 1999 and were refrigerated till complete analysis. Details of soils and sites of collection are presented in Table 1. The physicochemical characteristics of soils were analysed by standard methods. To obtain CLPP of various soils, seven sole nitrogen sources and fifteen sole carbon sources were used. List of various substrates used for CLPP is shown in Table 2.

Table 1: Description of the soil samples collected from Banaskantha district.

Soil sample number	Type of management practice	Location
3, 4, 5, 6, 7, 8 farming soil	Non-organic conventional	Tharad village
1, 2, 9	Organic farming soil	Tharad village
10	Uncultivated barren soil	Tharad village
11	Virgin soil	Tharad village
15, 16, 17	Non-organic conventional farming soil	Bhuria village
14	Virgin soil	Bhuria village
19, 20, 21	Organic farming soil	Baluntri village
18	Virgin soil	Baluntri village
12	Virgin soil	Ahmedabad
13	Botanical garden soil	Ahmedabad

Community level physiological profile assay

CLPP assay was performed in test tubes with 4 ml Davis broth along with a redox indicator dye (The Himedia Manual, 1998). For the assay of nitrogen and carbon substrates, ammonium sulphate or glucose in the medium was replaced by the particular nitrogen or carbon substrate as their sources. The substrates used can be categorised into different guilds such as amino acids, carboxylic acids, polymers, carbohydrates and miscellaneous.

Soil suspensions were prepared by transferring 10 g of soil into 90 ml sterile Ringer's salt solution in 250 ml Erlenmeyer flask (Alef and Nannipieri, 1995). All the flasks were placed on Newtronic environmental orbital shaker (125 rpm) for 30 minutes and then allowed to settle for another 30 minutes. All the substrates were inoculated with 100 µl of desired dilution of the supernatant from each soil sample. The tubes were incubated at 32±2° C for 10 days on

Newtronic environmental orbital shaker at 170 rpm. The degree to which a particular substrate is utilised was quantified by measuring the intensity of colour change caused by the redox dye.

Table 2: Various substrates used for the CLPP assay.

Amino acids	*Carboxylic acids*
Alanine (s1)	Acetic acid (s8)
Arginine (s2)	Citric acid (s10)
Asparagine (s3)	Formic acid (s12)
Glutamic acid (s4)	Lactic acid (s15)
Leucine (s5)	Malic acid (s16)
Phenylalanine (s6)	Succinic acid (s17)
Threonine (s7)	*Miscellaneous*
Carbohydrates	Cyclic AMP (s9)
Fucose (s13)	Creatine (s11)
Xylitol (s22)	Glycerol (s14)
Polymers	Thiamine (s18)
Tween 20 (s20)	Toluene (s19)
Tween 80 (s21)	

Note: Substrate labels are given into brackets.

Data analysis

The substrate utilisation data obtained were applied to Principal Component Analysis (PCA) and Hierarchical Cluster Analysis using the statistical package SPSS version 7.5 (1996) for windows.

Shannon Weiner diversity index was calculated for each sample using the following equation (Zak *et al.*, 1994).

$$H' = \Sigma \text{ pi } (\ln \text{ pi})$$

Where pi is the ratio of activity on particular substrate to the sum of activities on all substrates.

Functional diversity value for each soil sample was also calculated using Hill equation (Kennedy and Smith, 1995).

$$D_{Hill} = e^{H'}$$

Index of evenness was calculated using E_{Pielou} equation (Kennedy and Smith, 1995).

$$E = \frac{H'}{\ln (S)}$$

Where S is number of substrates utilised.

Richness was calculated using $R_{Menhinick}$ equation (Kennedy and Smith, 1995).

$$R = \frac{S}{\sqrt{n}}$$

Where n is the sum of total activity for each soil.

RESULTS AND DISCUSSION

At the time of sample collection, the ambient temperature ranged between 40-44° C. Physicochemical characterisations of soil viz. pH, texture, conductivity, organic carbon and soluble phosphorus is presented in Table 3. The studied parameters for all the soils were found to be within the normal range for agricultural soils but showed considerable diversity.

Table 3: Physico chemical characteristics of soil samples.

Sample number	pH	Soil texture	Conductivity (milli-moze/ cm)	Organic carbon (%)	Soluble phosphate (Kg/ha)
1.	7.7	Loamy	0.18	0.75	38
2.	7.6	Sandy	0.10	0.31	24
3.	7.6	Sandy	0.13	0.37	28
4.	7.6	Loamy	0.18	0.72	34
5.	7.7	Loamy	0.48	0.47	32
6.	8.2	Sandy	0.20	0.37	34
7.	8.0	Loamy	0.38	0.69	38
8.	8.0	Sandy with little loamy	0.10	0.51	34
9.	7.9	Sandy with little loamy	0.20	0.61	36
10.	7.5	Sandy	0.81	0.75	36
11.	7.9	Sandy	0.23	0.50	36
12.	7.5	Sandy	0.14	0.58	36
13.	8.1	Muck	0.24	1.00	40
14.	7.7	Sandy	0.16	0.94	38
15.	8.0	Sandy	0.34	0.61	34
16.	8.1	Sandy	0.35	0.64	34
17.	8.2	Sandy	0.36	0.43	32
18.	8.1	Sandy	0.15	0.44	34
19.	8.0	Sandy	0.10	0.39	32
20.	7.8	Sandy	0.10	0.52	34
21.	8.0	Sandy	0.11	0.44	34

Normal ranges : pH : 6.5 to 8.2; Electrical conductivity : <1.0; Organic carbon : 0.51 to 0.75; soluble phosphorus : 26 to 60.

The exceptions are soluble potassium and organic carbon. Soluble potassium was found to be above 450 Kg/h for all the soil samples which in spite of being above the normal range for agricultural soils, no adverse indications for the same were given by the Government soil testing laboratory, Gandhinagar, Gujarat. On the other hand, organic carbon was below the normal range for 8 soil samples. According to the standards mentioned by Government soil testing laboratory, Gujarat, the organic carbon of all of the soil samples except the botanical garden soil was below 1%. This could be due to the semi-arid soils collected near desert region. Similar level of organic carbon, has been reported for desert soils by Forster (Forster, 1995).

Analysis of soil functional diversity carried out on the basis of 21 different carbohydrates utilisation patterns has been reported elsewhere (Soni *et al.*, 2000). Twenty-two substrates used were divided into five guilds. Out of the seven amino acids used, glutamic acid was utilised to a greater extent by the soil microbial communities. The microbial community only from sample number 7 was able to utilise all the amino acids tested.

All the soil microbial communities failed to respond to creatine, formic acid, thiamine and toluene out of the substrates tested. Out of the different guilds of substrates selected for the assay, carboxilic acids showed maximum response of which malic acid was preferably used followed by lactic acid, succinic acid and citric acid (Graph 1). Other preferable substrates were tween 80, glycereol, tween 20 and xylitol respectively.

Graph 1: Amenability of substrates to various soil microbial communities

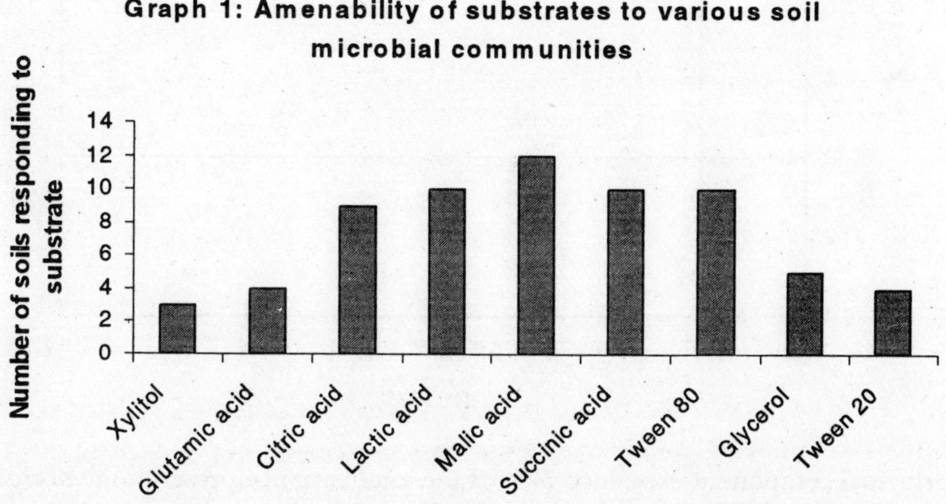

PCA of the soil samples and the substrates used were performed. In PCA, each PC extracts a portion of the variance in the original data, with the greatest amount of variance extracted by the first axis. Relationships among the samples are readily observed by plotting samples in two dimensions on the basis of their scores for the first two PCs (Jollife, 1996). Such relationships are difficult to observe when examining the original variables in multidimensional space (in this case 22 dimensional space) but PCA of the colour responses of the substrates used allows for the comparison of microbial samples on the basis of differences in the pattern of sole substrate utilisation.

PCA of substrate response was able to group the substrates (Graph 2) where all the amino acids except glutamic acid, which were not utilised by many soil samples were grouped together. Citric acid, glycerol, succinic acid and tween 80 formed one group with little distance from glutamic acid, lactic acid and malic acid. Cyclic AMP was distinctly placed in PCA of substrates as, it was used by only one soil microbial community and was also the only substrate used by that soil. The basis for such type of response is not clear at this junction.

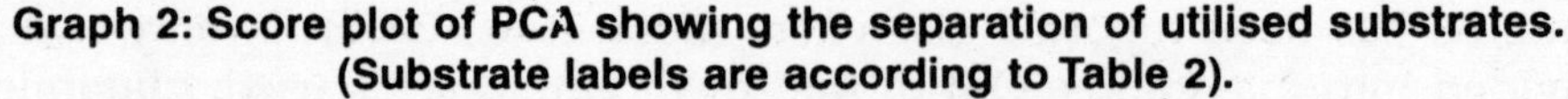

Graph 2: Score plot of PCA showing the separation of utilised substrates. (Substrate labels are according to Table 2).

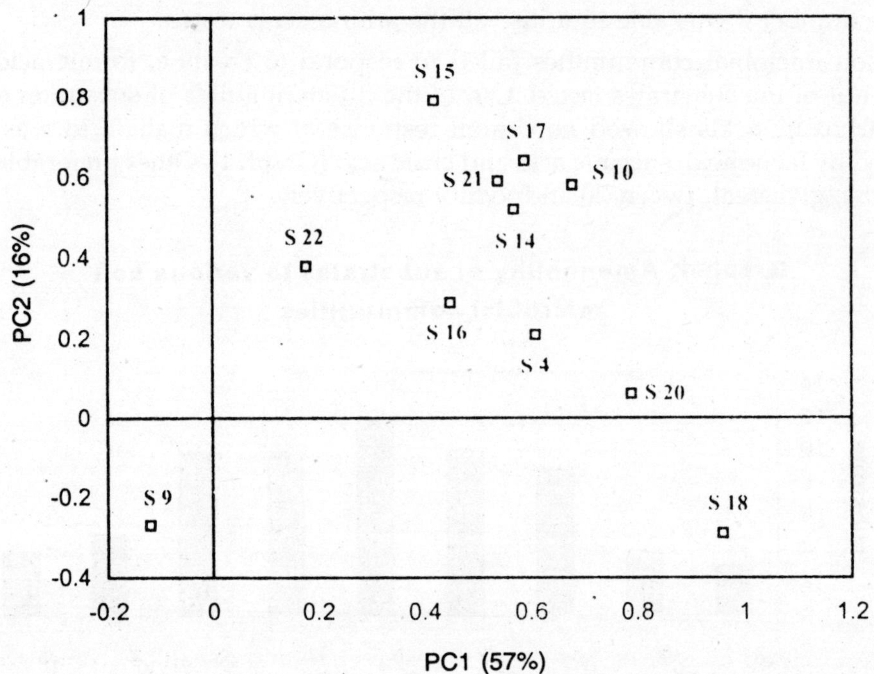

First principal component explained 57% of the total variance present in the original data followed by the second PC, which explained 16% of the total variance in the data. When examining the PCA of soil samples, first PC was able to separate soil sample number 7 with maximum distance from rest of the samples (Graph 3). Same observation is seen in Hierarchical Cluster Analysis where sample 7 is completely distinct from rest of the samples (Graph 4). The distinct placement of this soil could be due to the utilisation of highest number of diverse substrates (77%) including all amino acids.

Sample number 1, 5, 8, 9, 10, 11, 13 and 19 formed one group in PCA having substrate richness more than 4, among this group sample number 5, 8, 10 and 11 were closely placed since their microbial communities utilised similar set of substrates. PCA was able to differentiate sample number 16 on the basis of utilisation of a unique substrate, cyclic AMP, where as Hierarchical Cluster Analysis grouped this soil with soils whose microbial communities utilised 0 to 3 substrates.

Graph 3: Score plot of PCA showing the separation of soil samples on the basis of community level physiological profile.

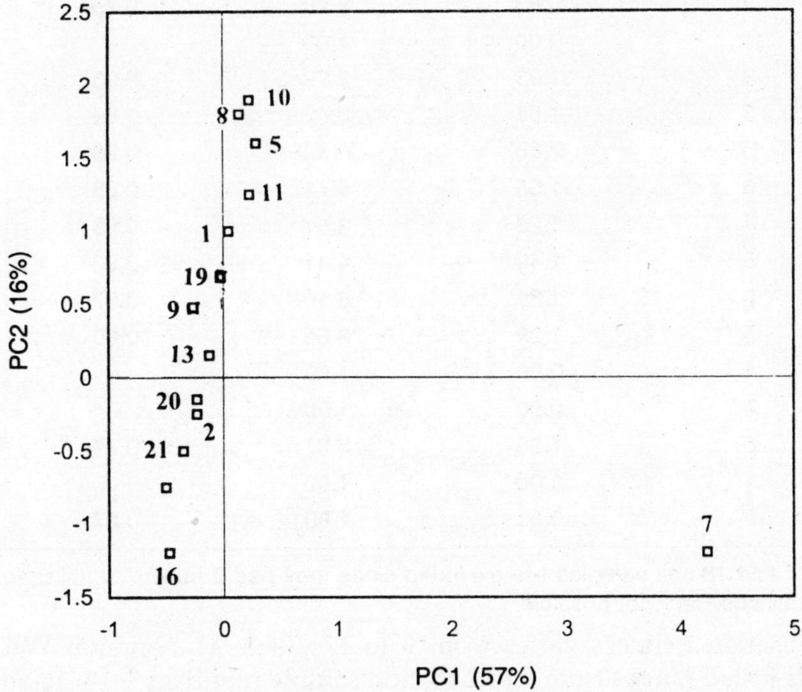

PCA as well as Hierarchical Cluster Analysis differentiate the samples on the basis of the similarities and differences in the substrate utilisation profiles of the samples but they do not give the account of the number of substrates utilised and the extent of their utilisation. This can best be understood by calculating the various diversity index values. There was found to be a high correlation between Shannon Weiner diversity index (H') and the principal component scores (r= 0.73) significant at 95% confidence level. Hence diversity values should be considered along with the PCA analysis for qualitative analysis of the soil samples which also highlight the basis for the differences observed in the samples.

Differences in the numbers and extent of utilised substrates among the soil microbial communities demonstrate a spatial dimension of functional diversity (Zak *et al.*, 1994). Microbial diversity index is a single value; thus it can not indicate the total make up of the community. For example, two communities may have same diversity index value but one may comprise low evenness and high richness, while the other may comprise high evenness and low richness. It is therefore important to consider evenness, richness and diversity collectively (Kennedy and Smith, 1995).

Table 4 : Richness, evenness and diversity values for microbial populations from various soils based on community level physiological profiles.

Sample number	Substrate utilisation richness (S)	Diversity indices			
		Shannon Weiner (H')	Hill (D_{Hill})	Evenness (E_{Pielou})	Richness ($R_{Menhinick}$)
1	5	1.45	4.26	0.90	2.38
2	3	0.83	2.28	0.75	3.56
3	1	0.00	1.00	-	2.31
4	3	1.03	2.79	0.93	3.16
5	8	1.86	6.42	0.89	3.47
7	17	2.68	14.63	0.95	4.87
8	6	1.55	4.71	0.86	2.36
9	4	1.28	3.61	0.93	2.18
10.	5	1.49	4.41	0.92	2.26
11	8	1.81	6.10	0.87	3.60
13	5	1.29	3.65	0.80	3.47
14	1	0.00	1.00	-	2.48
16	1	0.00	1.00	-	1.48
19	6	1.38	3.97	0.77	3.35
20	1	0.00	1.00	-	1.98
21	2	0.61	1.83	0.87	2.42

Note: 6, 12, 15, 17 and 18 soil samples are excluded since they had 0 substrate utilisation richness and further calculations were not possible.

Substrate utilisation richness varies from 0 to 17 (Table 4). Shannon Weiner diversity index for the soils tested ranges from 0 to 2.68. Soil sample numbers 3, 14, 16 and 20 have H' value of 0 which suggests that only one substrate utilising microbial community was present and hence no diversity or 0 diversity was there.

Sample number 7 showed highest Shannon Weiner and Hill diversity values followed by sample number 5 and 11. This was because sample number 11 was a virgin soil and 7 and 5 were from conventional farms where crop rotation with vegetable cultivation was practised through out the year whereas other samples were from the fields where only seasonal crops were harvested. Moreover, sample number 7 had the most diverse microbial communities capable of utilising 17 different substrates responsible for high diversity value. Richness and evenness indices were also highest for sample number 7. Thus we can say that cultivated soils specifically with mixed type of crop rotation have high diversity as compared to virgin soils. Similar results were obtained where diversity of prairie and cultivated soils were studied (Kennedy and Smith, 1995).

Significant correlation was not obtained between diversity and various physicochemical parameters of the soils. Diversity values were not able to classify the samples in to different guilds on the basis of different management practices. But one general observation was that diversity value of 0 was found to be less frequent in organic farming soils (one sample) as compared to conventional farming soils (5 samples). Soils where substrate utilisation richness is 0 indicate degraded soil health and they require further investigation coupled with proper management practices.

Graph 4: Dendrogram showing relationship among soil samples based on squared Euclidean distance using Hierarchical Cluster Analysis of CLPP data.

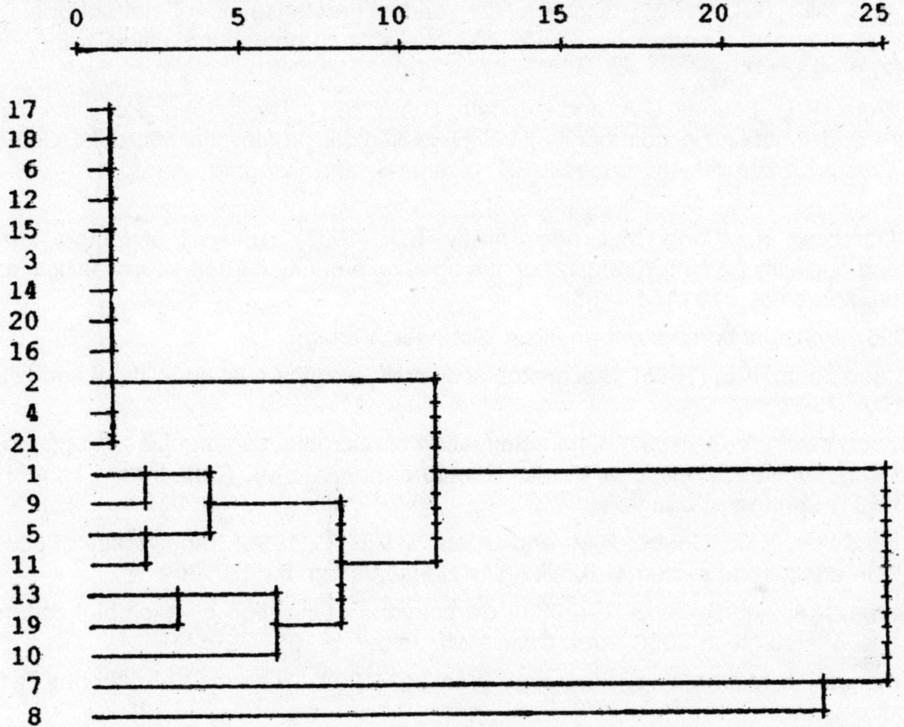

In summary, community level physiological profile patterns of soil samples is an easy and apt method for differentiating soils and for determination of the soil health. However, the use of diversity measurements to assess management impacts may be limited, therefore to determine the extent of functional microbial diversity in agroecosystems we need to increase our knowledge of the functional roles of microbes in agroecosystem quality and productivity.

ACKNOWLEDGEMENT

We acknowledge Government Soil Testing Laboratory, Gandhinagar, Gujarat, India for physicochemical characterisation of our soil samples.

REFERENCES

Alef, K. and Nannipieri, P. (1995). *Methods in Applied Soil Microbiology and Biochemistry*. Academic Press, London.

Forster, J.C. (1995). Soil sampling, handling, storage and analysis: Organic carbon. In *Methods in Applied Soil Microbiology and Biochemistry* (*Ed.* Alef K. and Nannipieri, P)., Academic Press, London pp 59.

Garland, J.L. (1996a). Analytical approaches to the characterisation of samples of microbial communities using patterns of potential C source utilisation. *Soil Biol. Biochem.* 28 : 213-221.

Garland, J.L. (1996b). Patterns of potential C source utilisation by rhizosphere communities. *Soil Biol. Biochem.* 28 : 223-230.

Garland, J.L. and Mills, A.L. (1991). Classification and characterisation of heterotrophic microbial communities on the basis of patterns of community-level sole-carbon-source utilization. *Appl. Environ. Microbiol.* 57(8) : 2351-2359.

Garland, J.L., Cook, K.L., Loader, C.A. and Hungate, B.A. (1997). The influence of microbial community structure and function on community-level physiological profiles. In *Microbial Communities : Functional Versus Structural Approaches* (Ed. Insam, H. and Rangger, A.).pp 171-183. Springer, Verlag.

Haack, S.K., Garchow, H., Klugg, M.J. and Forney, L.J. (1995). Analysis of factors affecting the accuracy, reproducibility and interpretation of microbial community carbon source utilisation profiles. *Appl. Environ. Microbiol.* 61 :1458-1468.

Jollife, I.T. (1996). *Principal component analysis.* Springer, Verlag.

Kennedy, A.C. and Smith, K.L. (1995). Soil microbial diversity and the sustainability of agricultural soils. *Plant Soil* 170 : 75-86.

Kennedy, A.C. and Lewin, V.G. (1997). Characterisation of microbial communities in agroecosystems. In *Microbial Communities : Functional Versus Structural Approaches.* (Eds. Insam, H. and Rangger, A.)., pp 121-131. Springer, Verlag,.

Pankhurst, C.E., Keller, K.O., Doube, B.M. and Gupta, V.V.S.R. (1996). Biodiversity of soil microbial communities in agricultural systems. *Biodiversity Conservation.* 5 : 197-209.

Soni, H.P., Haque, N.A. and Dave, S.R. (2000). Carbohydrate utilisation by microbial communities of semi-arid soils. Microbiotech 2000. *Ann. Conf. AMI*, Jaipur. p 165. (*Abstr.*)

The Himedia manual for microbiology laboratory practice. (1998). Himedia Laboratories Pvt. Limited, Mumbai, India.

Winding, A. (1994). Fingerprinting soil communities using Biolog microtitre plates. In *Beyond the Biomass : Compositional and Functional Analysis of Soil Microbial Communities* (*Ed.* Ritz, K., Dighton, J. and Giller, K.E.)., pp 85-94. John Wiley and Sons, Chichester, UK.

Zak, J.C., Willig, M.R., Moorhead, D.L. and Wildman, H.G. (1994). Functional diversity of microbial communities : A quantitative approach. *Soil Biol. Biochem.* 26(9) : 1101-1108.

Microbiology and Biotechnology for Sustainable Development (Ed. P.C. Jain),
CBS Publishers & Distributors, New Delhi (2004), pp. 225–234.

B-5

New Strategies in Organic Waste Utilization and its Management for Sustainable Agriculture

R. P. Thakre and A. A. Fulzele*
*Post Graduate Department of Botany, Nagpur University Campus,
Nagpur, (MS) – 440 010. India.*
** Shri M. Mohota College of Science, Nagpur. (MS) – 440 009. India.*

Abstract

Crop residues, rural and urban garbage and organic wastes from agro- industries have a great potential to be recycled in the field to increase the soil fertility and crop productivity. However, the traditional method presently employed in the rural areas for the production of organic manure is insufficient, time consuming and involves substantial loss of major nutrients. Attempts have been made to evaluate the potential of some of common weeds and crop plants as substrates for composting.

A simple and efficient method for the conversion of leafy biomass into bio- dung or organic manure within a short span of 15-20 day and 30-60 days for other wastes has been evolved. The degrading substrates were pretreated with water, cow urine and biogas slurry in different proportion as inoculum while urea as additive to enhance the composting process. Changes in temperature, pH and reduction in total solids during the process was studied at regular intervals. Mesophilic and thermophilic fungi involved during the process of composting were isolated at frequent intervals.

Effect of organic manure was compared with chemical fertilizers and FYM on the growth of crop plants. Further, it was observed that instead of using chemical fertilizers alone, combined application of prepared organic manure plus chemical fertilizers was found to be more promising.

Keywords: Biodegradation, composting, agriculture, biomass.

INTRODUCTION

Wastes are customarily considered from time immemorial as an auxiliary byproduct or refuse resulting from any economic activity. From ecological and economical viewpoint organic wastes are resources. Each and every kind of waste obviously contains matter and energy. Organic wastes are produced in agricultural milieu. There are enormous opportunities to develop new technologies as well as set up industries with wastes to improve upon quality of life. In this context instead of waste disposal, waste utilization shall be our prime concern. With the over production of grains in the country (200 M tones, 1999-2000) there is a continuous depletion in the fertility of soil. Due to indiscriminate use of chemical fertilizers, salinity of the soil increased in many parts of the country is well known, which is causing serious consequences over time and to avoid or to improve the soil condition, it is necessary to find alternative which must be environmental friendly, cost effective and productive. Organic manure produced by composting play vital role in maintenance of sound physical, chemical and biological condition of the soil, that means increased fertility of farming soil.

MATERIALS AND METHODS

In the present study attempts have been made to evaluate the potential of some common weeds and crop plants namely *Parthenium hysterophorus, Lantana camara, Leucaena leucocephala, Legacea mollis, Cassia tora, Xanthium strumarium, Clerodendum inerme,* and waste leaves of *Saccharum officinarum* and *Musa paradisiaca.* These substrates were used for the preparation of organic manure (Bio-dung). The methods developed and described by Das and Ghatnekar (1979), Joshi, et al., (1989) and Joshi and Thakre (1991) was adopted to achieve the aerobic biodegradation to the substrates under study. These substrates were collected from the fields. Banana and sugarcane leaves as waste materials were collected after the harvest. These were chopped of the size 5-6 cm and soaked well in water and placed in polythene bags of the size 12 × 16 inch of 150 gauze. Besides the polythene bags, pits of size 195 × 120 × 45 cm were prepared for large scale composting. To avoid leaching of nutrients in soil, polythene sheet was spread at the bottom of the pits, and on the top (Plates 3 and 4 on pages 235 and 236).

Following different types of treatments were given to each of the biodegrading biomass
500 g of biomass + Water 200 ml (Control)
500 g of biomass + Dry cattle dung 100 g
500 g of biomass + Cow urine 200 ml
500 g of biomass + *Trichoderma viride* inoculant.
Each treatment was performed in triplicates.

The experiments were performed in Sun Shade of trees and in room condition.

The bags and pits were regularly monitored to maintain required moisture and aeration. pH and temperature of the biodegrading substrates were noted at regular intervals. Associated mesophilic, thermotolerent and thermophilic fungi were isolated and identified to note the role of fungi in composting process. Final product (Organic manure) was analyzed for the total nitrogen and organic carbon percentage by microkjeldahl method. Pellett and Young (1980) and Walkley and Black (1934) methods were used to estimate nutrient contents of the organic manure prepared.

The pot culture experiments were carried out to study the effect of biodung manure on the growth of crop plants. Effect of different concentrations of manure was compared with that of FYM and chemical fertilizers, all the experiments were performed in triplicates.

The crop plants *Amaranthus paniculatus* and *Trigonella foenum graceum* were selected for these studies.

RESULTS AND DISCUSSION

Biodegradation of green leaves completed earlier as compared to other crop residues because the leaves contain less total solids than other substrates. Young and succulent tissues are metabolized more readily than mature plant residues. Degradation of biomass in polythene bags as well as in shallow pits covered with polythene sheets, were noted to be completed within short span of 20 days for green leaves and 10-20 weeks for other substrates. Biomass kept under shade and room conditions showed rapid and better decomposition as compared to that kept in direct sunlight.

Initially pH of the biomass was slightly acidic in the range of 6-7 but later on it became alkaline and remained in the range of 8-9 till the end of the process (Table 1a, 1b and 1c).

Table 1a: Changes In PH of Sugarcane Leaves Biomass Before and After Degradation

Treatments	Exposures								
	Sun			Shade			Room		
	8 am	1 pm	6 pm	8 am	1 pm	6 pm	8 am	1 pm	6 pm
CD	6.7	7.2	6.8	6.4	6.8	6.5	6.0	7.1	6.8
	(7.7)	(7.8)	(7.7)	(7.3)	(7.5)	(7.4)	(7.3)	(7.7)	(7.5)
U	6.0	7.1	6.8	5.7	6.3	5.8	5.9	6.8	6.0
	(7.9)	(8.0)	(7.9)	(7.3)	(7.6)	(7.4)	(7.8)	(7.9)	(7.8)
CD-U	7.1	7.4	7.3	6.2	7.4	6.5	6.3	7.6	6.99
	(7.8)	(8.0)	(7.8)	(7.5)	(7.9)	(7.7)	(7.3)	(8.0)	(8.2)
T	6.6	6.9	6.7	6.1	7.1	6.6	5.6	6.8	5.7
	(7.2)	(7.7)	(7.5)	(7.2)	(7.3)	(7.3)	(7.4)	(7.5)	(7.5)
C	6.3	6.9	6.6	5.5	7.0	5.8	5.8	6.9	6.8
	(7.3)	(7.6)	(7.5)	(7.3)	(7.8)	(7.6)	(7.4)	(7.5)	(7.5)

Note : i) Values of **first** day and in parantheses values of **last** day.

ii) **CD** = Cattle dung, **U** = Cow urine, **CD-U** = Cattle dung + Cow urine,

T = *Trichoderma viride* inoculum and **C** = Control

Temperature at the initial stage of decomposition was recorded to be in the range of 20-30 °C, in room condition and in shade conditions, while inn direct sun exposure it was 40-45 °C and reached to the peak 45-50 °C during 10th day. This was thermophilic phase of biodegradation. After this temperature declined and started mesophilic phase. In room condition temperature remained constant almost throughout the process of decomposition (Table 2a and 2b).

Table 1b: Changes in pH of Banana Leaves Biomass Before and After Degradation

Treatments	Exposures								
	Sun			Shade			Room		
	8am	1pm	6pm	8am	1pm	6pm	8am	1pm	6pm
CD	7.3	8.3	7.8	7.2	7.7	7.6	6.5	7.1	7.4
	(8.5)	(8.7)	(8.6)	(8.3)	(8.6)	(8.5)	(8.7)	(8.5)	(8.5)
U	6.7	7.8	7.3	7.3	8.0	7.7	7.1	7.6	7.6
	(8.2)	(8.4)	(8.3)	(8.6)	(8.5)	(8.5)	(8.4)	(8.5)	(8.4)
CD-U	7.1	7.8	7.3	7.5	7.7	7.6	6.6	7.2	6.7
	(8.4)	(8.6)	(8.3)	(8.6)	(8.7)	(8.7)	(8.2)	(8.3)	(8.1)
T	7.0	7.4	7.2	7.1	7.5	7.4	6.5	6.8	6.6
	(8.2)	(8.3)	(8.1)	(8.6)	(8.7)	(8.7)	(8)	(8.2)	(8.1)
C	7.1	7.9	7.3	6.7	8.0	7.7	6.6	7.6	7.0
	(8.1)	(8.4)	(8.2)	(8.7)	(8.8)	(8.8)	(8)	(8.2)	(8.3)

Note: i) Values of **first** day and in parantheses values of **last** day.

ii) **CD** = Cattle dung, **U** = Cow urine, **CD-U** = Cattle dung + Cow urine, **T** = *Trichoderma viride* inoculum and **C** = Control

Table 1c: Changes in pH during Biodegradation

Treatments	Initial	Days				
		1	3	5	10	15
Clerodendrum inerme						
Lvs+Water	5.8	6.5 (7.0)	7.7 (7.2)	7.4 (7.8)	7.5 (7.6)	8.4
Lvs+CD slurry+Urea	6.1	7.7 (7.8)	8.2 (8.1)	8.0 (8.0)	7.4 (7.5)	8.8 -
Parthenium histerophorus						
Lvs+Water	7.8	8.2 (7.9)	9.1 (8.3)	8.4 (7.8)	8.1 (7.8)	9.2 -
Lvs+CD slurry+Urea	7.5	8.2 (8.4)	9.0 (8.9)	8.4 (9.0)	8.1 (7.6)	9.3 -

(Contd.)

Treatments	Initial	Days				
		1	3	5	10	15
Lantana camara						
Lvs+Water	7.4	7.9 (8.2)	8.4 (8.4)	8.4 (7.8)	7.8 (7.5)	- -
Lvs+CD slurry+Urea	7.8	8.3 (8.1)	8.2 (8.4)	8.4 (8.3)	8.0 (7.9)	- -
Leucaena leucocephala						
Lvs+Water	5.2	7.5 (7.7)	8.2 (7.4)	8.1 (7.9)	7.7 (7.6)	9.4 -
Lvs+CD slurry+Urea	7.4	7.7 (7.8)	8.6 (8.8)	8.1 (8.4)	8.2 (7.6)	9.3 -

Note: Values in parenthesis shows pH in shade

Lvs. : Leaves

CD : Cattle dung slurry

Table 2a: Temperature range of degrading biomass at different hours in a day under Sun, Shade and Room condition during 16 days of degradation.

Light exposure	sample * leaves	Temperature °C at different hours in a day				
		7 AM	11 AM	3 PM	6 PM	11 PM
Sun	1	20-24	45-52	43.55	28-39	24-28
	2	20-24	42-55	40-55	29.38	23-29
Shade	1	20-26	35-41	34-44	27-34	24-29
	2	20-27	34-40	34-42	26-34	24-30
Room	1	20-27	28-36	30-37	29-31	28-31
	2	24-30	28-37	30-38	27-33	26-32

*1 - Clerodendrum inerme

2 - Leucaena leucocephala

During the process of degradation of biomass large number of fungi were isolated and identified. Thick fungal growth was observed over the surface of the leafy biomass as white mycelial mesh and powdery spore dust.

It was observed that thermophilic fungi were mainly responsible for cellulose and hemicellulose degradation during the thermophilic phase, prominent fungi include *Humicola* spp., *Talaromyces dupontii, Sporotrichum thermophile, Thermoascus aurantiacus, Torula thermphila, Absidia corymbifera, Mucor pussilus* etc. Similar results were reported by Cooney and Emerson (1964) during the mesophilic phase. Dominant fungi recorded were *Aspergillus fumigatus, Fusarium* spp., *and* Curvularia sp. Along with large number of other mucoraceous and deuteromycetous fungi (Table 4).

Table 2b: Temperature Range of the Degrading Biomass at different hours in a day under Sun, Shade and Room Condition during 60 days of Biodegradation

Light Exposure	Substrate	Temp. °C at different Hours of Days		
		8am	1pm	6pm
Sun	S	13-42	28-50	25-46
	B	13-40	30-48	26-45
Shade	S	13-38	24-45	26-45
	B	13-36	23-43	20-42
Room	S	20-36	20-40	21-38
	B	20-37	21-40	21-39

Note: S – Sugarcane leaves

B – Banana leaves

Table 3: Nutrient Estimation

Treatments	% C	%N	%P	%K	C/N Ratio
Clerodendrum inerme					
Lvs+Water	2.69	2.8134	1.95	1.075	9.842
Lvs+CD slurry+Urea	30.13	3.472	2.55	1.100	8.67
Parthenium histerophorus					
Lvs+Water	23.19	2.552	2.1	1.5	11.29
Lvs+CD slurry+Urea	26.66	4.220	2.02	1.95	6.317
Lantana camara					
Lvs+Water	25.49	4.038	2.10	0.9	6.312
Lvs+CD slurry+Urea	28.97	5.384	2.10	0.975	5.352
Leucaena leucocephala					
Lvs+Water	27.34	3.645	1.7	0.7	7.50
Lvs+CD slurry+Urea	27.68	3.645	1.8	0.9	7.59

Note: Lvs. : Leaves, CD Slurry : Cattle dung slurry

Treatment with cattle dung plus cow urine was found to be more efficient to hasten the process than other treatments. Cattle dung treatment alone was also found effective because it provides extra source of nitrogen to microbial development. Individual inoculant of *Trichoderma viride* and treatment with cow urine was inefficient for rapid degradation.

Table 4: Fungi Isolated from Composting Leafy Substrates

Absidia corymbifera	*Fusarium oxysporum*
Aspergillus flavus	*F. solani*
A.fumigatus	*F. dimerum*
A.niger	*Fusarium sp.*
Aureobasidium sp.	*Gonatobotrys sp.*
Botrytis sp.	*Humicola grisea*
Cheatomium sp.	*H. insolans*
Coprinus sp.	*H. lanuginosa*
Cunnighamella sp.	*Mucor pusillus*
Curvularia lunata	*Mucor sp.*
Dresclera sp.	*Nigrospora sp.*
Penicillium sp.	*Rhizopus nigricans*
Phytopthora sp.	*Sporotrichum thermophila*
Phoma sp.	*Torula thermophila*
Peyronellaca sp.	*Phythium sp.*

Table 5: Reduction in Total Solid After Biodegradation.

	% Total Solid	% Moisture	% Reuction in Total Solid
Clerodendrum inerme			
Lvs+Water	13.12	86.26	59.06
Lvs+CD slurry+Urea	17.11	82.89	48.95
Parthenium histerophorus			
Lvs+Water	11.71	88.28	33.08
Lvs+CD slurry+Urea	13.27	86.73	24.20
Lantana camara			
Llvs+Water	16.465	83.43	32.960
Lvs+CD slurry+Urea	14.78	85.22	39.82
Leucaena leucocephala			
Lvs+Water	20.67	79.33	41.14
Lvs+CD slurry+Urea	14.60	85.40	58.42

Note: Lvs. : Leaves, CD Slurry: Cattle dung slurry

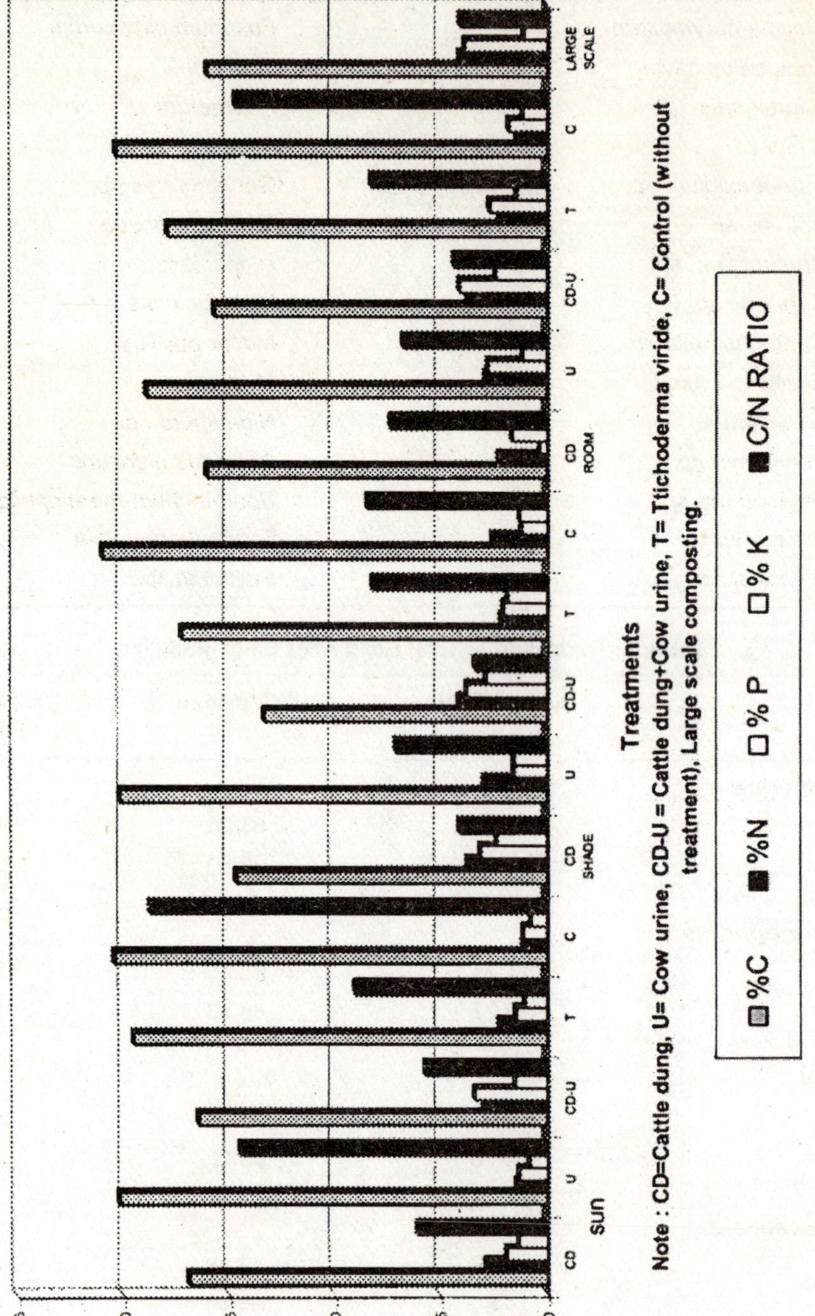

Fig. 1. Estimation of Nutrients of organic manure prepared from Sugarcane leaves

Nutrient analysis of prepared compost showed high percentage of nitrogen and low percent of carbon. C/N ratio and NPK calculated with various treatments for namely *Clerodendum inerme, Parthenium hysterophorus, Lantana camara, Leucaena leucocephala* presented in Table 3. For sugarcane and banana leaves Better nutrient composition was observed in the cow urine plus cattle dung treated manure as compared to other treatments. Concentration of nutrients was more in shade and room condition than direct sunlight exposure (Fig. 1). Reduction in total solid after biodegradation was observed in various substrates *Clerodendum inerme, Parthenium hysterophorus, Lantana camara, Leucaena leucocephala* with different treatment and cattle dung slurry plus urea gave best result as compared to control (Table 5).

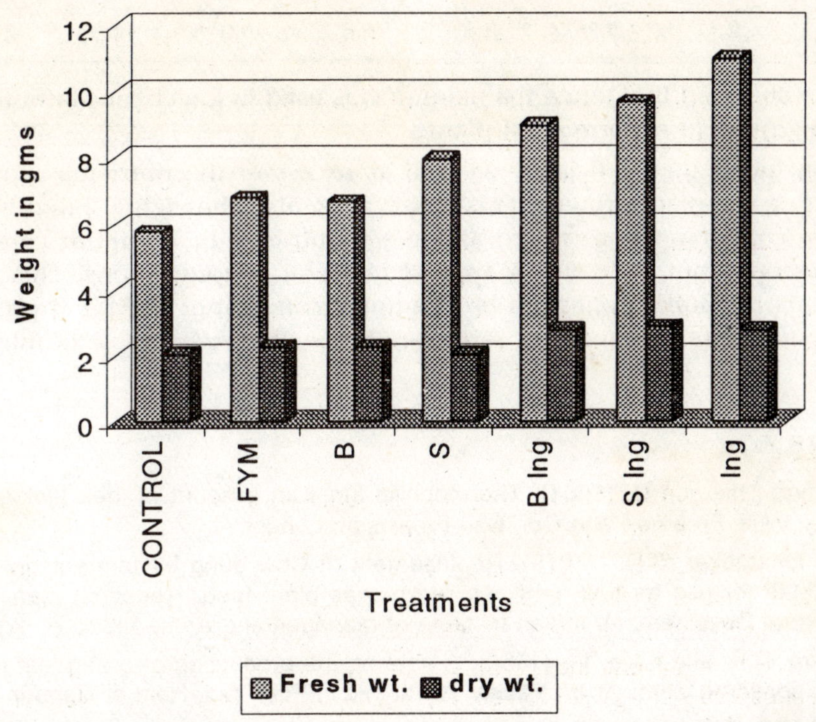

Control: Without fertilizer; **FYM:** Farm Yard Manure, **B:** Banana leaves Compost; **S:** Sugarcane leaves compost; **B-Ing:** Banana leaves compost + Inorganic fertilizers; **S-Ing:** Sugarcane leaves fertilizer + Inorganic fertilizers and **Ing:** Inorganic fertilizers.

Fig. 2. Effect of organic manure prepared from sugarcane and banana leaves on *Trigonella foenum graecum* and its comparison with FYM, inorganic fertilizer and mix effect of compost with inorganic fertilizers.

Experiments were conducted to evaluate the effect of prepared organic manure (biodung) on the growth of crop plants. *Trigonella* plant exhibited near about 30% more vegetative growth and dry weight as compared to control (Fig. 2). Maximum height in growth of

Amaranthus paniculatus was observed in 25 days with the treatment of soil plus bio-dung i.e. 29.9 cm on compared with 15.5 cm with control soil (Table 6).

Table 6: Effect of Different Manures on the Vegetative Growth of *Amaranthus paniculatus.* *(Height of plants in cm).*

Sample	Duration in Days							
	2	4	6	8	10	15	20	25
Soil (Control)	2.11	2.3	3.1	3.86	4.33	5.7	12.1	15.5
Soil + FYM	2.1	3.3	3.5	5.1	7.2	10.3	17.1	18.5
Soil + inorganic ferililizer	2.3	3.5	3.8	6.8	9.1	14.1	22.4	26.8
Soil + biodungl	2.1	3.1	3.8	6.6	9.9	14.8	27.3	29.9

It was also observed that when the manure was used in lower concentration (2%) it gave best result on growth of experimental plants.

It was concluded that deficiency as well as excess of the nutrients causes limiting or harmful effect on the plant growth. This observation also shows that bio-dung is a concentrated manure containing both micro and macronutrients in optimum concentration and therefore gives optimum yield when applied in lower concentrations. This in turn would help in reducing the bulk application of traditional compost or FYM and provide economically feasible substitute for inorganic fertilizers to develop sustainable farming system.

REFERENCES

Cooney, D.G. and Emerson R. (1964). Thermophilic fungi an account of their biology, activities and classification. W.H. Freeman and Co., San Fransisco. London.

Das, C.R. and Ghatnekar, S.D. (1979). Replacement of Cow dung by fermentation of aquatic and terrestrial plants for use as fuel, fertilizer and biogas plant feed. Research planing workshop on Energy for Rural Development. Indian Institute of Management, Ahmedabad P. 1-19.

Joshi, P., Thakre, R.P. and Kate, T. (1989). A note on the production of green leaf manure proc. All India UGC Sponsored Seminar on Recent Advances in Plant Sci. Held at Nagpur.

Joshi, P and Thakre, R.P. (1991). Composting of leafy biomass into farm manure. Proc. VIIth International conference on solid waste management and secondary materials, 3B, Philadelphia, P.A., U.S.A.

Pellett, L.P. and Young, R. (1980). Nutritional evaluation of protein foods, UN Univ. Publ.

Walkely, A.J. and Black, I.A. (1934). Estimation of soil organic carbon by chromic acid titration method. Soil Sci., 37 : 29-38.

PLATE 3

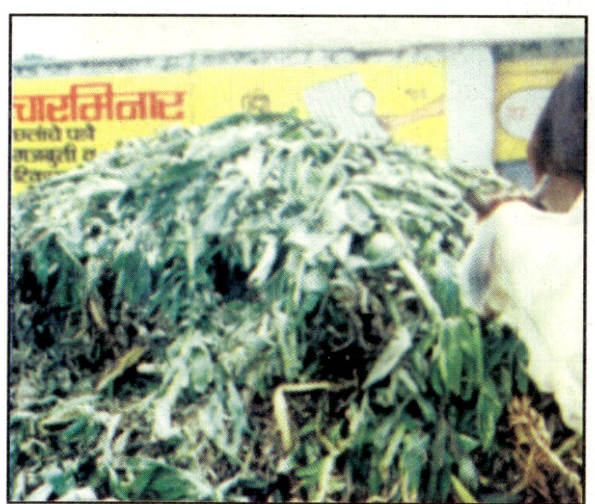

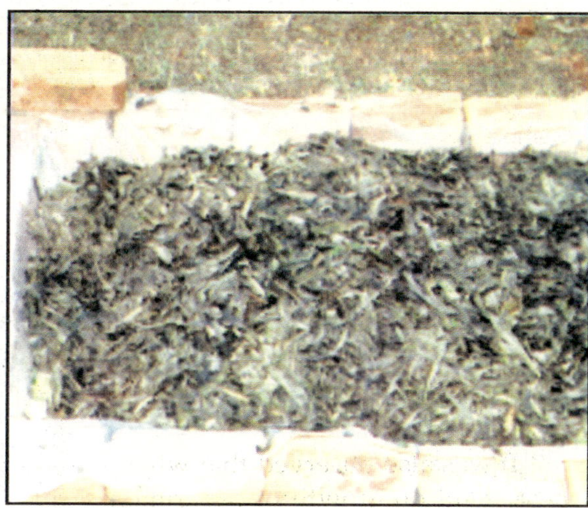

Biodegradation of waste banana leaves on large scale.

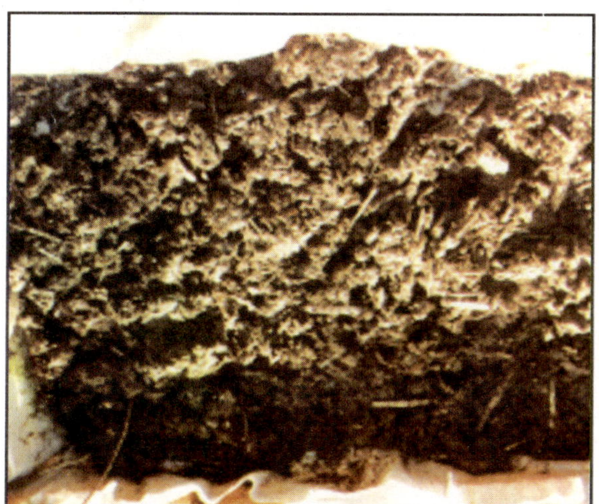

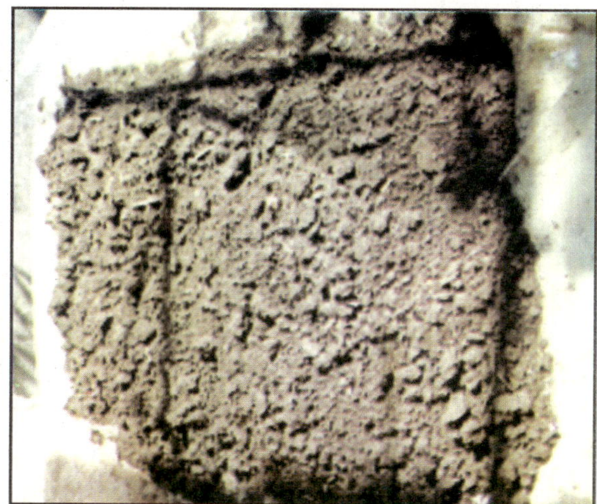

Biodegradation of waste sugarcane leaves on large scale.

PLATE 4

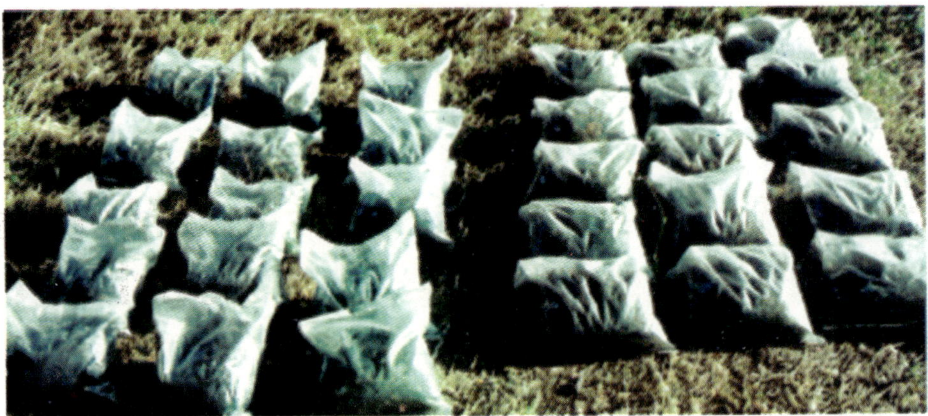

Process of composting in direct sunlight.

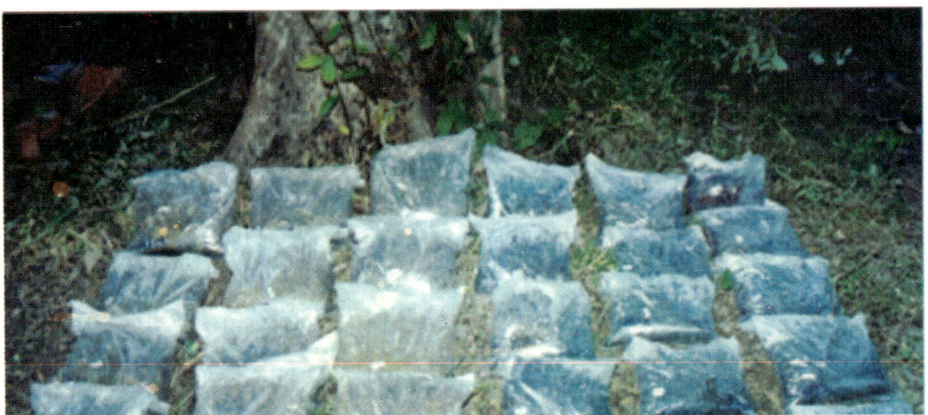

Process of composting under the shade of tree.

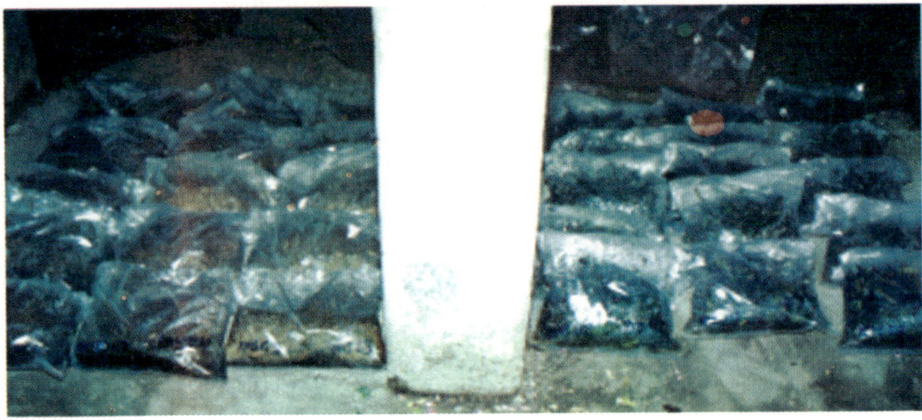

Process of composting in room.

Microbiology and Biotechnology for Sustainable Development (Ed. P.C. Jain),
CBS Publishers & Distributors, New Delhi (2004), pp. 237–247.

B-6

Bioremediation of Copper and Mercury by Plant and Microbial Biosorbent

S.R. Dave and B.D. Atodaria
Department of Microbiology, School of Sciences, Gujarat University, Ahmedabad 380009.

Abstract

Biosorption of heavy metal ions by dead biomass has been recognized as a potential alternative to existing metal removal technologies applied to wastewater treatment. Selective washed microbial and plant biomass was tested for bioremediation of copper and mercury from the aqueous solution. Among the selected biomass tested, the maximum metal removal was observed within first 60 minutes and then remained almost constant for next 3 hours. Among the biomass studied the microbial showed 1.24 times more copper removal as compared to the best plant biomass, under experimental conditions. Influence of metal solution pH was studied and pH 4.0 was found to be optimum for copper removal both for plant and microbial biomass. When reaction temperature was less than the ambient temperature the copper removal was negatively influenced and resulted in 40% reductions. Various pretreatments of biomass with acids, alkali and organic solvent showed considerable influence on copper removal. Only NaOH treatment was found to be beneficial. Mercury removal showed almost similar trend to that of copper except for the pretreatment, which resulted in drastic loss of mercury removal ability of the plant biomass. In case of microbial biomass only the acid treatment proved to be detrimental. The pH of reaction mixture between 2.0-6.0 showed mercury removal in the range of 62.5-78.75%. Wide range of pH tolerance for mercury removal was observed for microbial biomass with only 20% decrease from highest mercury removal between pH 2.0-6.0. both plant and microbial biomass under experimental study follow Langmuir isotherm for copper and mercury removal. The metal bioremediation study carried out in the laboratory proved the potential of selected plant and microbial biomass as effective copper and mercury scavenging agents from wastewater. The detailed results will be discussed.

Key words: Plant Biomass. Microbial biomass. Biosorption. Copper. Mercury.

Corresponding author: S.R.Dave E-mail:shaileshrdave@hotmail.com

INTRODUCTION

Bioremediation is a pollution treatment technology that uses biological systems to catalyze the destruction, or transformation or removal of various chemicals to less harmful forms (Atlas, 1995). In the last decade industrialized nations have placed greater emphasis on restoring the environment. Much awareness has been directed toward the preservation of water quality and the restoration of contaminated surface and groundwaters (Brierly, 1991). Thus where applicable, bioremediation proved to be a cost-effective means of restoring environmental quality. Its cost effectiveness as compared to the chemical and physical treatment technologies, especially for dilute contaminants, is the main driving force for the use of bioremediation. Although treatment of industrial effluents to remove organic contaminants has received the greatest emphasis, attention is now focused on treatment of metals since last two decades (Brierly, 1991). As metals are a nonrenewable, finite natural resource, the challenge is not limited only to their removal from the water streams, but also extends to finding efficient and economical ways of recovery and recycling. Some of the major sources of heavy metal pollution are electroplating, pigment producing, metal finishing, printed board manufacturing, and other electrical equipment manufacturing industries. When wastewaters emanating from such industries are released into rivers or other natural water bodies, they prove to be harmful to the biota. While passing along the food chain, these metals get bioaccumulated in small aquatic animals and finally reach humans by the process of biomagnification. A majority of heavy metals are toxic even at low concentration and, as such, pose serious health hazards to humans and live stocks (Alexander, 1994). Copper is an essential micronutrient for most, if not all, living organisms since it is the constituent of many metalloenzymes and proteins involved in electron transport, redox and other important reactions (Cervantes and Corona, 1993). In contrast, copper present at higher levels in its free ionic form (Cu^{2+}) is toxic (Cervantes and Corona, 1993). Copper toxicity causes Wilson's disease and nephrosis in human beings (Verma and Rehal, 1996). Mercury is a natural component of the environment occurring as metallic mercury and mercuric sulphide (HgS). Additional contributions are made to this "Background level" by a whole range of industries. The effects of mercury poisoning in man and its mobility through food chains are dramatically illustrated by what is known as the "Minamata Incident" (Higgins and Burns, 1975). Moreover, both copper and mercury are phytotoxic.

A number of physical and chemical methods have been developed to scavenge heavy metal ions from industrial wastewaters. However, these methods are industrially impractical due to either high operational cost or the difficulty of treating the secondary contaminants generated (Verma and Rehal, 1996). The use of biological materials for heavy metal removal or recovery has gained importance in recent years due to their good performance and low cost (Brierly, 1991; Volesky, 1987; Gadd, 1992; Macaskie, 1990, Mattuschka and Straube, 1992). Among various sources, both live and inactivated biomass of microorganisms exhibit interesting metal-binding capacities (Kuyucak and Volesky, 1988). The use of dead biomass eliminates the problem of toxicity not only from metal ions but also from adverse operating conditions as well as the trouble with maintenance and nutrient supply to living cells (Matis and Zouboulis, 1994). Bioconcentration, i.e., uptake without transformation, also can be used to treat heavy-metal contaminated soils and waters. This forms the basis for phytoremediation in which plants are used to extract metals from contaminated soils and waters (Atlas, 1995). The commercial applicability of microbial metal removal processes could be increased by a combination of different approaches including the use of waste biomass from industry and either chemical or physiological manipulation of biomass to improve its metal biosorption abilities (Simmons and Singleton, 1995).

In this context the present work was carried out with microbial and plant biomass for the removal and optimization of copper and mercury in the aqueous synthetic waste.

MATERIALS AND METHODS

Biomass: (Dried Plant and Microbial biomass)

Fresh stem bark was obtained from neem trees. The bark was dried in oven at 60°C. It was then ground to desired mesh size particles. The powder was washed with distilled water several times till it was free from color-causing substances and supernatant was clear. It was then again dried at 60°C (Ansari, 2000). Similarly, microbial biomass was washed thoroughly with distilled water and sun dried. Dried biomass was ground to desire mesh size particles. Both these biomass were then used for copper and mercury removal studies.

Pretreatment of glassware:

The glassware to be used for biosorption study was pretreated with con HNO_3 in water to remove contaminants, which would adversely affect the experiment under study. Glassware was then subsequently washed with several rounds of distilled water and then used for batch experiment.

Metal Solution:

Stock solutions containing 1mg/ml of copper and mercury were prepared by dissolving analytical grade $CuSO_4.5H_2O$ and $HgCl_2$ in distilled water adjusted to pH 4.0 with con. HNO_3.

Batch Experiment:

Experiments were conducted in 250ml Erlenmeyer flasks with total system of 50ml of synthetically prepared $CuSO_4.5H_2O$ and $HgCl_2$ solution at optimum pH. Flasks were agitated for 1hour after adding 500mg plant and microbial biosorbents. Samples were centrifuged and supernatant was taken and analyzed for the residual metal ion concentration.

Analytical Determination:

Equilibrium copper and mercury concentrations were estimated spectrophotometrically using diethyldithiocarbamate and malachite green indicators (Vogel, 1962). The difference between the initial and final metal ion concentration was reported as the metal ion adsorbed by the adsorbents. Metal loading capacity (mg/g removal) was calculated by amount of metal sorbed by unit weight of biomass (mg of metal / g of biomass).

Optimization of parameters:

Various parameters like reaction pH (2.0-6.0), contact time (1hour, 3hour, 17hours), temperature (10-60^{0}C) initial metal concentration (20-240 mg/l) were optimized by studying the effect of these particular parameters on metal remediation from the solutions.

Adsorption isotherm:

The metal biosorption data obtained were plotted using Langmuir [$C_{eq}/Q = 1/(bQ_{max}) + C_{eq}/Q_{max}$] equations to understand the metal removal pattern and mechanisms where:

C_{eq} = liquid phase concentration of metal.

b = Langmuir constant.

Q = metal uptake (mg/g biomass).

Q_{max} = maximum metal uptake.

Pretreatment of biomass:

Both plant and microbial biosorbents were treated with 50ml of acids (1NHCl, 1NHNO$_3$), alkali (1NNaOH, 1NKOH) and organic solvents (methanol, formaldehyde and ethyl alcohol) for 1 hour under agitation condition. The biomass was then subsequently washed with distilled water using centrifugation method (5000rpm, 30mins). These pretreated biomass were then used for batch experiment.

RESULTS AND DISCUSSIONS

Effect of pH:

The influence of pH on copper and mercury sorption by plant and microbial biosorbents are shown in Fig. 1 and Fig. 2. Under experimental conditions, less than 15% of copper was adsorbed at pH 2.0 by both biomasses studied. There was no significant influence of pH on biosorption of copper between pH 3.0 and 5.0. The observed marginal increase in copper sorption at pH 6.0 could be due to auto precipitation of copper as copper hydroxide. Thus, further experiments were carried at pH 4.0. In case of mercury, maximum removal of 162.5 mg/g was observed at pH 4.0 with plant biosorbent and on either side of the optimum pH there was considerable decrease in mercury removal. While in case of microbial biomass wide range of optimum pH was observed. The mercury removal was in the range of 62.5-78.75% for microbial biomass. There was only 20% difference noticed between mercury removal at optimum and lowest/highest pH under the study. The difference in pH range between plant and microbial biomass could be due to difference in the chemical composition of the biosorbents. The obtained data indicate the utility of microbial biomass in wide range of the pH for the treatment of the waste.

Effect of Temperature:

The influence of temperature on copper and mercury sorption by plant biosorbent is as shown in Fig. 3 and Fig. 4. When reaction temperature was less than the ambient temperature both copper and mercury removal was negatively influenced and resulted in 40% and 25% reductions for copper and mercury respectively. The observed difference could be due to the influence of temperature on the physiochemical mechanism of biosorption process between temperatures (10-60^{0}C). The temperature above the ambient temperature showed no significant influence on metal biosorption. These results are opposite to that of Nickel where Ni removal was largely independent of temperature in the range of 4^0 to 37^0 C.

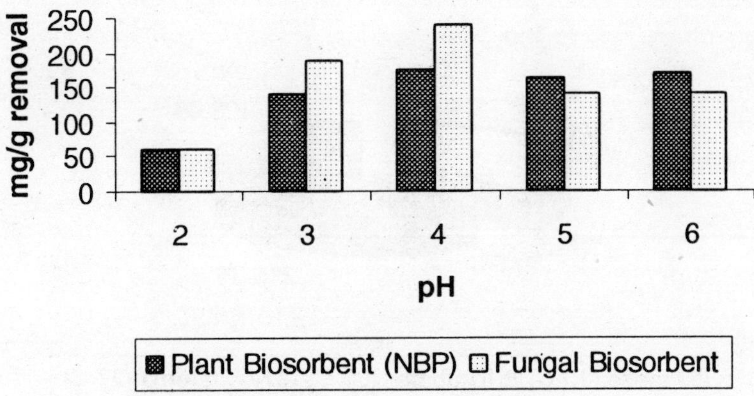

Fig. 1. Effect of pH of copper sorption

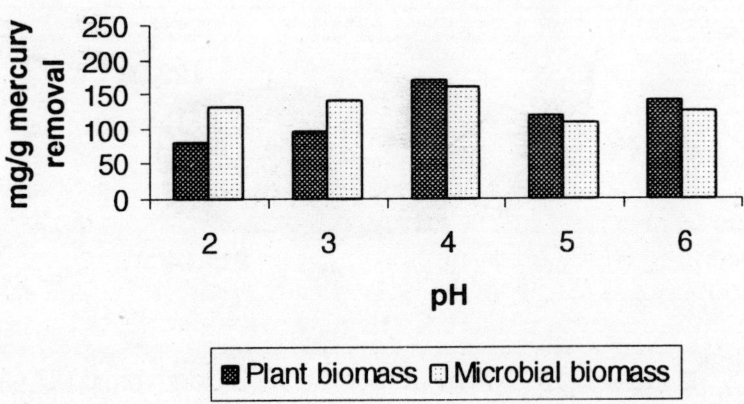

Fig. 2. Effect of pH on mercury sorption

Effect of Concentration:

Influence of initial concentration of bioadsorbate is depicted in Fig. 5a-b and Fig. 6a-b. As can be seen from the results the %copper sorption was found to be decreasing above 75mg/l of initial copper but when sorption was considered in terms of mg/g removal the copper sorption was increased up to 200mg/l of initial copper concentration. Thereafter there was gradual decrease. Similar trend in terms of mg/g removal was observed for mercury also. This could be due to less available metal ions or scarcity of available sorption sites below and above the optimum initial metal concentration respectively. When sorption was considered in terms of %sorption removal, almost complete mercury removal was observed at 20mg/l and below initial concentration. On the other hand even with 20mg/l of initial copper concentration complete removal was not observed. The observed difference could be explained on the basis of higher affinity of mercury for sorption to the biomass under study.

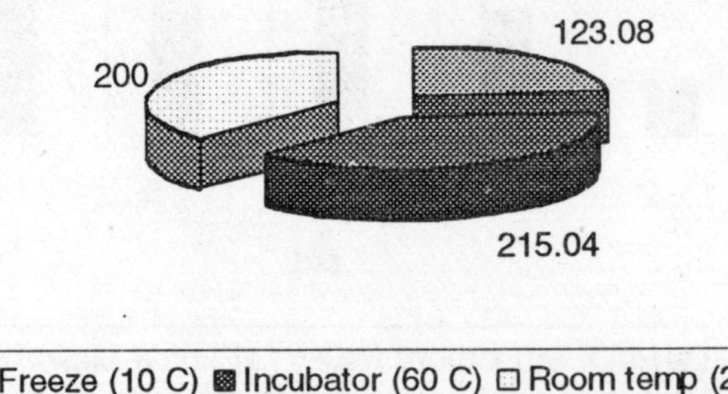

Fig. 3. Removal of copper by plant biomass (mg/g)

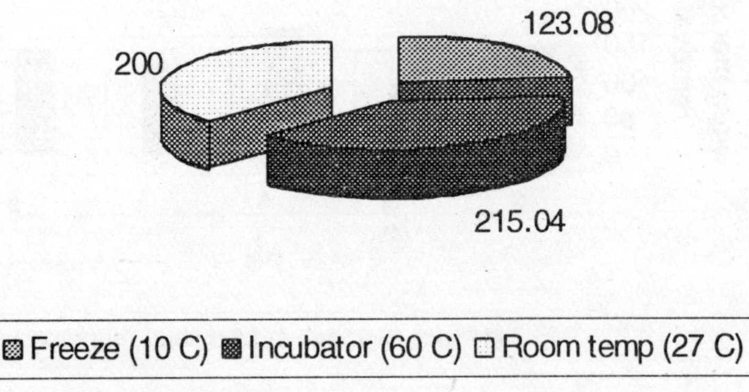

Fig. 4. Removal of mercury by plant biomass (mg/g)

Adsorption Isotherm:

Adsorption isotherm was drawn using the Langmuir equation (Fig. 7). Both the metals followed the Langmuir isotherm.

Influence of contact time:

The influence of contact time on metal sorption is shown in Table. 1. In case of both the metals the contact time of 1 hour was found to be sufficient for the lion shares of metal removal. The further incubation of two more hours showed no increase in removal. The observed maximum removal in first hour of incubation indicates the dominance of physiochemical mechanism of sorption.

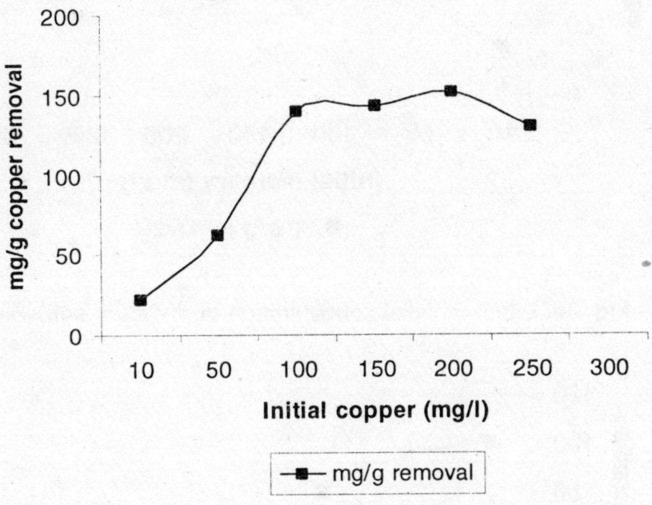

Fig. 5a. Effect of initial concentration on copper sorption

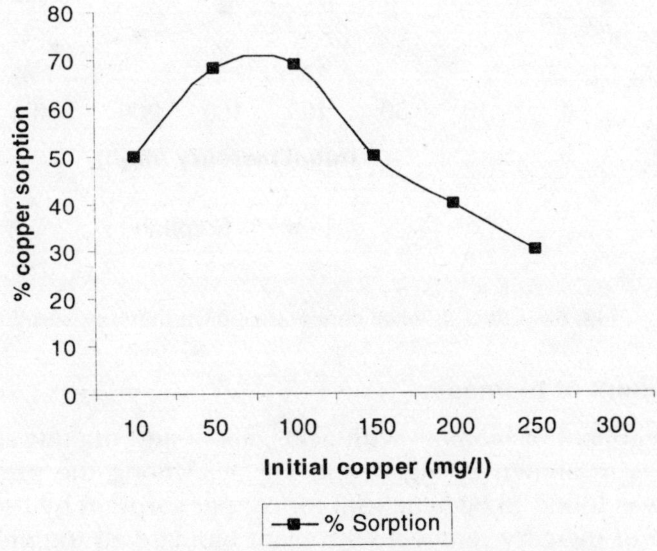

Fig. 5b. Effect of initial concentration on copper sorption

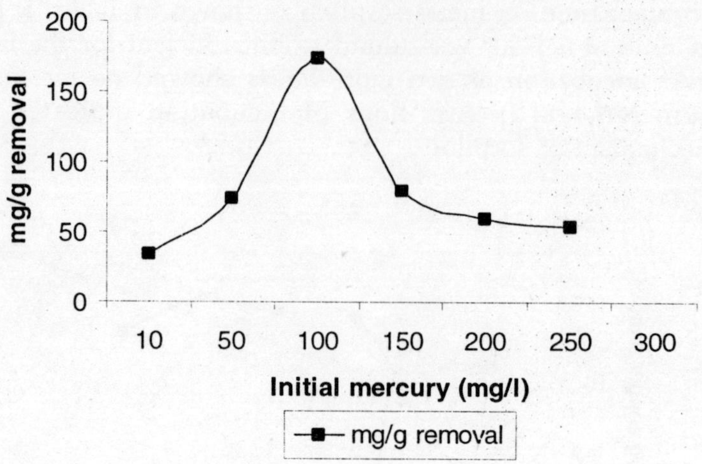

Fig. 6a. Effect of initial concentration on mercury sorption

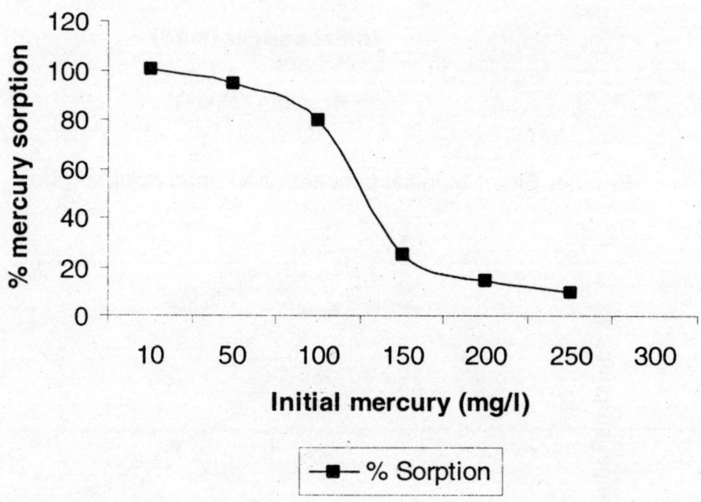

Fig. 6b. Effect of initial concentration on mercury sorption

Effect of pretreatment of biomass:

The effect of pretreatment of biomass with acids, alkali and organic solvents on copper and mercury sorption is as shown in Fig. 8 and Fig. 9. Among the pretreatments given only NaOH treatment was found to be beneficial for copper sorption by both plant and microbial biosorbent. In case of mercury removal with plant biomass all the pretreatments resulted in more than 40% decrease while in microbial biomass the drastic negative effect was observed with formaldehyde, 1N HCl and 1N HNO_3 treatment. The variation in the influence of different pretreatments could be explained on basis of loss of specific sorption sites for mercury from the biomass while the NaOH treatment showed beneficial influence for copper remediation. The observed considerable variations due to treatment require detailed study to elucidate the mechanism of biosorption.

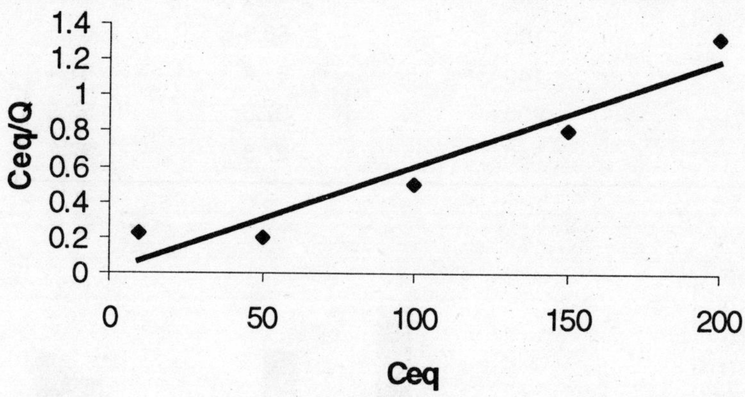

Fig. 7. Langmuir adsorption isotherm

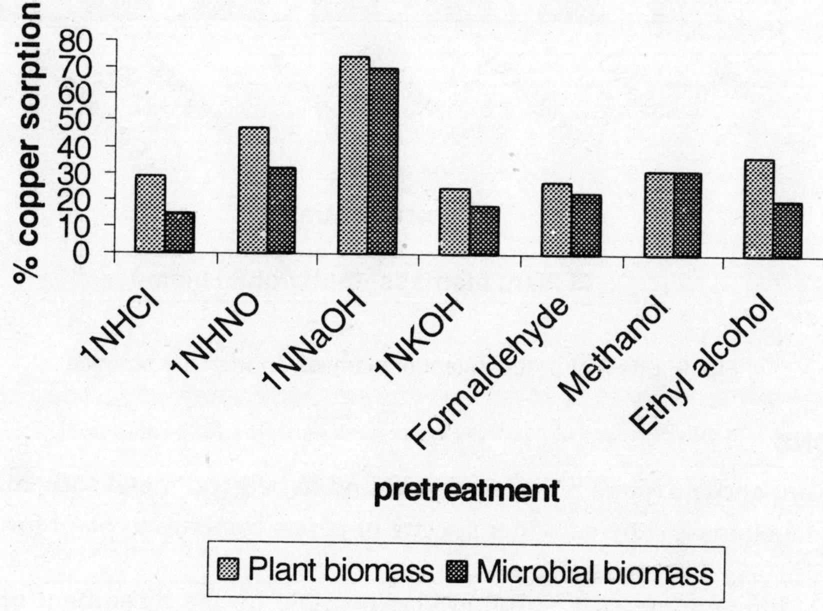

Fig. 8. Effect of pretreatment of biomass on copper sorption

Table 1: Effect of contact time on Copper Sorption by Plant Biosorbent.

No.	Initial concentration of copper (mg/l).	Copper sorption(%) in hours.		
		1	3	17
1	20	50	50	50
2	40	65.4	65.4	65.4
3	100	68.5	68.5	68.5
4	140	51.4	51.4	51.4
5	200	37.5	37.5	43.7
6	240	27.3	27.3	47.6

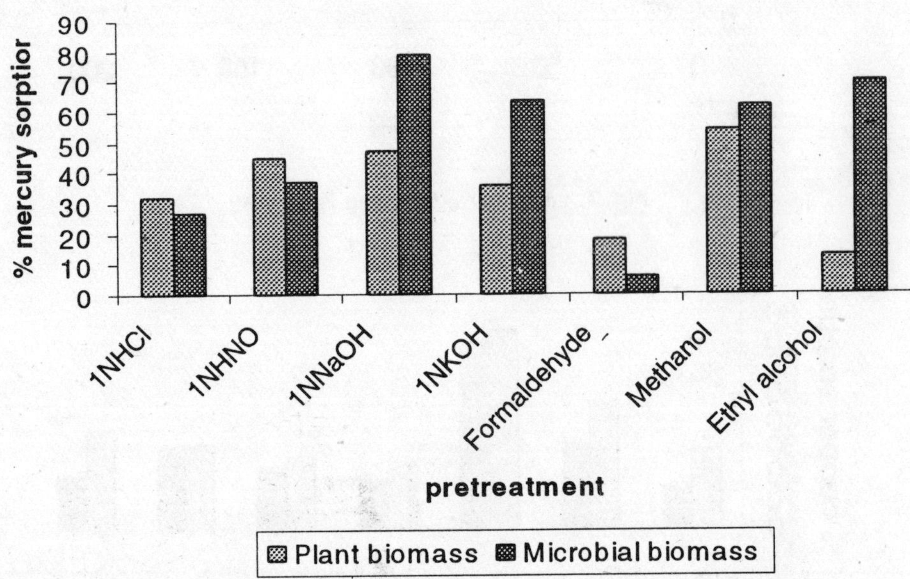

Fig. 9. Effect of pretreatment of biomass on mercury sorption

CONCLUSIONS

- Both plant and microbial biomass were found to be good metal sorbents.
- Microbial biomass showed wider spectra of pH as compare to plant for mercury metal sorption.
- Almost complete mercury sorption was possible by the biosorbent up to 20mg/l of initial mercury concentration.
- Contact time of 1 hour was found to be sufficient for the process.

- Metal sorption was found, to be directly influenced from refrigerator temperature to 25^0C, thereafter the influence was marginal.
- Except NaOH treatment all other treatments were found to be detrimental.
- Both the metals follow the Langmuir isotherm.
- The obtained results are very much encouraging for the application of biomass as biosorbent for copper and mercury remediation.

REFERENCES

Alexander, M. (1994). Biodegradation and Bioremediation. Academic Press, San Diego, Calif. pp. 16-38.

Ansari, M.H. (2000). Neem (*Azadirachta indica*) Bark for Removal of Mercury from Water. *J. IAEM*. 27: 133-137.

Atlas, R.M. (1995). "Bioremediation". *Chem. Eng. News*. 3: 32-42.

Brady, D. and Duncan, J.R. (1994). Bioaccumulation of metal cations by *Saccharomyces cerevisiae*. *Appl Microbiol Biotechnol*. 41: 149-154.

Brierly, C. (1991). Bioremediation Of Metal–Contaminated Surface and Ground waters. *Geomicrobiol. J*. 8: 201-223.

Cervantes, C and Corona, F.G. (1993). Copper resistance mechanisms in bacteria and fungi. *FEMS Microbiol.Rev*. 14: 121-138.

Gadd, G.M., (1992). In Microbial Control of Pollution. Cambridge Uni.Press, Cambridge. 59 pp.

Higgins, I. J and Burns, R.G. (1975)."Metals". *In the Chemistry and Microbiology of Pollution*. Academic Press. New York. 189-210.

Kuyucak, N. and Volesky, B. (1988). Biosorbents for recovery of metals from industrial solutions. *Biotechnol. Lett*. 10: 137-142.

Macaskie, L.E., (1990). An immobilized cell bioprocess for the removal of heavy metals from aqueous flow. *J. Chem. Tech. Biotechnol*. 49: 357-379.

Matis, K.M. and Zouboulis, A.I. (1994). Flotation of Cadmium-Loaded Biomass. *Biotechnol Bioeng*. 44: 354-360.

Mattuschka, B. and Straube, G. (1992). Biosorption of metals by a waste biomass. *J. Chem. Tech. Biotechnol*. 58: 57-63.

Norberg, A. and Rydin, S. (1984). Development of a continuous process for metal accumulation by *Zoogloea ramigera*. *Biotechnol Bioeng*. 26: 265.

Shah, M.P., Vora, S.B and Dave, S.R. (1999). Copper Remediation by Waste *Streptomyces* Biomass. *I JM*. 39: 109-112.

Simmons, P. and Singleton, I. (1995). A method to increase silver biosorption by an industrial strain of *Saccharomyces cerevisiae*. *Appl. Microbiol. Biotechnol*. 45: 278-285.

Verma, N and Rehal, R. (1996). Sorption of Cu (II) Ions From Industrial Waste Water by *Albizia lebbeck* Pods. *Current Researches in Plant Sciences*. 2: 259-262.

Vogel, A.I. (1962). A textbook of Quantitative Inorganic Analysis ELBS and Longman, London.

Volesky, B. (1987). Biosorbents for metal recovery. *TIBTECH*. 5: 96-101.

Microbiology and Biotechnology for Sustainable Development (Ed. P.C. Jain),
CBS Publishers & Distributors, New Delhi (2004), pp. 248–253.

B-7

Role of Potassium on the Occurrence of Vesicular–Arbuscular Mycorrhizal Spores in the Rhizosphere of *Lantana* Species

O.P. Dwivedi, R.K. Yadav, D. Vyas* and K.M.Vyas
*Department of Botany, Dr. H.S. Gour Vishwavidyalaya,
Sagar 470003 (M.P.) India*

Abstract

Present study deals with the effect of potassium on the occurrence of VAM fungi. We have found that out of three soil samples collected from rhizosphere of three Lantana species i.e. L. camara, L. indice and L. aculeato. Soil samples belonging to L. camara and L. indice showed presence of VAM fungi where as in L. aculeato there was no VAM fungi. The absence of VAM fungi in L. aculeato is attributed to the presence of higher concentration of potassium in the soil where as soils of L. camara has low concentration of K and has large number of VAM fungi followed by L. indice which has comparatively high K than L. camara and has only two VAM species.

Keywords: VAM, *Lantana* sp., Mycorrhizae & Potassium.

INTRODUCTION

The term mycorrhiza literally means "Fungus root" and is commonly used to denote the symbiotic relationship between feeder plant root of crop plant and fungal mycelia (Subba Rao, 1995). Mycorrhizae are ubiquitous in nature and their use in biofertilizer technology is well known for sustainable development of agriculture, horticulture, floriculture, forestry, plant protection, waste land reclamation and afforestation, mining areas, eroded soils, degraded forests, saline soil, sand dunes and deserts. About 95% of vascular plant species are reported to harbour mycorrhizae.

* Corresponding author email: dvyas1 @.rediffmail.com dvyas@sancharnet.in

The Vesicular arbuscular Mycorrhizal fungi are intercellular, obligate endosymbionts, which have not yet been grown in pure culture (Mosse, 1973). These fungi are classified on the basis of their spore morphology. Recently (Bentivenga and Morton, 1994) grouped them in a single order, Glomales, encomparing six genera with 149 species.

Mycorrhizal plants increase the surface area of their root system for better absorption of nutrients from soil especially when the soils are deficient in phosphorus. VAM is a type of endomycorrhiza, which possesses special structures known as vesicles and arbuscules, the latter helping in the transfer of nutrients from soil into root system (Subba Rao, 1995). The quality of the soil not only supports the growth and development of the plants but also attracts and provides niche to many soil microbes. Mosse (1973) reported that all soils contain either spores of VA mycorrhizal fungi or mycorrhiza formed by them. McCully (1999) suggested that the chemical, physical and biological interactions that occur between roots and the surrounding environment of the soil are highly complex. Harrison (1999) gave detailed information about the molecular and cellular aspects of VAM symbiosis.

Sagar university campus is situated on the hills of vindhyan ranges surrounded by well-developed forest. The university department of Botany also has a good Botanical garden consisting of diverse plants. The above mentioned, facts prompted us to undertake the present study around the university campus. Therefore, we selected three different *Lantana* spp. growing in three different soil types.

MATERIALS AND METHODS

Soil samples were collected from rhizosphere of *Lantana* plants from three different localities of the Sagar university campus. In each case, soil from 10-15 cm depth was dug out. The soil samples were collected and processed by techniques of Gerdemann and Nicolson (1963) using wet sieving and decanting, and using sucrose centrifugation to isolate VAM spores. The different species of VAM fungi were identified on the basis of extermatrical spores present in the soil following the key of Schenck and Perez (1987).

Physicochemical studies of soil samples

Physical Properties

The texture, colour and odour of the soil were recorded as per method of Mishra (1968) and pH and conductivity were determined as per method of Cromwell (1955).

Chemical Properties

Nitrogen and potassium were analyzed by the method of Jackson (1973). Phosphorus and base deficiency were measured by the method of Mishra (1968). Organic carbon was estimated by the method of Piper (1944).

RESULT AND DISCUSSION

Out of three *Lantana* spp. only two spp. *Lantana camara* and *Lantana indice* showed well-developed VAM association. The VAM species identified were *Acaulospora scrobiculata,*

Glomus mosseae, Glomus tenue, Sclerocystis pachycaulis from the rhizosphere of soils of *Lantana* spp. In case of *Lantana aculeato* VAM fungi were not found. Data on soil pH, conductivity, texture, colour, odour, N, P, K, organic carbon and base deficiency are presented in Table 1. Soil pH of the three localities was almost equal, i.e., 7.3, 7.2 and 7.4; conductivity varied from 0.30 to 0.49 sm^{-1}, lowest in the soil sample of *Lantana camara* and highest in the soil sample of *Lantana aculeato.* N concentration was same in the soil samples of *Lantana camara* and *Lantana indice,* i.e., 328.5 kg/hec. While in the soil sample of *Lantana aculeato,* N was found to be 267.0 kg/hec. Phosphorus concentration was same in case of *L. camara* and *L. indice* (8.0 kg./ hec.) soil samples. P (11.2 kg/hec.) was found to be very high in *L. aculeato.* Similarly K concentration (596.0 kg/hec.) was very high in the soil samples of *L. aculeato.* On the other hand, it was found to be 134.4kg/hec. and 196.0 kg/hec. in the soil samples of *L.camara* and *L. indice,* respectively. Organic carbon was also high in the case of soil samples of *L. aculeato,* i.e., C 5.5 kg/hec. followed by 4.0 kg/hec. in *L. indice* and lowest in the soil sample of *L. camara* (1.5 kg/hec.). In the case of *L. camara,* soil was found to be highly base deficient, but soil of *L. aculeato* and *L. indice* were found to have little or no base deficiency.

A plant is considered VA mycorrhizal when its root contains characteristic structures like an internal hyphal system, intercellular arbuscules and vesicles (Brundrett et al. 1985, Jagpal and Mukerji 1988). It is established that VAM fungi grow under the phosphorus limiting condition and form symbiotic association with the host plant (Mago and Mukerji, 1994). According to Mosse and Boweny (1968), Hayman (1970) Powell (1977) the population of VAM spores varies considerably from place to place according to the physical and chemical nature of soil. Manjunath *et al.* (1983) have also reported that VAM colonisation, infection grading and spore count in the root region soils differ in different soils. According to them fewer mycorrhizal fungi occur in clayey soil as compared to sandy soil. Suresh kumar *et al.* (1995) have reported influence of edaphic factors such as P,organic carbon, soil pH and soil moisture on the occurrence of VAM symbiosis with pigeonpea. VAM colonization was more in pigeonpea grown in coastal sandy where a low level of available soil P was recorded. A proportionate reduction in VAM colonization was observed in plants grown in grayish onattukara and laterite soil where the available soil P was comparatively high. However, data obtained from our study suggests that in spite of the presence of a good amount of phosphorus (8.0 kg/hec.) in the rhizosphere soil of *Lantana camara* and *Lantana indice,* VAM fungi occur in the soil. In the case of rhizosphere soil of *Lantana aculeato,* phosphorus was much higher (11.2 kg/hec.) in comparison to soil samples of *L. camara* and *Lantana indice.* These results showing absence of VAM fungi in the soil may be due to the presence of phosphorus, but here we emphasize the role of potassium, which is very high in the soil of *Lantana aculeato* (596.4 kg./hec.). This high amount of potassium is enough to suppress the occurrence/growth of VAM fungi in soil considering the ratio of N, P, in the soil of *Lantana camara* and *L. indice,* where the amount of N and P is same (328 kg/hec. N and 8 kg/hec. P) in both the soils, one would expect the same number of VAM fungi, which we did not find. The reason behind it is a significant difference in the amount of potassium (K for *L. camara* 134.4 kg/hec. and K for *L. indice* 196.0 kg/hec.). The presence of the higher amount of K in the soil of *Lantana indice* resulted in occurrence of lesser number of VAM fungi in comparison to *Lantana camara* soils. However earlier Mathur and Vyas (1994) reported the occur-

Table 1: Occurrence of VAM Fungi associated with *Lantana sp.* in soil samples collected From University Campus, Sagar

Lantana plant species.	Soil analysis										Total No. of VAM fungal species	VAM species
	pH (sm^{-1})	Conductivity (kg/ha)	N (kg/ha)	P	K (kg/ha)	C (%)	Base Deficiency	Texture	Colour	Odour		
Lantana camara	7.3	0.30	328.5	8.0	134.4	1.5	+++	Gravel sand	Brown	Volatile	4	A. scrobiculata G. mosseae G.Tenue *S. pachycaulis*
Lantana indice	7.4	0.38	328.5	8.0	196.0	4.0	-	Clay sand	Black	Ammonium	2	G. mosseae *G. tenue*
Lantana aculeato	7.2	0.49	267.0	11.2	596.4	5.5	+	Coarse sand	Black	Ammonium	None	None

Note: The values of N, P, K, are given in kg/ha. In S.I. metric units.

+++ Highly base deficient, + Less/little base deficiency, - No base deficiency.

K Potassium, P Phosphorus, N Nitrogen, C Organic carbon.

rence of VAM fungi in association with *Simmondsia chinensis* in soils of eight different localities in which N, P and organic carbon was measured, but they did not measure potassium in the soils.

Recently, Sastry and Johri (1999) studied the occurrence of VAM fungi in 18 different types of soils of Bailadila, Bastar, (M.P.) having 10 different plant species including one species of *Lantana*. They have found association of VAM fungi in all the soil samples tested except two types of soils having high iron ore slates and white mineral strata. They have also measured N, P, C. Thus, considering the above facts, we can say that phosphorus is not a sole factor for occurrence of VAM fungi in the soil but potassium can also play an important role in the occurrence/absence of VAM fungi in the soil. Lower concentration of K favours occurrence of VAM fungi whereas a high concentration of potassium inhibits the occurrence of VAM fungi in the soils.

ACKNOWLEDGEMENT

Authors are thankful to Incharge, soil testing laboratory, Sagar for their help in analyzing soil samples. Authors are also thankful to the Head, Department of Botany, Dr. H.S. Gour Vishwavidyalaya, Sagar for providing lab facilities.

REFERENCES

Abbott, L.K. and A.D. Robson (1982). The role of vesicular-arbuscular mycorrhizal fungi in agriculture and the selection of fungi for inoculation. Aust. J. agric. Res. 33: 389-392.

Bentivenga, S. P. and Morton J.B. (1994). Systematics of glomalean endomycorrhizal fungi: current views and future direction. In mycorrhizae and plant health. FL Pfleger, R.G. Linderman. (ed.), St. Paul, MN: APS Press, pp. 283-308.

Brundrett, M.C., Piche, Y. and R.L Peterson (1985). A developmental study of the early stages in vesicular-arbuscular mycorrhiza formation. Can. J. Bot. 63: 184-193.

Cromwell, B.T. (1955). The alkaloids : A General Introduction, In : Modern Methods of Plant Analysis p. 367-374, K. Paech and M.V. Tracey, (eds.). Springer-verlag. Berlin-Gottingen Heidelberg.

Gerdemann, J.W. and, Nicolson T.H. (1963). Spores of mycorrhizal *Endogone* species extracted from soil by wet sieving and decanting. Trans. Brit. Mycol. Soc. 46: 235-244.

Harrison , M.J. (1999). Molecular and cellular aspects of the arbuscular mycorrhizal symbiosis, Annu Rev. Plant Physiol. Plant mol. Biol. 50: 361-89.

Hayman, D.S. (1970). Endogone spore numbers in soil and vesicular-arbuscular mycorrhiza in wheat as influenced by season and soil treatment. Trans. Brit.Mycol.soc. 54: 53-63.

Jackson, M.L. (1973). Soil chemical analysis. Prentice Hall of India (Pvt. P. Ltd.). New Delhi.

Jagpal, R. and, Mukerji K.G. (1988). Distribution of VA mycorrhizal association in old Delhi ridge; In mycorrhiza round table, IDRC Canada MR Zole; A.K. Verma, A.K. Oka, K.G. Mukerji, KVBR Tilak and Raj (eds.). Madras, India : Alamau Printing works, pp. 257-267.

Mago, P. and Mukerji, K.G. (1994). Vesicular-arbuscular mycorrhiza in Lamiaceae. I Seasonal variation in some members. Phytomorphology. 44: 83-88.

Manjunath, A., Mohan, R. and Bagyaraj, D.J. (1983). Response of citrus to vesicular- arbuscular mycorrhizal inoculation in unsterile soil. Can.J. Bot. 61: 2729-2732.

Mathur, N. and Vyas, A. (1994). Vesicular-arbuscular mycorrhizal relationship of *Simmondsia chinensis.* Phytomorphology. 44: 11-14.

McCully, M.E. (1999). Roots in soil, unearthing the complexities of roots and their rhizospheres. Annu. Rev. Plant Physiol.Plant Mol. Biol. 50 : 695-718.

Mishra, R. (1968). Ecological workbook, Oxford and IBH Publishing Co. Calcutta.

Morton, J.B. and Benny, G. L. (1990). Revised classification of arbuscular mycorrhizal fungi (Zygomycetes) : a new order, glomales, two new suborders, glomineae and igasporineae, and two new families, aculosporaceae and gigasporaceae, with an amendation of glomaceae. Mycotaxon. 37: 471-91.

Mosse, B. and Boweny G. D. (1968). The distribution of endogone spore and in some Australian and Newzealand. soils, and in an experimental field soil at Rothamsted. Trans.Brit. Mycol. Soc. 51: 485-492.

Mosse, B. (1973). Advances in the study of vesicular-arbuscular mycorrhiza. A Rev. Phytopath. II: 171-196.

Piper, C.S. (1944). Soil and plant analysis. Hassel-Press Adelaide Australia.

Powell, C.L. (1977). Mycorrhiza in hill country soil. II. Spore bearing mycorrhizal fungi in 37 soil. N. Z. Fl. agric. Res. 20 : 53-57.

Sastry, M.S.R. and Johri B.N. (1999). Arbuscular mycorrhizal fungal diversity of stressed soil of Bailadila iron ore sites in Bastar region of Madhya Pradesh. Current Science. 77: 1095-1100.

Schenck, N.C. and Perez, Y. (1987). Manual for identification of VAM fungi; Synergistic Pub. Gainesville; F1, U.S.A.

Smiths, C.W. and Skipper H.D. (1979). Soil, Sci. Soc. Amer. J. 43. 722-725.

Subba Rao, N.S. (1995). Mycorrhizal fungi in biofertilizer in agriculture and forestry. 3rd ed. Oxford and IBH Pub. Co. Pvt. Ltd., New Delhi. p. 134-151.

Suresh Kumar, K.V., Harikumar, V.S. and Gopalakrishnan, P.K. (1995). Influence of host variet and edaphic factors on vesicular – arbuscular mycorrhizal (VAM) association in Pigeonpea. Acta. Botanica Indica. 23: 81-85.

Microbiology and Biotechnology for Sustainable Development (*Ed.* P.C. Jain),
CBS Publishers & Distributors, New Delhi (2004), pp. 254–260.

B-8

Enumeration and Characterization of Acidophilic Metallurgical Useful Bacteria from Lignite and Copper Mine

S.R. Dave, D.R. Tipre and K.P. Ladhawala
Department of microbiology, school of sciences
Gujarat University, Ahmedabad 380 009
E-mail : shaileshrdave@hotmail.com

Abstract

The microbiology of extremely acidic metal rich environments was studied with reference to lignite and copper mines. The studied mining environments were found to be extreme in terms of pH as low as 1.44, ORP more than 600 mV, and total solids above 100 g/lit. The presence of microbial life in such extreme environment is known. Many of these microorganisms are responsible for metal extraction. Efforts were therefore made to isolate and characterize the native acidophilic metallurgical useful bacteria from this acid mine waters but universally accepted obstacles in quantifying the bioleaching autotrophic bacteria are problems with their growth on solid medium. Thus most probable number (MPN) and serial dilution techniques were used to enumerate iron-oxidizing bacteria. Sensitivity of conventional MPN technique was enhanced by certain modification viz. concentration of ferrous and incorporation of indicator dye in the medium. The modified MPN technique showed good correlation with serial dilution method. Isolation of iron and sulphate oxidizers were performed using ferrous and thiosulphate as substrate. Among the eleven isolates, majority of the isolates were identified T. ferrooxidans, T. thiooxidans and L. ferrooxidans. The isolates T. ferrooxidans was found to be unique in its tolerance to osmotic pressure, presence of metal ions and acidity of the medium. The obtained results showed that microbial bioleaching consortium rather than single organisms are found in acid mine environments. The finding will give new insight in biologically mediated metal extractions processes from sulphidic ores and concentrates.

Key words: Acidophilic bacteria, bioleaching, lignite, copper mine.

INTRODUCTION

Extremely acidic environments (pH<3) occur in nature, e.g. in geothermal and costal ores, particularly where mining of coals and metals are carried out. The biotic components of these environments are predominantly microbiological, and it is now recognized that acid tolerant and obligate acidophilic microorganisms, which inhabit these, are a highly diverse group of microorganisms (Johnson, 1995; 1996). Archaea, bacteria, fungi, algae and protozoa have been isolated from, and have been shown to be active in extremely acidic sites (Johnson, 1995; Johnson, 1996; Ehrlich, 1999). Of these, most research interests have focused on-applied side of these organisms and pollution aspects. Iron and sulphur oxidizing bacteria have metal mobilizing abilities which are exploited in the biological processing of sulphidic ores and their oxidation of mineral sulphides is a primary cause of acid mine drainage (Rawlings and Simon, 1995). Although these organisms are exploited extensively throughout the world, the scientists have overlooked the systematic diversity studies of these extremophilic bioleaching bacteria. Few literatures are available regarding this aspect. D.B.Johnson has studied the biodiversity and ecology of extremophilic organisms of extremely acidic environment (Johnson, 1996) and Gomez *et al.* (1993) have isolated and characterized novel bioleaching organisms from Rio-tinto river. In India, S.R. Dave and K.A.Natarajan did preliminary systematic study on microbial ecology of sulphidic mines of India (Dave and Natarajan, 1989). One of the reasons for scarce studies on biodiversity of these organisms is the technical difficulty in growing them on solid media. To facilitate the study of acidophilic microorganism, it is necessary to grow them on solid media. Numerous media have been reported, for the isolation of these biotechnologically useful organisms (Karavaiko, 1988a; Johnson and Robert, 1991; Johnson, 1995) but none of the single medium has proved efficient to grow all the organisms. So, the enumeration of acidophilic bacteria based on viable plate count method has little success. Direct microscopic count using Petroff-Hauser counting chamber, number of PCR molecules and immunological method like fluorescent antibody staining method give inaccurate measures as they count both, the dead and the live cells (Lafleur, *et al.,* 1993; Escobar and Godoy, 1999). So, to determine active cell number most probable number method was employed but its limitation of low enumeration potential coupled with limitation of 3 weeks long incubation period leads to the development of modified methodology of most probable number. The modified MPN method has high enumeration potential to enumerate the active microbial population with the capacity to detect oxidized Fe (II) and reduced sulphur compounds (Karavaiko, 1988b; Lafleur, *et al.,* 1993; Escobar and Godoy, 1999).

This paper summarizes details of lignite and copper mines samples, enumeration of iron and sulphur oxidizers and the existing organisms with their characteristics.

MATERIALS AND METHODS

Collection and characterization of sample

Acid mine drainage samples were collected in sterile screw capped bottles from lignite and copper mine. Bottles were immediately closed after collection and brought to the laboratory as soon as possible. pH, mV and conductivity of the samples were determined at the site by portable instruments. Specific physico-chemical properties of the samples were determined by using standard methods as described in APHA (Eaton *et al.* 1995). All samples were microscopically examined by hanging drop preparation using phase contrast microscope (Metzer).

Enumeration

Iron oxidizers were enumerated by conventional 3 tubes MPN method and by serial dilution method. The medium used was 9K basal salt with 2% $FeSO_4$. Later on, conventional MPN method was modified by using diluted medium and positive results were confirmed by using 1% solution of potassium thiocyanate as an indicator (Karavaiko, 1988b; Lafleur, *et al.*, 1993; Escobar and Godoy, 1999).

Heterotrophic iron and sulfur oxidizers were enumerated by using viable plate count method. For this purpose, yeast extract was used as an organic source with 9K medium and Starkey's basal salt medium supplemented with 1% thiosulphate / 1% sulphur/ 1% tetrathionate (w/v) for iron and sulphur oxidizers respectively (Karavaiko, 1988a; Johnson and Robert, 1991; Johnson, 1995).

Isolation

Isolation of the various iron oxidizers and sulphur oxidizers were carried out on the same above mentioned media. Media were solidified with 0.8% w/v washed agar as gelling agent.

Preservation

The purified isolates were transferred in respective liquid medium in sterile screw capped tubes and all the isolates were preserved at –4° C temperature.

Identification

Selected isolates were characterized and identified using their specific features such as Gram's staining reaction, morphology, microscopy and substrate utilization (Starr *et al.*, 1981; Krieg *et al.*, 1989; Asmah *et al.*, 1999).

RESULTS AND DISCUSSION

Both, lignite and chalcopyrite mine showed the presence of all extremities with the parameters studied such as pH, redox potential, conductivity, total solids etc.. Results are shown in table 1. Looking to extreme prevailing condition, only organism having extreme tolerance can grow in this ecosystem. In normal media hardly any growth was seen.

The enumeration of iron oxidizers was carried out in liquid media and results are depicted in table 2. The conventional MPN method showed nearly five fold less count as compared to serial dilution method. Then, the MPN method was modified, by diluting the medium nutrients and positive results were confirmed by addition of potassium thiocyanate indicator. The count was enhanced by 1.5 to 4.0 fold as compared to serial dilution method and nearly 10 folds as compared to conventional MPN method. Moreover, the incubation period was reduced as compared to conventional MPN method. This could be due to the better efficiency of ferric detection by the application of dye and better growth of the organisms is due to the dilution of nutrients of the medium. When the counts of two samples were compared, copper mine showed nearly 5 to 10 fold higher counts as compared to lignite mine water sample. This could be due to diversity of the sites and could be specifically linked with the presence of left out ferrous in copper mine water sample which is the sole nutrient source for the iron oxidizers. Lignite mine water sample showed almost zero ferrous which could be one of the reasons for low count and gradual death in this environment.

Table 1: Characteristics of AMD water samples

Parameter	Samples	
	Lignite mine	Chalcopyrite mine
Color	Yellowish brown	Brown
pH	1.64	1.40
Redox potential (mV)	640	674
Conductivity (mS)	17.20	19.20
Total solids (g/l)	100	150
Dissolved solids (g/l)	50	100
Suspended solids (g/l)	50	50
Ferrous (mg/l)	0	87.7
Sulphate (g/l)	10	23

Table 2: MPN and serial dilution counts from AMD water (After 17 days incubation)

Sample	MPN count (cells/ml)		Serial dilution (Cells/ml)
	Conventional Method	Modified Method	
Lignite mine water	23	240	10^2
Chalcopyrite mine water	390	1500	10^3

The acidophilic heterotrophs were also enumerated and once again except StY medium all the media showed higher count from copper mine water. The count varies from 0 to as high as 450 cells/ml. The acidophilic fungi were very low and maximum two varieties were recorded in StY medium, while SsY and SteY medium showed one variety. When the count was considered in terms of incubation hours, the interesting data was seen in SteY medium where organism were required longer time to grow and substantial very high increase was seen after 96 hours of incubation. Compared to other medium tetrathionate medium requires longer incubation time for more than 90% of the population.

Attempt was also made for the enumeration of heterotrophic, autotrophic, facultative anaerobic and aerobic iron metabolizing organisms. The results are shown in table 4. Water from the copper mine showed growth only on citrate and 9K agar while water from lignite mine showed growth on all the media. This indicates anaerobic iron metabolizing organisms were absent in copper mine water while they were present in considerable number in lignite mine water. This may be due to the comparative more organic matters available in lignite mine water as compared to copper mine. Mostly, lignite contains 'S' in the form of organic and inorganic which may facilitate the growth of these group of organisms. The iron precipitator- *Sphaerotilus* spp. was isolated from citrate agar with considerable iron precipitation.

Table 3: Total viable counts for acidophilic heterotrophs

Site	After 48 hours (cells/ml)				After 96 hours (cells/ml)			
	9KY	StY	SsY	SteY	9KY	StY	SsY	SteY
Lignite	20	20	100	20	20	20	110	450
Mine water	1B	2B	3B+1F	1B	1B	2B	3B+1F	1B
Copper	20	180	270		60	180	270	280
Mine water	1B	5B+2F	2B+1F		1B	5B+2F	2B+1F	1B+1F

Y – yeast extract, S – starkey's basal salt medium,

t – thiosulphate, s – sulphur, te – tetrathionate.

B – bacterial variety. F – fungal variety.

Table 4: Enumeration of hetrotrophic, autotrophic, facultative anaerobic and aerobic iron metabolizing organisms

Sample	No. of CFU/ml			
	Citrate agar	Iron sulphite agar	Sulphite agar	9k agar
Lignite mine	20 (2F)	70 (3B)	130 (3B)	11 (4B)
	110	-	-	15 (7B)
Chalcopyrite Ore mine	(1F+3B)			

F: Fungal variety, B: Bacterial variety

The identification of the selected isolates represented the presence of *T. ferrooxidans* and *T. thiooxidans* from both the sites and *L.ferrooxidans* from copper mine site. This may because it requires ferrous for its growth that was present in copper mine site and absent in lignite mine. The other properties such as substrate oxidized, colony characteristics, Gram's reaction, cell shape and growth on solid media are summarized in table 5.

Table 5: Morphological, physiological and biochemical characteristic of bacterial isolates from AMD water samples

Isolate	Substrate Oxidized		Colony character				Growth on solid media			Identified Org.
	S^0	Fe^{+2}	Color	Shape	Dia. mm.	Gram's reaction	Cell Shape	Ferrous	Thio-Sulphate	
Lignite 1	+	-	WC	P	0.5-1	-	SR	-	+	T.t.
Lignite 2	+	+	YOC,Y	C, IR	0.5-1	-	SR	+	+	T.f.
Chalco 1	+	+	YOC,Y	C, IR	0.5-1	-	SR	+	+	T.f.
Chalco 2	+	-	WC	P	0.5-1	-	SR	-	+	T.t.
Chalco 3	-	-	-	-	-	-	CR	-	-	L.f.

WC – whitish cream, YOC – yellowish orange with dark center, Y - yellow,

P - punctiform, C – circular, IR – irregular, SR – straight rod, CR – curved rod,

T.t. – *Thiobacillus thiooxidans*, T.F. – *Thiobacillus ferrooxidans*, L.f. – *Leptospirillium ferrooxidans*

CONCLUSION

- Both the mining site showed high extremities for pH, mV, iron, sulphate and solids.
- Copper mine's environment was found to be more extreme in all the parameter studied.
- Extremities of pH and dissolved solids found to be one of the detrimental factors for the normal life.
- Modified method showed nearly ten fold higher counts then conventional MPN method and 1.5 to 4.0 fold higher than serial dilution method. Thus, modification in MPN method was found beneficial.
- Ferrous and sulphur oxidation activity was found to be sustainable under this extreme environment.
- The major sustainable organisms were,

  T.ferrooxidans

  T. thiooxidans

  L. ferrooxidans

  Sphaerotilus spp.

ACKNOWLEDGEMENT

We are thankful to DBT, New Delhi for the project grant and fellowship to K.P.L. and Research Associate ship to D.R.T.

REFERENCES

Asmah, R.H., Bosompem, K.M., Osei, Y.D., Rodrigues, F.K., Addy, M.E., Clement, C., Wilson, M.D. (1999). Isolation and characterization mineral oxidizing bacteria from the Obuasi gold mining site,

Ghana. *In biohydrometallurgy and the environment toward the mining of the 21st century.* (Eds. Amils, R. and Ballester, A.). Part – A: Elseveir, Amsterdam, p 657-662.

Dave, S.R. and Natarajan, K.A. (1989). Microbial ecology of some Indian sulphidic mines. *In transaction of the Indian institute of metals.* 40: 315.

Eaton, Clesceri, L.S. and Greenberg, A.E. (1995). *Standard methods for the examination of water and waste water* ed.19. APHA, U.S.A.

Ehrlich, H.L. (1999). Past, present and future of biohydrometallurgy. *In biohydrometallurgy and the environment toward the mining of the 21st century.* (Eds. Amils, R. and Ballester, A.). Part – A: Elseveir, Amsterdam, p 3-12

Escobar, B., and Godoy, I. (1999). Determination of sulfur and iron oxidation bacteria by the most probable number (MPN) technique. *In biohydrometallurgy and the environment toward the mining of the 21st century.* (Eds. Amils, R. and Ballester, A.). Part – A: Elseveir, Amsterdam, p 681-687.

Gomez, E., Lopez, A. I., Marin, I. and Amils, R. (1993). Isolation and characterization of novel bioleaching microorganisms from Rio Tinto. *In biohydrometallurgical techniques.* (Eds. Torma, A.E., Apel, M.L., and Brirely, C.L.). Elseveir, Amsterdam, 2: p 479-486.

Johnson, D.B. (1995). Selective solid media for isolating and enumerating acidophilic bacteria. *Journal of microbiological methods.* 23: 205-218.

Johnson, D.B. (1996). Biodiversity and ecology of acidophilic microorganisms. *In FEMS Microbiol. Ecol.*, 27 : 307-317.

Johnson, D.B., and Robert, F.F. (1991). Heterotrophic acidophiles and their roles in bioleaching of sulfide minerals. *In biomining: theory, microbes and industrial processes.* (Eds. Rawlings, D.E.). Landes biosciences-Austin, p 259-279.

Karavaiko, G.I. (1988a). Methods of isolation, evaluation and studying of microorganisms. *In biotechnology of metals. Center for international projects GKNT,* Moscow. p 59-70.

Karavaiko, G.I. (1988b). Microorganisms and their significance for biogeotechnology of metals. *In biotechnology of metals. Center for international projects GKNT,* Moscow. p 8-45.

Krieg, N.R., Sneath, P.H.A., Staley, J.T. and Williams, S.T. (1989). In *Bergey's Manual of Systematic Bacteriology.* 8th ed., 1-4. Williams and Wilkins.

Lafleur, R., Roy, E.D., Couillard D. and Guay, R. (1993). Determination of iron oxidizing bacteria numbers by a modified MPN procedure. *In biohydrometallurgical techniques.* (Eds. Torma, A.E., Apel, M.L., and Brirely, C.L.). 2 Elseveir, Amsterdam, p 433-441.

Lopez-Archilla, A.I., Marin, I. and. Amils, R. (1995). Microbial ecology of an acidic river. *In biohydrometallurgical techniques.* (Eds. Torma, A.E., Apel, M.L., and Brirely, C.L.). 2, Elseveir, Amsterdam, p 63.

Rawlings, E. D., and Simon Silver (1995). Mining with microbes. *In biotechnology.* 13: University of Illinois, Chicago, p 773-778.

Starr, P.M., Stolp, H., Truper, G.H., Balows, A. and Schlegel, G.H. (1981). *The prokaryotes* 1-2. Springer-Verlag, NY.

Microbiology and Biotechnology for Sustainable Development (*Ed.* P.C. Jain),
CBS Publishers & Distributors, New Delhi (2004), pp. 261–266.

B-9

Production of a Hyperthermostable α-Amylase by an Extreme Thermophile *Geobacillus thermoleovorans*

Ritu Malhotra, Sonali Narang, J.L.Uma Maheswar Rao and T.Satyanarayana
Department of Microbiology, University of Delhi South Campus,
New Delhi-110 021.

Abstract

Among starch hydrolysing enzymes that are produced on an industrial scale, thermostable α-amylase is of considerable commercial interest. α-Amylases randomly hydrolyse α-1,4–glucosidic linkages in starch or its hydrolysis products. Bacteria belonging to the genus Bacillus have been widely used for the commercial production of thermostable α-amylases. The α-amylases presently used in starch saccharification require Ca^{2+} for activity and/ or stability. The continuing need for novel α-amylases which do not require Ca^{2+} has been emphasized.

Geobacillus thermoleovorans produced 36 and 15 U per ml α-amylase in optimized chemically defined and synthetic media, respectively. The enzyme exhibited optimum activity at 100 °C and pH 8.0, and $t_{½}$ of 3h at 100 °C. Both α-amylase activity and production were Ca^{2+} independent. This enzyme can find application in starch saccharification due to its high thermostability and lack of Ca^{2+} requirement for its activity and/ or stability.

Key words: *Geobacillus thermoleovorans*, Ca^{2+} independent, Thermostable α-amylase.

INTRODUCTION

α-Amylases hydrolyse α-1,4–glucosidic linkages in starch and related substrates in an endo-fashion liberating linear and branched oligosaccharides of varied length (Antranikian 1992). Thermostable enzymes are essential for industry because of their high stability and longer shelf life (Crabb and Mitchinson 1997, Niehaus *et al.*, 1999). The α-amylases currently used in starch saccharification requires Ca^{2+} for activity and/or stability (Douglas *et al.*, 1989), and therefore, need extensive use of ion–exchangers for their removal from the product steam. A need for novel α-amylases with out requirement for Ca^{2+} has been emphasized (Antranikian 1992, Malhotra *et al.*, 2000, Narang and Satyanarayana, 2001). A chemically defined medium permits understanding of the specific requirements for growth and product formation by systematically adding or eliminating chemical components from the formulation, with minimal complicated medium interactions (Cano and Colome, 1988). The production of metabolites in a fermenter provides several advantages over production in a shake flask (Humphrey, 1998). In this investigation, α-amylase production by *Geobacillus thermoleovorans* was carried out in chemically defined and synthetic media, followed by partial purification and characterization. The scale up of production was also attempted in shake flasks as well as in a laboratory fermenter.

MATERIALS AND METHODS

Bacterial strain

The bacterial strain used in this investigation was isolated using enrichment culture by directly inoculating hot-spring water samples from Waimangu Volcanic valley, New Zealand into Castenholz medium (Castenholz, 1969).

Production of α-amylase

The bacterium was grown in the amylase production medium that contained (w/v) starch 2%, tryptone 0.3%, yeast extract 0.3%, K_2HPO_4 0.1%, NaCl 0.1% and $MgSO_4.7H_2O$ 0.02%. The chemically defined medium was prepared by substituting starch, yeast extract and tryptone with glucose (2%), riboflavin (50μ/ml), equimolar proportion of nitrogen in the form of amino acid (cysteine), respectively. The production was carried out at 65 °C for 12h with 200 rpm. The culture fluids for assaying α-amylase were obtained by centrifugation of the culture broth at 8000 xg for 20 min in a Sorvall centrifuge at 4 °C, and decanting the supernatant fluid.

Scale up in shake flasks

The bacterial strain was grown in 50, 100, 200, and 400 ml of the production medium in 250 ml, 500ml, 1-1 and 2-1 Erlenmeyer flasks, respectively. A 2% inoculum (6-h-old) was used to inoculate the medium, and incubated at 65 °C and agitated at 200 rpm.

Batch fermentation in a laboratory fermenter

The bacterial strain was grown in a 22-1 fermenter containing 10-1 of the production medium. The 6h- old 2% (v/v) inoculum was directly transferred to the production medium whose pH was adjusted to 7.0 after sterilization in the fermenter. The fermenter was operated at 60 °C, 200 rpm and 1 vvm aeration.

Partial Purification of α-amylase and enzyme kinetics

The enzyme was precipitated from crude culture filtrate by adding chilled acetone to 80% (v/v) saturation. The precipitate was centrifuged at 12000 xg for 20 min, dissolved in 0.1M phosphate buffer, and dialysed overnight against the same buffer. This partially purified enzyme preparation was used for finding out the effects of temperature, pH, substrate concentration and various cations on the enzyme activity.

End product analysis

The products liberated by the action of amylase on starch were identified by spotting the starch digest and standard sugars (glucose, maltose and maltotriose) on a silica gel plate activated at 110 °C for 2h. The plates were developed in the solvent contains butanol: ethanol: water in the ratio of (5:3:2) and dried overnight at room temperature. The individual sugars were visualized by spraying with aniline-diphenyamine reagent (Hansen, 1975).

Assay of α-amylase

The saccharogenic α-amylase activity was determined by the modified method of Bernfeld as described earlier (Babu and Satyanarayana 1993) using dinitrosalicylic acid reagent. One saccharogenic α-amylase unit is defined as the amount of enzyme required for the liberation of one μmole reducing sugar as glucose per minute under the assay conditions.

RESULTS AND DISCUSSIONS

The production levels of amylase in synthetic medium were 15U/ml, which are much less as compared to that in chemically defined medium. In the chemically defined medium, glucose serves as carbon source. When yeast extract was replaced with different vitamins, it was observed that riboflavin alone increased the enzyme yield, followed by that in the medium containing all vitamins. Niacin, pantothenate and pyridoxine also supported enzyme production (Table 1). When tryptone was replaced with different amino acids, it was observed that cysteine, agrinine, asparagine, serine and proline showed a positive effect on amylase production (Table 2). The addition of cysteine supported a high amylase secretion. Enzyme production was negligible when there was no vitamin in the medium, whereas an increase in enzyme production was recorded when the medium was supplemented with riboflavin, this vitamin caused a two-fold increase in enzyme production. This observation suggests that the organism required growth factors for its growth and maximum enzyme secretion by *Bacillus thermooleovorans* (Narang and Satyanarayana, 2001). Hence a chemically defined medium was formulated for the growth and amylase production that consisted of glucose (2%), riboflavin (50μ/ml), cysteine(0.3%), $MgSO_4.7H_2O$ (0.02%), K_2HPO_4 (0.1%) and NaCl (0.1%).

Enzyme Production in Shake flasks

The production levels of α-amylase increased with increasing volumes of the medium when the ratio of the volume of the medium to that of the flask was kept constant. The production of α-amylase increased from 14780 Ul^{-1} in a 250-ml flask to 22510 Ul^{-1} in 200-ml medium in a 1liter flask. A slight decline in amylase production was recorded in a 2-liter flask containing 400 ml medium. This could be due to improper mixing of the nutrients or inadequate aeration on increasing the volume of the medium.

Table 1: Effect of vitamins on growth and α-amylase production in chemically defined glucose mineral salts medium in 12h

Vitamin	Growth *(A600nm)*	Amylase activity *(U/ml^{-1})*
All vitamins*	0.3	25.1
Biotin*	0.2	11.8
Cyanocobalamin*	0.1	08.8
Folic acid*	0.1	16.5
Niacin*	0.1	17.0
No vitamin	0.1	03.0
Pantothenate*	0.2	17.6
Pyridolxine*	0.1	17.4
Riboflavin*	0.4	26.4
Thiamine*	0.3	11.8
ControlØ	0.2	14.0

*Vitamins. Yeast extract as vitamin source.

Tryptone as nitrogen source. (Mean of 3 values, SD within 10%)

Table 2: Effect of amino acids on growth and α-amylase production in chemically defined glucose mineral salts medium in 12h

Amino acid	Growth *(A600nm)*	Amylase activity *(U/ml^{-1})*
Cysteine#	0.6	28.0
Alanine#	0.6	25.8
Arginine#	0.8	27.6
Asparagine#	0.6	26.0
Histidine#	0.3	25.0
Leucine#	0.4	25.6
Phenylalanine#	0.3	25.0
Proline#	0.2	27.0
Serine#	0.2	27.6
Threonine#	0.3	19.7
Tyrosine#	0.2	26.2
Control	0.6	27.3

Amino acids. Tryptone as nitrogen source.

Amino acids used in equimolar proportions of nitrogen present in glucose mineral salts medium.

(Mean of 3 values, SD within 10%)

Production of α-amylase in a laboratory fermenter

The age and amount of inoculum is one of the most significant factors to affect the growth and enzyme production. The addition of 5% inoculum reduced the lag phase and also the optimal time for enzyme production. The pH of the medium dropped from 7.0 to 5.20 after 6h incubation. As compared with production in shake flasks, the optimal production time of the enzyme reduced from 12 to 8h and enzyme levels increased from 15000 to 24050 Ul^{-1}. When the pH was maintained, the lag phase reduced to 50 min and an increased enzyme production (33360 Ul^{-1}) was attained with in 5h in optimal conditions. When fermentation was carried out at 300 rpm the lag phase extended up to 100 min and enzyme secretion was reduced up to 20930 Ul^{-1}). The optimal temperature for growth and enzyme production in the fermenter was 60 °C. The optimal temperature in shakes flasks for growth and enzyme production was at 70 °C (Malhotra *et al.,* 2000). This might be due to improper heat transfer in a shaker. The main products of starch hydrolysis by the enzyme action were maltose, maltotriose and some maltodextrins, suggesting that the enzyme produced by the strain is a α-amylase.

Partial purification of amylase with acetone led to a 43.7% recovery of enzyme with 6.2-fold purification. The enzyme was optimally active at 100 °C at pH 8.0. The enzyme exhibited a half-life of 3h at 100°C. The K_m and V_{max} (soluble starch) values were 0.83-mg ml^{-1} and 250 μ moles/min/ml. A slight stimulation of enzyme activity was observed with 5 m mol l^{-1} by $Fe^{2+}$and NH_4^+ ions, while inhibited by Cu^{2+}, $Mg^{2+}$and Mn^{2+}ions. Similar effect has been reported in *Bacillus subtilis* (Takasaki 1982), and *B. coagulans* (Babu and Satyanarayana 1993). The presence or absence of 5 m mol l^{-1} Ca^{2+} did not affect enzyme activity. The α-amylase of *G. thermoleovorans,* being calcium independent and thermostable (Narang and Satyanarayana 2001), it could be useful in starch hydrolysis (Malhotra *et al.,* 2000).

REFERENCES

Antranikian, G. (1992). Microbial degradation of starch. In Microbial Degradation of Natural Products ed.Winkel,. Weinhein, V.C.H., Germany, G. pp. 27-51.

Babu, K.R. and Satyanarayana, T. (1993). Extracellular calcium inhibited α-amylase of *Bacillus coagulans* B49. Enzyme Microbial Technology 15: 1066-1069.

Bernfeld, P. (1955). Amylases, α and â. Methods in Enzymology 1: 149-158.

Cano, R.J. and Colome, J.S. (1988) Essentials of Microbiology. St. Paul, MN: West Publishing Company.

Castenholz, R.W. (1969). Thermophilic blue green algae and the thermal environment. Bacteriological reviews 33: 476-504.

Coolbear, T. (1992). The enzyme from extreme thermophiles: Bacterial sources, thermostabilities and industrial relevance. Advances in Biochemical Engineering and Biotechnology 45: 57-97.

Crabb, W.D. and Mitchinson, C. (1997). Enzyme involved in the processing of starch to sugars. Triends in biotechnology 15: 349-352.

Douglas, S. Bush, Liliane Sticher, Robert van Huystee, Doris Wangeer. (1989). The Calcium Requirement for Stability and Enzymatic Activity of Two Isoforms of Barley Aleurone α-Amylase. The Journal of Biological Chemistry. 264: 19392-19398.

Hansen (1975). Thin layer chromatographic method for identificaion of oligosaccharides in starch hydrolyzates. Journal of chromatography 105: 388-390.

Humphrey, A. (1998). Shake flask to fermenter: What have we learnt? Biotechnology Progress 14: 3-7.

Malhotra, R., Noorwez, S.M. and Satyanarayana, T. (2000). Production and partial characterization of thermostable and calcium independent α-amylase of an extreme thermophile *Bacillus thermo-oleovorans* NP54. Letters in Applied Microbiology 31: 378-384.

Narang, S. and Satyanarayana, T. (2001). Thermostable α-amylase production by an extreme thermophile *Bacillus thermooleovorans*. Letters in Applied Microbiology 32: 32-35.

Niehaus, F., Bertoldo, C.,Kahler, M. and Antranikian, G.(1999). Extremophiles as a sources of novel enzymes for industrial application. Applied Microbiology and Biotechnology 51: 711-729.

Takasaki,Y.(1982). Production of maltohexaose by α-amylase from *Bacillus circulans* G6. Agricultural and Biological Chemistry 46: 1539-1547.

Microbiology and Biotechnology for Sustainable Development (Ed. P.C. Jain),
CBS Publishers & Distributors, New Delhi (2004), pp. 267–276.

B-10

Comparison of Amino Acid Sequence of Active Site of L-Arginase Enzymes

P.A. Wadegaonkar*, Priti Dodiya, A.P. Ramteke, N.J. Chikhale and M.K. Rai
Department of Biotechnology, Amravati University,
Amravati (Maharashtra) 444602

Abstract

Three Arginase signatures were obtained from motif database PROSITE. The largest Arginase signature having 22 amino acids was subjected to BLASTp and similarity was present in all the arginases reported in GeneBank. Arginase signature of 33 arginases, were aligned using ClustalW and physico-chemical analysis was carried out using GeneDoc software. Ten amino acids were conserved in this region and the predicted active site was S-[X]-D-[D]-[X]2-D-P-[X]3-P-[X]2-G-T-[X]-V-[X]-G-G. Three Aspartic acid residues, two each of Glycine and Proline residues and one each of Threonine and Valine were conserved. Out of three only one Aspartic acid residue was having net negative charge while other two did not show any charge since these two aspartic acid residues were sandwiched between hydrophobic amino acid residues. The secondary structure predicted from SOPM software suggests that the active site of arginase consists of beta- turns, extended strands and no helical structure and located towards C-terminal end. The Aspartic acid residues (pKa value 3.86) may be responsible for the broad pH optima (from pH 3.5 to 8.0) of L-Arginase of Penicillium citrinum.

Key words: L-Arginase, active site, Sequence analysis

INTRODUCTION

Protein retains a certain pattern of residues for its function. This may be diagnostic of short sequence that is known as active site or binding region of protein. These are regarded as clefts or cervices or pockets occupying a small region in a big molecule. (Paulin and Corey, 1951; Levitt and Chothia, 1976; Lehninger, *et al.*, 1993). The existence of active site is due to the tertiary structure of protein resulting in three-dimensional native conformation. This 3

* *Corresponding author. Email: prasadwadegaonkar@rediffmail.com*

dimensional entity is formed by groups that comes from different parts of linear amino acid sequence -indeed residues far apart of sequences may interact strongly than adjacent residue in the amino acid sequence. These recognize the specific intern receptors or motifs & hence possible to predict the functional utility (Satyanarayan, 1999). However, it does provide an experimentally testable hypothesis as to protein functions. Since conserved sequences can be found around the active site, site of post-translational modification, binding site for co-factors, protein sorting signals etc. A number of bio-informatics resources have been developed both to build database of conserved pattern & to search of such patterns in sequences. (Rost *et al.*, 1994; Thompson *et al.*, 1994; Gevurjan and Deleage, 1995; Higgins *et al.*, 1996; Brass, 1997; Nicholas and Nicholas, 1997; Schular, 1998).

L-Arginase (E.C. 3.5.3.1) is a urea cycle enzyme. It is present in almost all the organism. Macrophages release L-arginase upon activation which cause, depletion of the free L-arginine content present in microenvironment, which ultimately resulted in killing tumour cells. Similarly, the contaminating mycoplasmas of the mammalian cell culture are known to release arginase in the system which effects an *in vitro* inhibition of tumour cell lines of human erythroleukemia, mouse fibrosarcomas, mouse thymoma and lymphoma cultures. Miyazaki *et al.,* (1990) subsequent studies confirmed the essentiality of L-arginine for various human tumour cell lines in culture. *Penicillium citrinum* and *P. spinulosum* have been found as potential organisms for production of L-arginase (Wadegaonkar *et al.,* 1992). L-arginase of *P. citrinum* has been purified by affinity chromatography and subsequently characterized (Wadegaonkar 1995). This enzyme has been reported to inhibit the multiplication of mouse myelomas, human cervix carcinoma and human larynx carcinoma *in vitro* (Joshi, 1995).

In present study an attempt has been made to locate and study the active site of L-arginase from various sources and compare it with characteristics of L-arginase of *P. citrinum*.

MATERIALS AND METHODS

Retrieval of Amino Acid Sequence of L-Arginase from DNA Database of Japan:

For the search and retrieval of amino acid sequence of L-Arginase from various organisms DNA Database of Japan was used. Search was made, by giving the key word "ARGINASE". The sequences of Translation were used for further analysis.

MULTIPLE SEQUENCE ALIGNMENT ANALYSIS:

1. ClustalW

For alignment of sequences ClustalW was used. The sequences to be aligned, were clubbed in one file of NBRF/PIR format as per requirement of the software in non-document mode of notepad.

The following multiple alignment parameters were selected to develop the alignments.

K-tupple size: it is kept one residue for nucleotide sequences.

Gap Opening Penalty: 10.00

Gap Extension Penalty: 0.05

Matrix: Blossum 30

The aligned sequences were save as *arg.aln* out put file.

2. Genedoc:

The *aln.aln* files so created by the program CLUSTAL W was imported in to GENEDOC. Aligned sequences were then further studied for conservation, physico-chemical properties, hydrophobic/ hydrophilic nature etc. of amino acids.

ACTIVE SITE PREDICTION OF L- ARGINASE:

Prosite:

Amino acid sequence of L-Arginase of *Mus musculus* obtained from DDBJ was submitted to ***PROSITE*** *http://expasy.hcuge.ch/sprot/prosite.html* for prediction of possible active site.

BLAST (Basic Local Alignment Search Tool):

For homologues search of active site of L- Arginase, the Arginase family signature 3 obtained from PROSITE was submitted to using BLASTp (Altschul *et al.*, 1997).

SECONDARY STRUCTURE PREDICATION:

SOPM A:

One of the ultimate goals of computer based sequences analysis is to predict protein structure. Amino acid sequences of various L-Arginases were submitted to SOPMA (http:// *www.ihcp.fripredict.html*). The SOPMA method was implied by submitting the query sequence itself in single letter format. The alignment was based on sequences similarity and each of the component i.e. amino acid were predicted for analysis of secondary structure (SOPMA : http: // *www.bcp.frlpredict.html*)

RESULTS AND DISCUSSION

GenBank is the NIH genetic sequence database, annotated collection of publicly available nucleotide and protein sequences. GenBank is built by National Center for Biotechnology Information at NIH, Maryland with its two partners, the DNA Database of Japan (DDBJ, Japan) and the European Molecular Biology Laboratory (EMBL) nucleotide database from European Bioinformatics Institute, England. Search for amino acid sequence of L-arginase enzyme was performed online using DDBJ using "L-Arginase" as a key word. Total 17 outputs were downloaded from DDBJ and their translations were used as amino acid sequence. DDBJ search gave information regarding the detail of source, locus, number of base pairs, accession number, and version along with detailed references.

The amino acid sequence of L-Arginase of *Mus musculues* from DDBJ was submitted to PROSITE by pasting the sequence in form for determination of possible active site or enzyme family signature. PROSITE database is a collection of protein signature (Bairoch, 1997).

Protein signature is short pattern that arises from tight constraints on three-dimensional structures of binding or active site. The PROSITE found total three signatures belonging to Arginase family. The largest one was 22 amino acid long and was from 249-270 amino acid position (Table 1).

Table 1: Prediction of active site using PROSITE

Sequence Submitted for predicton :

ScanProsite - Protein against PROSITE

MFLRSSASRL	LHGQIPCVLT	RSVHSVAIVG	APFSRGQKKL
GVEYGPAAIR	EAGLLKRLSR	LGCHLKDFGD	LSFTNVPQDD
PYNNLVVYPR	SVGLANQELA	EVVSRAVSGG Y	SCVTMGGDH
SLAIGTIIGH	ARHRPDLCVI	WVDAHADINT	PLTTVSGNIH
GQPLSFLIKE	LQDKVPQLPG	FSWIKPCLSP	PNIVYIGLRD
VEPPEHFILK	NYDIQYFSMR	EIDRLGIQKV	MEQTFDRLIG
KRQRPIHLSF	DIDAFDPKLA	PATGTPVVGG	LTYREGVYIT
EEIHNTGLLS	ALDLVEVNPH	LATSEEEAKA	TARLAVDVIA
SSFGQTREGG	HIVYDHLPTP	SSPHESENEE	CVR

Out put - Predicted sequences :

[1] *PDOC00135 PS00147* ARGINASE_1

Arginase family signature 1

116-129 MGGDHSLAIGTIIG

[2] *PDOC00135 PS00148* ARGINASE_2

Arginase family signature 2

139-147 VIWVDAHAD

[3] *PDOC00135 PS01053* ARGINASE_3

Arginase family signature 3

249-270 SFDIDAFDPKLAPATGTPVVGG

Multiple molecular sequence alignment are among the most important tools for analyzing biological sequences. Homologues sequence alignment is a powerful tool in bioinformatics (States and Boguski, 1991). Multipe sequence align-ment of many DNA or Protein sequence is among the most important & most challenging tasks in computational biology. There are several approaches to multiple alignment, (Schular *et al.*, 1990; Mehta *et al.*, 1995; Anbarasu, 1999). Global alignment methods are most appropriate to sequence that are small (<500 residues), approximately equal in length & share a global but perhaps, relationship (Lipman *et. al.*, 1989). Local alignment methods, on the other hand are preferable for longer sequences that vary greatly in length & may share only isolated regions of similarly separated by variable length segments of little or no sequence conservation (Posfai *et. al.*, 1989). Finally the progress alignment strategy is the only one i.e. practical for large number of sequences. A major advantage of local alignment methods is that a new theory for estimating the statistical significance of sequence similarities can be applied to the un-gapped homology blocks obtained. However global alignment methods using dynamic programming are superior for determining the locations & extents of insertion & deletion mutations (Lipman *et.al.,* 1989).

Table 2: Search of Arginase family signature in proteins present in protein data banks

BLASTP 2.0.10 [Aug-26-1999]

Query= (22 letters)

Database: Non-redundant GenBank CDS translations+PDB+SwissProt+SPupdate+PIR 437,022 sequences; 134,330,735 total letters

Distribution of 47 Blast Hits on the Query Sequence

Examples :

sp|O08691|ARG2_MOUSE ARGINASE II PRECURSOR (NON-HEPATIC ARGINASE) (KIDNEY-TYPE ARGINASE)

Length = 354

Score = 49.6 bits (116), Expect = 3e-06

Identities = 22/22 (100%), Positives = 22/22 (100%)

SFDIDAFDPKLAPATGTPVVGG 22

SFDIDAFDPKLAPATGTPVVGG

Sbjct: 249 SFDIDAFDPKLAPATGTPVVGG 270

sp|P40906|ARGI_COCIM ARGINASE >gi|1078615|pir||JC4033 arginase (EC 3.5.3.1) -

Coccidioides immitis >gi|550472

Length = 322

Score = 39.1 bits (89), Expect = 0.005

Identities = 16/22 (72%), Positives = 19/22 (85%)

Query: 1 SFDIDAFDPKLAPATGTPVVGG 22

SFD+DA DP+ AP+TGTPV GG

Sbjct: 245 SFDVDALDPQWAPSTGTPVRGG 266:

The sequence of 22 amino acids obtained from the PROSITE as Arginase signature III was submitted to BLASTp and online search was made for homologous sequences in the database of GeneBank. From the query of 22 amino acids sequence, 47 hits were found on the BLASTp distributed database, which have 437,022 sequences with over 13x10 7 letters. BLASTp showed % identity and probability along with positive and score of matching the desire sequence with BLASTp (Table 2). With high level of conservedness, out of 47 sequences 33 sequences were used for further analysis. These sequences were aligned using ClustalW and then analyzed using GENEDOC software, a tool of analysis of multiple sequence alignment. Table 3 and 4 indicate the conserved sequence in the active site of L-arginase, serine is the first amino acid in this sequence, and is conserved in the 32 out of 33 sequences. Similarly, three aspartic acid residues, two proline residues, three glycine residues and three threonine residues are conserved. The formation of bends in the polypeptide chain can be determined by precious location of specific bend producing amino acids residue such as proline, threoinine, serine, (Stryer, 1985). Proline was shown to be conserved at 9 and 13

Table 3: Multiple Sequence Alignment (Conserved Sequence)

Arginase Signature

	* 20	
p1_Mus_mus	: SFDIDAFDPKLAPATGTPVVG---G	: 22
p2_Mus_L	: SFDVDGLDPAFTPATGTPVLGG---	: 22
p3_Rattus	: SFDIDAFDPKLAPATGTPVVGG---	: 22
p4_hepatic	: SFDVDGLDPVFTPATGTPVVG--G-	: 22
p5_HumanKl	: SFDIDAFDPTLAPATGTPVVGG---	: 22
p6_HumanHe	: SFDVDGLDPSFTPATGTPVVGG---	: 22
p7__3_Afri	: SFDIDAFDPALAPATGTPVIG-G--	: 22
p8__2_Afri	: SFDIDAFDPALAPATGTPVIGG---	: 22
p9__1_Afri	: SFDIDAFDPALAPATGTPVIGG---	: 22
p10_Rana_c	: SFDIDGLDPSVAPATGTPVPG-G--	: 22
p11_Rana_c	: SFDIDGLDPSVAPATGTPVPGG---	: 22
p12_Rana_c	: SFDIDGLDPSVAPATGTPVPGG---	: 22
p13_Binucl	: SFDVDGLDPVFTPATGTPVVGG---	: 22
p14_ARGINA	: SFDVDGLDPVFTPATGTPVVGG---	: 22
p15_Coccid	: SFDVDALDPQWAPSTGTPVRG--G-	: 22
p16_Africa	: SFDIDGLDPSIAPATGTPCPGG---	: 22
p17_Neuro4	: SFDVDALDPMWAPSTGTPVRG-G--	: 22
p18_Neuro3	: SFDVDALDPMWAPSTGTPVRGG---	: 22
p19_Emeric	: SFDVDALDPQWVPSTGTPVRGG---	: 22
p20_Schizo	: SFDVDACDPIVAPATGTRVPGG---	: 22
p21_Leishm	: SYDVDTIDPLYVPATGTPVRG-G--	: 22
p22_YEAST	: SYDVDGVDPLYIPATGTPVRGG---	: 22
p23__Deino	: SFDADALDPGVCPGVGTPVPGG---	: 22
p24__NON-H	: SFDIDALDSNVAPSTGTAVRGG---	: 22
p25_B.subt	: SLDLDGLDPNDAPGVGTPVVG-G--	: 22
p26_Rhodob	: SFDVDFLDPGIAPAVGTTVPGG---	: 22
p27_B.cald	: SLDLDGLDPSDAPGVGTPVIGG---	: 22
p28_Brucel	: SLDVDFLDPSIAPAVGTTVPG-G--	: 22
p29_A.tume	: SLDVDFLDPAIAPAVGTTVPGG---	: 22
p30_S.aure	: SLDVDALDPLETPGTGTRVLG-G--	: 22
p31_S.aure	: SLDVDALDPLETPGTGTRVLGG---	: 22
p32_A.tume	: SLDVDFLEPSIAPAVGTTVPGG---	: 22
p33_Synech	: TIDMDGFDPGFMPGVGTPEPGG---	: 22
	s D D dp P GT v G	

PROPOSED ACTIVE SITE

[S]-X-[D]-X-[D]-X2-[D]-X-[P]-X3-[P]-X2-[G]-[T]-X3-[G]-[G]

Table 4: Multiple Sequence Alignment Analysis (Physicochemical Properties) Arginase Signature

	* 20	
p1_Mus_mus	: SFDIDAFDPKLAPATGTPVVG---G	: 22
p2_Mus_L	: SFDVDGLDPAFTPATGTPVLGG---	: 22
p3_Rattus	: SFDIDAFDPKLAPATGTPVVGG---	: 22
p4_hepatic	: SFDVDGLDPVFTPATGTPVVG--G-	: 22
p5_HumanKl	: SFDIDAFDPTLAPATGTPVVGG---	: 22
p6_HumanHe	: SFDVDGLDPSFTPATGTPVVGG---	: 22
p7__3_Afri	: SFDIDAFDPALAPATGTPVIG-G--	: 22
p8__2_Afri	: SFDIDAFDPALAPATGTPVIGG---	: 22
p9__1_Afri	: SFDIDAFDPALAPATGTPVIGG---	: 22
p10_Rana_c	: SFDIDGLDPSVAPATGTPVPG-G--	: 22
p11_Rana_c	: SFDIDGLDPSVAPATGTPVPGG---	: 22
p12_Rana_c	: SFDIDGLDPSVAPATGTPVPGG---	: 22
p13_Binucl	: SFDVDGLDPVFTPATGTPVVGG---	: 22
p14_ARGINA	: SFDVDGLDPVFTPATGTPVVGG---	: 22
p15_Coccid	: SFDVDALDPQWAPSTGTPVRG--G-	: 22
p16_Africa	: SFDIDGLDPSIAPATGTPCPGG---	: 22
p17_Neuro4	: SFDVDALDPMWAPSTGTPVRG-G--	: 22
p18_Neuro3	: SFDVDALDPMWAPSTGTPVRGG---	: 22
p19_Emeric	: SFDVDALDPQWVPSTGTPVRGG---	: 22
p20_Schizo	: SFDVDACDPIVAPATGTRVPGG---	: 22
p21_Leishm	: SYDVDTIDPLYVPATGTPVRG-G--	: 22
p22_YEAST	: SYDVDGVDPLYIPATGTPVRGG---	: 22
p23__Deino	: SFDADALDPGVCPGVGTPVPGG---	: 22
p24__NON-H	: SFDIDALDSNVAPSTGTAVRGG---	: 22
p25_B.subt	: SLDLDGLDPNDAPGVGTPVVG-G--	: 22
p26_Rhodob	: SFDVDFLDPGIAPAVGTTVPGG---	: 22
p27_B.cald	: SLDLDGLDPSDAPGVGTPVIGG---	: 22
p28_Brucel	: SLDVDFLDPSIAPAVGTTVPG-G--	: 22
p29_A.tume	: SLDVDFLDPAIAPAVGTTVPGG---	: 22
p30_S.aure	: SLDVDALDPLETPGTGTRVLG-G--	: 22
p31_S.aure	: SLDVDALDPLETPGTGTRVLGG---	: 22
p32_A.tume	: SLDVDFLEPSIAPAVGTTVPGG---	: 22
p33_Synech	: TIDMDGFDPGFMPGVGTPEPGG---	: 22

PROPOSED ACTIVE SITE

[S]-X1-[D1]-X2-[D2]-2X3-[D3]-[P]-2X4-X5-[P]-2X6-[G]-[T]-3X7-[G]-[G]

Where [S] - Serine

X1, X2, X3, X5 - Hydrophobic amino acids

[D1,2] - Asp (No net charge), [D3] Asp (Net negative charge)

[P] - Pro

[G] - Gly

position. It prevents the helix formation. This could possibly explain, as nitrogen atom in proline is the part of rigid ring and have no relation of the ring N-C bond is thus possible. More over there is no substitute hydrogen on the nitrogen atom of proline residue in the can be determined by precious location of specific bend producing amino acids residue such as proline, threoinine, serine, (Stryer, 1985). Proline was shown to be conserved at 9 and 13 formation of peptide bond (Lehninger *et al.*, 1993). Thus no inter-chain hydrogen bonds can form within the proline peptide bond as a partner. The consequence is that where ever the proline residue occur in the polypeptide chain it will cause a bend. The helix formation is also prevented by Threonine. This is due to the fact that when threonine occurs close together with proline due to its bulky side and shape of R group (Satyanaryan, 1999). Threonine was resulted to be conserved at 19 position and also serine was founded to be conserved due to its hydrophobic nature (Stryer, 1985).

Table 5: Secondary structure prediction of L-arginase

10 20 30 40 50 60 70

MFLRSSASRLLHGQIPCVLTRSVHSVAIVGAPFSRGQKKLGVEYGPAAIREAGLLKRLSRLGCHLKDFGD
eeecccccccettccceeeeeccceeeeecccccttccceeeeecchhhhhhhhhhhhhhttcchttccc
LSFTNVPQDDPYNNLVVYPRSVGLANQELAEVVSRAVSGGYSCVTMGGDHSLAIGTIIGHARHRPDLCVI
ceeeecccccccteeeeeccthhhhhhhhhhhhhhhhhtttceeeeeeccccceeeeeeeectttcctteeee
WVDAHADINTPLTTVSGNIHGQPLSFLIKELQDKVPQLPGFSWIKPCLSPPNIVYIGLRDVEPPEHFILK
eeettccttcceeeeeccccttccceehhhhhtttcccccttceeeetccccccceeeeeecccccccthhheec
NYDIQYFSMREIDRLGIQKVMEQTFDRLIGKRQRPIHL*SFDIDAFDPKLAPATGTPVVGG*LTYREGVYIT
ttteeeeeeecttchhhhhhhhhhhhhhhhccccccceeecccccccttcctttccceecccccctteeee
EEIHNTGLLSALDLVEVNPHLATSEEEAKATARLAVDVIASSFGQTREGGHIVYDHLPTPSSPHESENEE
ccccccthhhhheeeeccccccchhhhhhhhhhhhhheeehccccccccttcceeeeccccccccccchhhhh
CVRI
hhee

Sequence length : 354

SOPM :

Alpha helix	(Hh)	:	83 is 23.45%	310 helix	(Gg)	:	0 is 0.00%
Pi helix	(Ii)	:	0 is 0.00%	Beta bridge	(Bb)	:	0 is 0.00%
Extended strand	(Ee)	:	90 is 25.42%	Beta turn	(Tt)	:	46 is 12.99%
Bend region	(Ss)	:	0 is 0.00%	Random coil	(Cc)	:	135 is 38.14%

Glycine moieties present at the end of the sequence were also found to be conserved. Since being smallest amino acid structurally with polar nature and non-symmetrical property. Hence, usually present in the region where shape (three dimensional) structure is conserved (Lehninger *et al.*, 1993).

Aspartic acid was found to be dominant at 3rd, 5th, and 8th position but physicochemically expressed only at 8 position while shows no charge in 3rd and 5th position. This suggest due to the surrounding hydrophobic amino acid. Due to hydrophobic surroundings they cannot have free R ionisable group and therefore no charge when present in the environment of adjacent amino acid. Thus there may be formation of secondary structure of amino acid present in the most probable active site design from different sources for L-Arginase. The secondary structure predicted from SOPM software suggests that the active site of arginase consists of beta- turns, extended strands and no helical structure and located towards C-terminal end (Table 5). The functional feature can be predicted directly from the protein sequence after analysis. That was very useful utility that allows to known the structure of the protein site by different properties of amino acids sequence present in the protein domain of active site pattern that arise form tight constraints on three dimensional structures of binding or active site.

ACKNOWLEDGEMENT

PAW is highly thankful to Prof. A.S. Kolaskar, Vice Chancellor, Pune University, Ms. Urmila Kale and Sangeeta Sawant, Scientists, Bioinformatic Centre, Pune for providing necessary softwares and guidance.

REFERENCES

Altschul, S.F., Gish, W., Miller W., Myers, E.W. and Lipman, D.J. (1990). Basic local alignment search tool. *J. Mol. Biol.* 2/5, 403-410.

Altschul, Stephen F., Thomas L. Madden, Alejandro A. Schäffer, Jinghui Zhang, Zheng Zhang, Webb Miller, and David J. Lipman (1997), "Gapped BLAST and PSI-BLAST: a new generation of protein database searchprograms", Nucleic Acids Res. 25:3389-3402.

Anbarasu A.L. (1999). Multiple Sequence Alignment using Parallel Genetic Algorithms. Workshop on 'Biomolecular Structure and Modeling', Bioinformatics Centre, Pune, 14-17 Dec.

Brass Andy (1997). DNA Sequencing from Experimental Methods To Bioinformatics, (Ed. Luhe Alphey) Bios Scientific Publishers. 12-16, 125-185.

Bairoch A., Bucher P. and Hofmann, K. (1997). The PROSITE database, its status in 1997. *Nucleic Acids Res.*, 25, 217-221.

Gevurjan, C. and Deleage, G. (1995). sopma: Significant improvement in proteins secondary structure prediction by consensus predictions from multiple alignments, *CABIOS//*.681-684.

Higgins, D.G., Thompson, J.D. and Gibson, T .J. (1996). Using Clustal for multiple sequence alignment .*Methods Enzymol.*266, 383-402.

Joshi, P.M. (1995). Effect of L-Arginase on the growth of cell in *in vitro*. M.Sc. dissertation submitted to Amravati University, Amravati.

Levitt, M. and Chothia, C. (1976): Structural Patterns in Globular Proteins .*Nature* 261, 552-558.

Lipman, D.J., Altschul, S.F. and Kececioglu, J.D. (1989): "A Tool for multiple sequence alignment". *Proc.Natl.Acad.Sci. USA*.82:3073-3077.

Lehninger, A.L., Nelson, D.L. and Cox, M.M. (1993): Principles of Biochemistry, II edition, C.B.S. Publishers and Distributors, New Delhi, p. 1013.

Mehta, P.K., Heringa, J., and Argos, P. (1995); A simple and fast approach to prediction of secondary structure from multiply aligned sequences with accuracy above 70%. *Protein Sci.* 4, 2517-2525.

Nicholas, K.B. and Nicholas, H.B. Jr. (1997): Gene Doc : A tool for editing and annotating multiple sequence alignments. *www.cris.com/~ketchup/genedoc.shtml*

Pauling, L., and Corey, R.B. (1951). The structure of protein : Two hydrogen bonded helical configurations of the polypeptide chain. *Proc. Natl. Acad. Sci. USA.* 37, 205-211.

Posfai, J., A.S. Bhagwat, G. Posfai and R . J. Roberts, (1989). "Predictive motifs derived from cytosine methyl transferase". *Nucleic Acids Res.* 17; 2421-2435.

Rost, B. Sander, C., and Schneider. R. (1994). PHD: A mail server for protein secondary structure prediction. *CABIOS*, 10, 53-60.

Satyanarayan, U. (1999): Biochemistry, 2, 64-67.

Schuler. D. Greregary (1998): Bioinformatics: A Practical Guide to the Analysis of Genes &Proteins, A.D. Baxevanis & B.F.F. Ouellette. John Wiley & sons, Inc., Publications. 7, 145-171.

States. J.D. and Boguski. S. Mark (1991) : Sequence Analysis Primer, Gribskov Michael & Devereux John, Stockton press, 3, 64-67.

Schuler, G.D., S.F. Altschul and D.J. Lipman (1990): "A Workbench for multiple alignment construction & analysis". *Protein Struct. Funct. Genet.*

Stryer Lubert, (1985): Biochemistry, Fourth edition, 2, 190-192.

Thomspon, J.D., Higgins, D.G. and Gibbson, T.J. (1994): CLUSTAL W; improving the sensitivity of progressive multiple sequence alignment through sequence weighting, position – specific gap penaulties and weight matrix choice. *Nucleic Acids Res.*22, 4673-4680.

Wadegaonkar, P.A.; Rai. V and Ali S.S. (1992). Affinity chromatographic method for rapid purification of fungal L-arginase. *Biome* 6(2), 88-91.

Wadegaonkar, P.A. 1995. Studies on amino acid metabolizing enzymes and their biotechnological prospects. Ph.D. Thesis, Pt. Ravishankar Shukla University, Raipur. Unpublished.

Microbiology and Biotechnology for Sustainable Development (Ed. P.C. Jain),
CBS Publishers & Distributors, New Delhi (2004), pp. 277–282.

B-11

Transfer of Drug Resistant Plasmid with Km^r Gene in *Vibrio cholerae* KB 207

Pratyoosh Shukla, Naveen Kango and Vijay P. Bondre*
Department of Applied Microbiology and Biotechnology,
Dr. H.S. Gour Vishwavidyalaya, Sagar (M.P.) – 470 003.
** National Institute of Virology (NIV), Pune (Maharashtra)*
e mail – pratyooshbio@rediffmail.com

Abstract

Transfer of drug resistant plasmid was carried out by the donor strain E. coli SM10 into Vibrio cholerae KB 207 strain. The selection was based on donor and recipient strains on Kanamycin and Streptomycin plates respectively. The isolated transconjugants carrying plasmid pRT291 were studied for slide agglutination by using anti KB207 serum of rabbit, which gave positive results. The plasmid isolated from transconjugants was compared with plasmid isolated from that of donor and recipient strain by agarose gel electrophoresis which showed bands of identical size indicating the plasmid pRT291 (Km^r) was transferred from the donor strain to recipient strain.

Key words: Drug Resistance, Transconjugant, Kanamycin, *Vibrio cholerae*.

INTRODUCTION

Conjugation is one of the natural methods for transfer of genetic elements in bacteria (Beadle and Tatum, 1941) while transformation is another mechanism for the transfer of genetic information among bacteria which is based on the principle of uptake of foreign DNA by cell (Bolivar *et al.*, 1977; Taylor and Trotter, 1967). For transformation the cells are usually exposed to high concentration of calcium (Ca^{++}) ions and higher temperature which causes the bacterial plasma membrane to admit foreign DNA (Sambrook *et al.*, 1982). Transfer of drug resistant plasmid was carried out by many workers (Niemi *et al.*, 1983; Hatha *et al.*, 1993; Bayer *et al.*, 2000). This work was initiated in the view of development of cross-resistance between some amino glycoside antibiotics (Onaolapo, 1994). The development of resistance among *Vibrio cholerae* was studied by Yamamoto *et al.*, (1994); Niemi *et al.*, (1983) etc. This drug resistance plasmid in *Vibrio cholerae* is a useful tool to carry out further investigations in designing medication strategies for new drugs against *Vibrio cholerae* infections. Bacterial conjugation has been selectively used to construct recombinant bacterial strains, which are used on industrial scale for the production of enzymes, antibiotics and for biodegradation of hazardous and recalcitrant environmental pollutants. Similarly, transformation technology is exploited for cloning, characterization and expression of various genes in self replicating plasmid vectors to identify various genetic characteristics (Bolivar *et al.*, 1977).

In the present work we have studied transfer of genetic material (plasmid vector, pRT291) encoding antibiotic resistance by conjugation between donor *E.coli* strain SM10 and the recipient *Vibrio cholerae* 01 El Tor strain KB 207. The transconjugants *V. cholerae* were selected and the plasmid vector encoding Km^r was isolated and transformed into *E.coli DH5α* and studied by agarose gel electrophoresis.

MATERIALS AND METHODS:

Bacteria used:

V.cholerae strain KB 207	:	01 El Tor, Sm^r
E.coli strain SM10	:	Carrying plasmid pRT 291, Kmr
E.coli strain DH5α	:	Host strain used for transformation of pRT 291

Media used:

All ingredients specified in the media were dissolved in milli-RO grade of distilled water (w/v) and sterilized by autoclaving at 121°C for 20 min.

Luria Bertani (LB) Broth : Tryptone, 1%; Yeast Extract, 0.5 % ; Sodium Chloride, 0.5 %

Luria Bertani (LB) Agar : 1.5 % of agar-agar was added in LB broth before sterilization.

Terrific Broth (TB) : Peptone, 1.2 % ; Yeast Extract, 2.4 % ; Glycerol,0.4 % (v/v)

To the above media 10 ml of phosphate buffer was added separately after sterilization.

Buffers and Solutions used for plasmid isolation:

Phosphate Buffer

K_2HPO_4 : 12.5 % ; KH_2PO_4 : 2.31 %

SDS-NaOH Solution

SDS :1 % ; NaOH : 0.2 N

Acetate Mixture

Sodium acetate :1M ; Ammonium acetate : 2.5 M

70 % Ethanol

Prepared by mixing 70 ml of double distilled absolute (96 %) ethanol in 30 ml of milli-Q water and stored at – 20°C. (Sambrook *et al.*, 1982).

TE Buffer

Tris-HCl (pH 8.0) :10 mM ; EDTA (pH 8.0) :1 mM

Buffers and Solutions used for Transformation:

Transformation buffer I (TfbI)

Morpholinopropane Sulphonic acid (MOPS-pH 7.0):10 mM ; Rubidium chloride:10 mM

Transformation buffer II (Tfb II)

MOPS (pH 6.5): 100 mM; Calcium chloride: 50 mM; Rubidium chloride:10 mM

Solutions used for Agarose Gel Electrophoresis:

TBE Buffer

Tris-(Hydroxymethyl)-aminomethane, 0.89 M; Boric Acid, 0.89 M; EDTA, 20 mM; PH, 8.2

Nutrient Broth

Peptone : 1.0 % ; Glucose : 0.2 %

Antibiotics used for selection of transformants:

Antibiotic solutions were prepared by dissolving the dehydrated powder in distilled water or phosphate buffered saline and sterilized by filtration through bacteriological filters (0.45 μm pore size). The antibiotics used were Streptomycin and Kanamycin with 100 mg/ml and 4.5 mg/ml as stock concentration i.e. 100 μg/ml, 45 μg/ml as final concentration and were stored at 4°C in dark.

General buffer :

Phosphate Buffered Saline :

K_2HPO_4 : 0.121 % ; KH_2PO_4 : 0.034 % ; NaCl : 0.8 % ; PH : 7.2

Buffers and Solutions used for Plasmid Preparation :

All the buffers and solutions were prepared in mili-Q grade of distilled water and sterilized by autoclaving at 121°C for 20 min. The solutions were stored at 4°C until use.

Glucose Tris EDTA (GTE) Buffer :

Tris HCl, pH 8.0 : 25 mM ; EDTA: 10 mM ; Glucose : 50 mM

Bacterial Conjugation

Bacterial conjugation was carried out on LB agar plates at 37°C. The freshly grown nutrient agar slant culture of donor *E.coli* strain SM 10 was inoculated on LB agar plate containing kanamycin (Km). The recipient *V.cholerae* 01 El Tor strain KB 207 was grown on LB agar plate containing streptomycin (Sm). A loopful of the donor as well as recipient cultures were harvested in sterile phosphate buffered saline (PBS). The PBS suspension of donor strain was streaked on LB agar plate with the help of inoculation needle and allowed to dry. Similarly the PBS suspension of recipient strain was streaked on the LB agar plate at right angle to the streak of donor strain, so as to form a cross between the donor and recipient strains. The mating mixture was allowed to conjugate by incubating at 37°C for 24 hrs.

A loopful from the centre of the mating mixture was suspended in LB broth and serially diluted in PBS. The PBS suspension was plated on LB agar plates containing 'Sm' and 'Km' and incubated at 37°C for 24 hrs. The colonies appearing on the 'Sm' and 'Km' plates were selected as transconjugants and further confirmed as *V.cholerae* by slide agglutination with rabbit anti KB 207 serum (Williams and Skuurray, 1980).

Preparation of Plasmid DNA: Plasmid DNA was prepared by alkaline lysis method. TB grown bacterial culture was centrifuged at 6,000 xg for 10 min. The cell pellet was suspended in GTE buffer by vortexing. Freshly prepared alkaline lysis solution (NaOH- SDS) was added to it and mixed homogeneously by gently rotating the tube in fingers. (Itakura,1982). It was incubated on ice for 15-20 min and centrifuged at 12,000 xg for 15 Min. at 4°C. The clear supernatant was transformed to fresh tube and the plasmid DNA was precipitated by adding 2 volumes of chilled 96 % ethanol followed by incubation at –20°C for 2 hrs. The plasmid DNA was pelleted by centrifugation at 12,000 xg for 20 min at 4°C. The DNA pellet was washed twice with 70% ethanol and finally with 96% ethanol. The DNA pellet was air dried and suspended in a appropriate amount of TE buffer.

Transformation of Plasmid DNA: Plasmid DNA was transformed in *E.coli DH5α* was inoculated in 5ml LB broth and incubated at 37°C or rotary shaker for 3 to 3.5 hr so as to reach the cell density of A_{600} = 0.3 (approximately 10^8 cfu/ml*)* *(*Hanahan, 1983). The culture was centrifuged at 6000 xg for 10 min and the cell pellet was suspended in Tfb I buffer. It was centrifuged at 6,000 xg for 10 min. at 4°C and the cell pellet was suspended in Tfb II buffer. The cell suspension was incubated on ice for 30 min. The competent cells were centrifuged at 6000 xg for 10 min at 4°C and re-suspended in 400 µl of Tfb II buffer. The plasmid DNA (100 ng to 1 µg) was directly added to the competent cell suspension and incubated on ice for 30 min. Heat shock was given at 43.5°C for 30 seconds in water bath and quickly transferred to ice. To the transformed cell suspension 2.6 ml of Z-broth was added and incubated at 37°C for 40 minutes.

The transformants were plated on LB agar plates containing Kanamycin as a selection marker and incubated at 37°C for 24 hr. The transformants carrying Km^r were selected for further studies.

Agarose Gel Electrophoresis: Agarose gel electrophoresis was carried out in horizontal gel electrophoresis apparatus (Johnston-Dow *et al.,* 1987). The dehydrated agarose powder was dissolved in TBE buffer by boiling and then cooled down to 48°C before pouring. It was poured in gel tray fitted with comb and allowed to solidify for 30 to 40 min at room temperature. The comb was removed and both the buffer reservoirs were filled with TBE buffer. The DNA to be electrophoresed was mixed with 6X tracking dye (bromophenol blue dye in TBE buffer) to the final concentration of 1X and loaded into the wells carefully. The electrophoresis was carried out at 100V and monitored on the basis of movement of the tracking dye. When the dye reached the bottom of gel, the electrophoresis was terminated and the gel was stained with ethidium bromide solution. The DNA in gel was visualized under UV light and photographed.

RESULTS AND DISCUSSION

In this work, we have studied transfer of drug resistant plasmid pRT 291 from the donor strain *E.coli* SM 10 into *V.cholerae* strain KB 207 by conjugation. The mating mixture was selected on LB agar plates containing selective antibiotics Km and Sm. Selection pressure of Sm allowed the growth of recipient strain KB 207 (Sm^r) receiving the plasmid pRT (Km^r) on Sm and Km plates while inhibiting the growth of donor strain. Therefore transconjugants carrying pRT 291 were selected while the growth of donor as well as recipient strains was inhibited.

10^{-2} dilution of the mating mixture was plated on LB agar plate containing Km and Sm. 3000 transconjugants/ml of this dilution were scored. Some of these transconjugants were studied for slide agglutination by using anti-KB 207 serum. The parent strain KB 207 (Sm^r) as well as the transconjugants carrying Sm^r gave positive results of agglutination within seconds.

The plasmid isolated by alkaline lysis method showed bands of identical size when analyzed by agarose gel electrophoresis. The plasmid isolated from the transconjugant was compared with the plasmid isolated from that of the donor strain *E.coli* SM 10, which showed bands of identical size indicating plasmid pRT 291 (Km^r) being transferred from the donor strain which was responsible for the Km^r phenotype of the transconjugants.

The plasmid isolated from transconjugants KB 207 (Sm^r, Km^r) was transformed into *E.coli DH5α* and the transformants were selected on LB agar plates containing Km as selective antibiotic. About 500 Km^r clones/ml of the transformation mixture was scored.

Plasmid isolated from some of the Km^r transformant was analyzed by agarose gel electrophoresis and was compared with the plasmid isolated from the donor strain *E.coli SM* 10 as well as the transconjugants KB 207 (Sm^r, Km^r). All these plasmid preparations showed DNA bands of identical size indicating that the same plasmid was carried by the donor strain *E.coli* SM 10 (Km^r), the transconjugants KB 207 (Sm^r, Km^r) as well as transformants *E.coli DH5α* (Km^r).

ACKNOWLEDGEMENTS

Authors are thankful to Director, CDRI, Lucknow for providing the laboratory facilities and to Prof. B.S. Srivastava for his valuable guidance.

REFERENCES

Bayer, M.; Bischof, K.; Noiges, R. and Koraimann, G. (2000). Subcellular localization and processing of lytic transglycosylase of the conjugative plasmid R1. FEBS Letters (In press).

Beadle, G.W. and Tatum, E.L. (1941). Genetic control of biochemical reactions in *Neurospora*. Proct. Natl. Acad. Sci. U.S.A., 27:499-506.

Bolivar, F.; Rodriguez, R.L.; Greene, P.J.; Betlach, M.C.; Heynecker, H.L. and Boyer, H.W. (1977). Construction and characterization of new cloning vehicles II : A multipurpose cloning system; Genes 2, 95-113.

Hanahan, D. (1983). Studies on transformation of E.coli with plasmids, J. Mol. Biol., 166: 557-580.

Hatha, A.A.M.; Gomathinayagam, P. and Lakshmanaprumalsn, P. (1993). Incidence of multiple antibiotic resistant *E. coli* in the Bhivani River. World J. Microbiol. Biotechnol. 9 : 605-610.

Itakura (1982). Chemical synthesis of Genes. TIBS, 7:442.

Johnston-dow, Mardis, L.E.; Heimer, C. and Roe, B.A. (1987). 'Optimized methods for fluorescent and radiolabelled DNA sequencing' Biotechniques, 5: 754-765.

Niemi, M.; Sibakav, M. and Niemala, S., (1983). Antibiotic resistance among different species of faecal coliforms isolated from water samples. Appl. Environ. Micorbiol. 45: 79-83.

Onaolapo, J. (1994). Cross-resistance between some aminoglycosides antibiotics. Afr. J. Med. Sci. 23: 209-215.

Sambrook, J., Fritsch, E.F. and Maniatis, T. (1982). Molcular Cloning : A laboratory manual, Cold Spring Harbour Publications, New York.

Taylor, A.L. and Trotter, C.D. (1967). Revised linkage map of *E. coli.* Bacteriol. Rev., 31 : 332-353

Williams, N. and Skuurray, R. (1980). The conjugation systems of F-like plasmids. Ann. Rev. Genet., 14 : 41-76.

Yamamoto, T., Nair, G. and Takeda, Y. (1994). Emergence of tetracycline resistance due to a multiple drug resistance plasmid in *Vibrio cholerae* 0139. FEMS Immunol. Med. Microbiol. 11: 106-131.

Microbiology and Biotechnology for Sustainable Development (*Ed.* P.C. Jain),
CBS Publishers & Distributors, New Delhi (2004), pp. 283–292.

B-12

Production of Industrially Important Alkaline Cellulases from Newly Isolated *Fusarium* spp.

Santosh Vyas, Absar Ahmad and Anil Lachke*
*Division of Biochemical Sciences, National Chemical Laboratory,
Pune 411008. India*

Abstract

Alkaline cellulases that are active and stable in an alkaline pH range are in demand because of their potential ecofriendly applications in textile, detergents and paper and pulp industries. However, microbial alkaline cellulases are very rare. We isolated an alkalotolerant fungus Fusarium sp. locally. It produces extracellular cellulolytic complex when grown in Reese (MI) medium containing 1% cellulose as the sole carbon source. The optimum pH and temperature for enzyme activity was 5.0 and 60°C respectively. The enzyme retained 60% activity at pH 8.5 and 20% at pH 10.0. The half-life of the enzyme at pH 8.5 and at 50°C was found to be 10 hrs. The pattern of decreasing viscosity of 1% solution of carboxymethyl cellulose and subsequent increase in reducing sugars during a viscometric assay confirmed the endo- type of hydrolytic action of the isolated endoglucanase component. The data indicated that enzyme can be useful for deinking operations during recycling of mixed office waste paper.

Keywords: Alkaline Cellulase, *Fusarium* spp., Viscometric characterization, Biodeinking

INTRODUCTION

Cellulase is a multicomponent enzyme system that is well studied because of its potential industrial applications (Bhat and Bhat, 1997). Conventionally cellulase complex has been utilized in the bioconversion of lignocellulosic materials into biofuels like ethanol (Wheals

* Author to whom all correspondence should be addressed: Ph: +91-20-5893034, Fax: +91-20-5894032 e-mail lachke@dalton.ncl.res.in

et al., 1999). Recently alkaline active and/or alkali stable cellulases have gained commercial importance because of their potential applications in textile, paper/pulp, and detergent industries. These enzymes are found useful in denim washing (Kierulff, 1997), 'Biopolishing' of textiles (Peterson *et al.* 1992), as well as in deinking operations during recycling of Mixed Office Waste Paper (MOW) (Jeffries *et al.*, 1994). Alkaline active cellulases also used as a component of detergents (Susumo, 1997). In all these applications the enzyme should be active and stable in alkaline environments and at elevated temperatures. Very few fungal sources are identified for the industrial production of cellulases. Here we describe production of alkaline cellulase from the alkalotolerant *Fusarium sp.* under various growth conditions. In addition to that some of the enzymic properties of the refined cellulase preparation are also presented.

MATERIALS AND METHODS

Chemicals:

Sodium salt of carboxymethyl cellulose (CMC), Oat spelt xylan, *p*-nitrophenyl-β-D glucopyranoside (*p*-NPG), *p*-nitrophenyl-β-D-xylopyranoside (*p*-NPX) were purchased from Sigma Chemical Co. U.S.A. Cellulose-123 was purchased from Carl Schleicher & Schull Company, Germany. All buffer salts and microbial media components were from standard commercial source and of highest quality available.

Microorganism

The alkalotolerant fungal strain was isolated locally and identified as *Fusarium sp.* on the basis of microscopic observations. It is maintained by periodic transfer on potato dextrose agar (0.5% dextrose), slants at 30°C.

Media and Culture conditions: The fungus was grown in M-I medium. (Reese and Mandels, 1963) The basal M-I medium contained (g/l of distilled water): KH_2PO_4, 2.0; $(NH_4)_2SO_4$, 1.4; $CaCl_2$, $2H_2O$, 0.3; $MgSO_4.7H_2O$, 0.3; urea, 0.3; Proteose peptone, 0.25; Yeast extract, 0.2, Cellulose-123, 10.0 and trace metal solution, 1ml [$FeSO_4.7H_2O$, 5 mg/l; $MnSO_4.7H_2O$, 5.6 mg/l; $ZnSO_4.7H_2O$, 3.34 mg/l; $CoCl_2.2H_2O$, 2 mg/l], Tween 80 – 1ml/l

The pH of the medium was adjusted after autoclaving by using separately sterilized 1M Na_2CO_3.

The M I medium supplemented with 0.5% wheat bran was inoculated with vegetative mycelia from 7 day old sporulating slant on PDA. The culture was grown for 3 days and used as the innoculum. Enzyme production was carried out in 250 ml Erlenmeyer flask containing 50 ml M I medium with cellulose powder (1%) as the sole carbon source .The culture was incubated at 30°C on a rotary shaker at 200 rpm. The samples were withdrawn at regular intervals and mycelium was removed by centrifugation at 7000 rpm at 4°C; clear supernatant was obtained. The enzyme was subjected to ultrafiltration using a (PM-10, Amicon) membrane. This preparation was used to study the physico-chemical and enzymatic properties.

Effect of culture conditions on enzyme production

The fungus was grown in M-I basal medium supplemented with different cellulosic substrate at 30°C and enzyme production and change in pH was monitored for 10 days. The effect of inorganic nitrogen source was studied replacing ammonium sulfate from the medium by different inorganic nitrogen sources. Effect of initial pH on production was also studied by growing culture at different pH (4-10) at 30°C.

Enzyme assays

The activities of CMCase, xylanase, FPase were measured in terms of release of reducing sugar by 3,5 dinitrosalicylic acid (DNSA) method. [Miller (1959), Miller *et al.*, (1960)]. An aliquot (0.5) ml of appropriately diluted culture filtrate was mixed with 0.5ml of 1% CMC in 0.05M sodium phosphate buffer, pH 7.0. The reaction mixture was incubated for 30 min at 60°C.The release of reducing sugars was estimated by DNSA reagent. For Filter paper activity (FPase) 50 mg (1X6cm) of Whatman No.1 paper was added to 1ml of phosphate buffer, pH 7.0 and 1ml diluted enzyme sample. The reaction mixture was incubated for 1 Hr and the released reducing sugars were estimated. The β-glucosidase and β-xylosidase activities were determined using synthetic substrates *p*-NPG, *p*-NPX, respectively at pH- 6.0 and 50 °C. (Lachke, 1988).

The buffers used for studying effect of pH on the enzyme activity were 50 mM citrate buffer (pH 3-6), Sodium phosphate buffer (pH 7- 8.0), Glycine-NaOH buffer (pH 8.5 to 10.00). For the determination of pH stability of the enzyme, it was pretreated in different pH buffers for 10 hrs at 50 °C and assayed at 60 °C at pH 7.0.

1 IU of enzyme activity was defined as amount of enzyme which liberates 1μ mole glucose/min (for CMCase, FPase) or xylose / min (for xylanases) under the standard assay conditions. 1 IU of β Glucosidase and β Xylosidase has been defined as the amount of enzyme, which liberates 1μ mol of *p*-nitrophenol/min under the standard assay conditions.

The endoglucanase activity was also confirmed by congo red staining of CMC Agar culture plate. (Teather. and Wood, 1982)

CMCellulose hydrolyzing activity of endoglucanase was determined by decrease in viscosity of 1.0% CMC solution. (Sadana *et al.*, 1984).

The reaction mixture contained 1.0% of CMC in 50mM sodium phosphate buffer pH 7.0 in an Ubbelohde viscometer at 60 °C. Diluted enzyme then added and changes in viscosity recorded at 3.0 min interval. Reducing sugar formation was subsequently estimated using ρ-HBAH (ρ-Hydroxy benzoic acid hydrazide) method (Hurst *et al.*, 1977).

For enzymatic deinking studies, the enzyme treatment was carried out in the presence of a surfactant (0.01% concentration) at 7.0% consistency in the pulper for 30 min. The enzyme dose of 200 IU/200 g pulp was selected. Each treatment was followed by 10-min floatation run at 1% consistency. A control run was taken under similar conditions replacing active enzyme by same volume of heat denatured enzyme preparation. After deinking trials handsheets were made and compared with standard run for following properties of the paper brightness, opacity, number of ink specks and strength properties like tensile strength, burst index, as well as tear index.

RESULTS & DISCUSSION

Characteristics of the fungal isolate

On the basis of morphology and microscopic observations the culture was identified as a *Fusarium* sp. The mycelium is septate, extensively cottony with some tinge of purple colour. Conidiophore is variable and short branched. Conidia are hyaline, variable and principally of two types. Microconidia are slightly curved and ovoid shaped. Macroconidia are large, several celled and typically canoe shaped. The cultural studies showed that the fungus grows best at 30°C. However the optimum growth was observed around pH 7.0. The culture grows luxuriously at pH 10, indicating its alkalotolerant nature.

Effect of different cultural conditions on production of enzyme

The yield of different activities, were depending on the composition of the medium. Higher xylanolytic enzyme units were observed when the MI medium was supplemented with 1% wheat bran. (Table 1) Experiments with different cellulosic substrates indicated that refined cellulosic substrates are best for induction of cellulases (Table 2) and the enzyme can also be produced on agricultural residues like bagasse pith, corncob, and wheat bran. Effect of inorganic nitrogen sources (Table-3a) on enzyme production showed that replacing $(NH\ )_2SO_4$ in the MI medium with $(NH\ )_2\ HPO_4$ increases enzyme production. There is substantial increase in the enzyme activity when the amount of complex nitrogen sources like yeast extract; peptone was doubled in the medium (Table-3b). The effect of initial pH of the medium showed that there is significant difference in the growth and yield of enzyme. The fungus grew well around neutrality and produced high amounts of enzyme in neutral to alkaline medium confirming alkalotolerant nature of the fungal isolate. Supplementing MI medium with salts like Co^{2+}, Mn^{2+} at 10 mM concentration increased enzyme production by 14% and 10%, respectively while Hg^{2+}, Cu^{2+} inhibited enzyme production by 70% and 8%, respectively. The maximum enzyme production was obtained on 8th day of cultivation. There was a slight decrease in the enzyme activity after 10th day. It seems that increase in the enzyme production is associated with drop in pH.

Table 1: Enzyme Activities in Culture Supernatant

Activity	IU / ml
CMCase [Endo (1 4)-β-D-glucan-glucano hydrolase (EC 3.2.1.4)]	8.80
FPase (Filter paper degrading activity)	0.52
1,4-β-D-glucan glucohydrolase (EC 3.2.1.21)	1.31
β- D-xylanase (EC 3.2.1.8)	0.72
β-1,4-D-xylan xylano hydrolase (EC 3.2.1.37)	0.32
Protease	N.D.

Properties of Enzyme

The enzyme CMCase is active in a broad pH range of 4 to 10 with a pH optima at 5.0 at 60°C

(Fig. 2) The enzyme showed maximum activity at 60°C. The enzyme showed 80% of the maximum enzyme activity at 70°C (Fig. 3). The enzyme is stable in an alkaline pH range of 8-10 at 50°C (Fig. 2). The half-life of the enzyme at pH 8.5 at 50°C was found to be 10 hrs.

Table 2: Effect of Cellulose Substrates on Enzyme Production

Cellulose Substrates (1 %)	Final pH	Growth	CMCase (IU / ml)	FPase (FPU / ml /)
Cellulose Powder	5.0	+++	7.44	0.59
Avicel	5.5	++	6.54	0.53
Solka flock (SW 40)	5.0	+++	6.99	0.51
Filter Paper	5.0	+	6.45	0.38
Roll Milled Cotton	5.0	+	6.87	0.39
CMC	6.5	++	6.27	0.49
Wheat Bran	8.0	+++	6.94	0.32
Rice Bran	6.5	+	5.85	0.32
Corn Cob	7.0	+++	7.44	0.51
Bagasse Pith	6.5	+	7.98	0.32
Jute Powder	7.0	+	5.22	0.32

Samples were withdrawn on 8th day and assayed at pH 7.0 at 60 °C

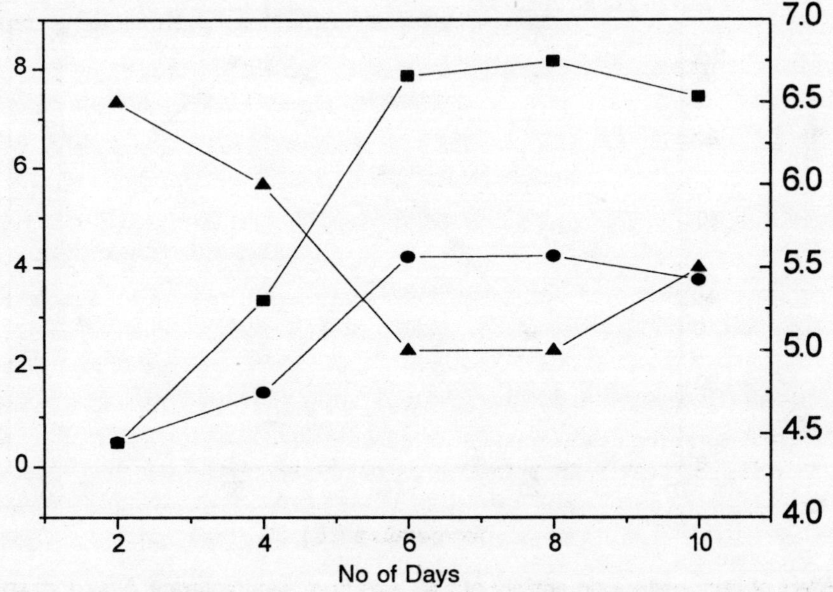

Fig . 1. Profile for Cellulase production by alkalotolerant *Fusarium* Sp. In submerged culture. Exracellular CMCase activity (■), FPase (●), pH (▲) . Samples were taken at regular intervals and assayed by standard assay procedure (see text.)

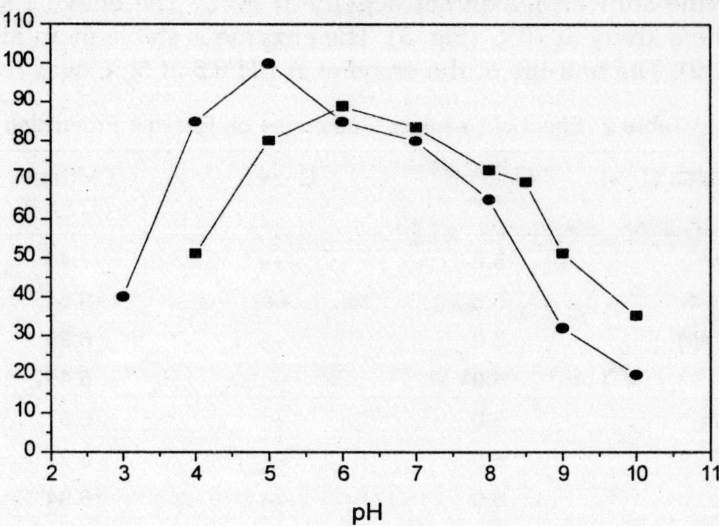

Fig. 2. Effects of pH on the activity (●) and stability (■) of CMCase. The buffers used for studying effect of pH on the enzyme activity were 50mM citrate buffer (pH 3-6), Sodium phosphate buffer (pH 7- 8.0), Glycine-NaOH buffer (pH 8.5 to 10.00). For the determination of pH Stability of the enzyme, it was pretreated in different pH buffers for 10 hrs at 50 °C and assayed at 60°C at pH 7.0.

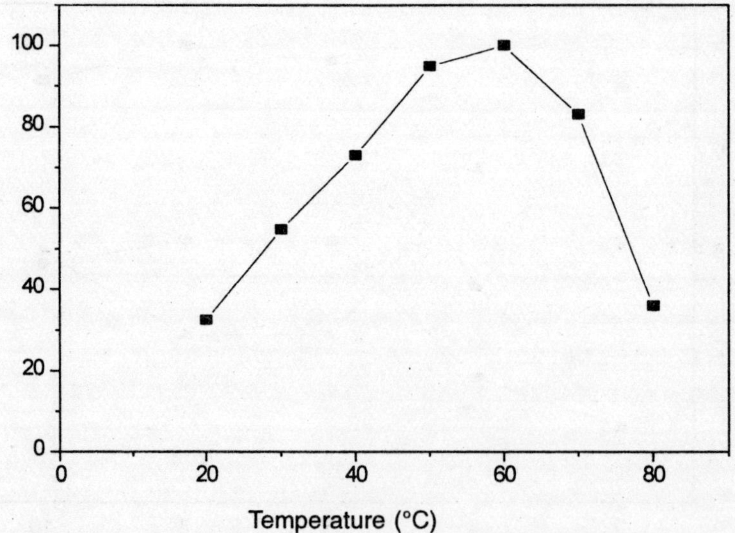

Fig. 3. Effect of temperature on activity of CMCase from alkalotolerant *Fusarium* sp.

The enzyme shows substantial decrease in viscosity of 1% CMC solution during the viscometric assay at 60°C (Fig 4a, 4b). The pattern of decreasing viscosity and subsequent increase in reducing sugars confirmed a random mode of attack of endoglucanase on the substrate. (Sadana *et al.*, 1984)

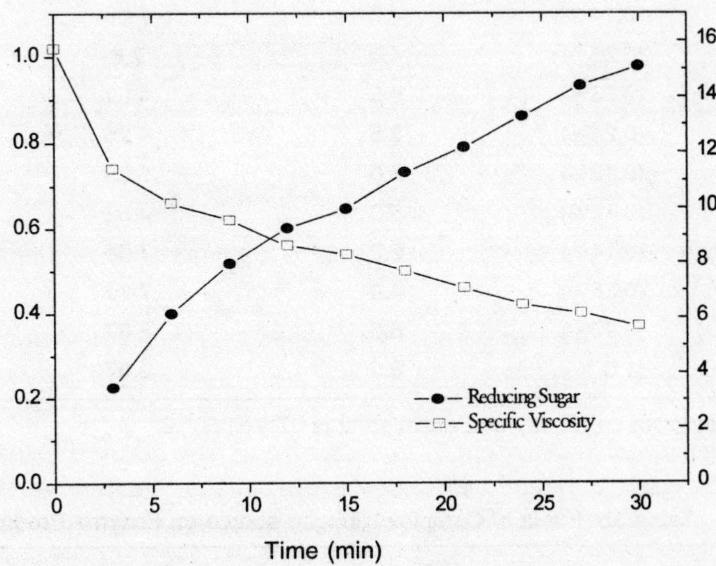

Fig. 4a. The time course hydrolysis of CMC by endoglucanase. CMC (10mg/ml) and endoglucanase (10μg) was incubated at 60°C. aliquots were removed for reducing sugar estimation using *p* HBAH Method periodically.

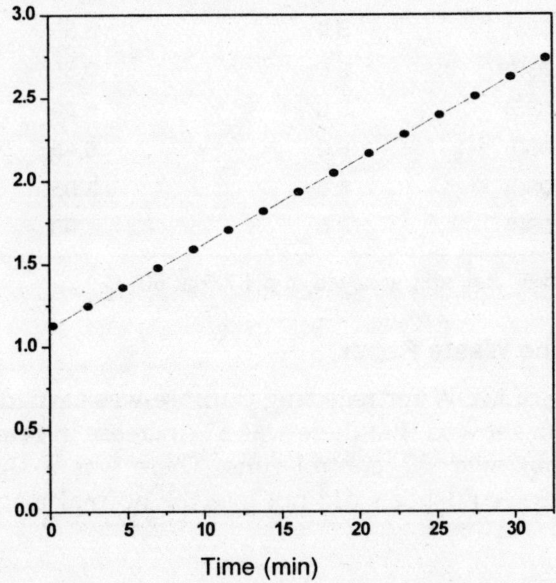

Fig. 4b. The relationship between increase in fluidity against time during enzymatic hydrolysis of corboxymethyl cellulose.

Table 3a: Effect of Inorganic Nitrogen source on Enzyme Production

Nitrogen source		Final pH (IU / ml)	CMCase (FPU /ml)	FPase
$(NH\ )_2SO_4$	(0.14 %)	4.0	7.04	0.45
$(NH\ )_2SO_4$	(0.28 %)	4.0	7.6	0.47
KNO_3	(0.23%)	8.5	4.62	0.17
$NaNO_3$	(0.28%)	8.5	4.25	0.18
$(NH\ )\ NO_3$	(0.18%)	5.0	5.03	0.22
NH Cl	(0.12%)	5.0	4.83	0.21
$(NH\ )_2\ HPO_4$	(0.14%)	5.0	7.05	0.41
$(NH\ )_2\ HPO_4$	(0.28%)	4.0	7.12	0.44
$(NH\ )_2\ HPO_4$	(0.70%)	6.0	8.07	0.53
$(NH\ )_2\ HPO_4$	(1.0 %)	6.0	8.07	0.52

Samples were withdrawn on 8th day and assayed at pH 7.0 at 60° C

Table 3b: Effect of Complex Nitrogen source on Enzyme Production

Nitrogen source		Final pH	CMCase (IU / ml)	FPase (FPU /ml)
Proteose peptone	(.025)	5.0	7.20	0.37
	(.050)	5.0	8.21	0.44
Yeast extract	(.025)	5.0	8.35	0.47
	(.050)	5.0	9.55	0.51
Soya meal	(.025)	5.0	6.20	0.36
	(.050)	6.0	6.45	0.37
Urea	(.030)	8.0	8.05	0.42
	(:060)	8.0	8.90	0.49

Samples were withdrawn on 8th day and assayed at pH 7.0 at 60° C

Deinking of Mixed Office Waste Paper

The enzymatic deinking of MOW for recycling purpose was carried out in a 10 liter capacity high density pulper. Data showed that there was 6% increase in brightness of the handsheets made from deinked pulp over the control runs. There was a significant decrease in the residual ink specks. These handsheets did not lose the normal mechanical strength.

DISCUSSION

Microbial cellulases are generally active in a pH range of 4-6. The deinking operations can be well performed under the alkaline conditions. The alkalotolerant *Fusarium* strain reported in this work secretes high amount cellulolytic enzymes when cultivated under submerged fermentation. The enzyme preparations in the present studies were found to be alkali stable indicating their potential for deinking process. The enzyme can be produced on cheap agricultural waste residues like wheat bran, corn cob and bagasse pith. Alkaline active cellulases are rare amongst fungi. Kang and Rhee, (1995) reported alkaline active carboxymethyl cellulases from *Cephalosporium* sp. *Humicola* sp. have been commercially exploited for production of alkaline cellulases. These endoglucanases are optimally active in a broad pH range of 6-10 but their thermal stability at alkaline pH is low. (Schulein, 1997). Although *Trichoderma* sp. and *Aspergillus* sp. produce high amounts of cellulase, their activities at alkaline pH are negligible (Hurst *et al.*, 1977). The enzyme reported by us is active and stable at pH 8.0 and at 50°C. These are the conventional processing conditions for the recycling process in paper and pulp industry.

Table 4: Quality Control Tests for Recycled Paper Handsheets made from Enzyme Deinked pulp

Q.C. Test	Control	Test Run -1	Test Run -2
Brightness %	68.6	74.0	74.2
Opacity %	86.6	84.2	83.7
Ink Specks/m²			
>220 μm	258	173	158
160μm	417	180	157
80-160 μm	167	56	63
10-80 μm	310	63	71
Breaking length (meters)	3228	3300	3320
Burst index (g scm/gsm)	21.4	22.8	22.7
Tear index	73	68.2	68.9

Handsheets were made after enzymatic treatment to the mixed office pulp. The treatment was carried out in the presence of surfactant (0.1%) concentration at 7% consistency in the pulper for 30 min. The enzyme dose of 200 IU was selected for treating 200 g of pulp sample.

Each treatment was followed by 10 min floatation run at 1% consistency.

Control run were taken under similar conditions replacing active enzyme by same volume of heat denatured enzyme preparation.

ACKNOWLEDGEMENT

The award of CSIR (New Delhi, India) Fellowship to SV is gratefully acknowledged.

REFERENCES

Bhat, M.K., and Bhat, S. (1997). Cellulose degrading enzymes and their potential industrial applications. Biotechnology Advances, 15, 583-620.

Hurst, P. K., Nielsen, J., Sullivan, P.A. and Shepherd, M.G. (1977). Purification and Properties of cellulase from *Aspergillus niger* Biochem.J. 165,33-41.

Jeffries, T. W., Klungness, J. H., Marguerite, S., and Cropsey, K. R. (1994). Comparison of enzyme enhanced with conventional deinking of xerographic and laser-printed paper Tappi. J. 77, No. 4, 173-179.

Kang, M. K. and Rhee, Y .H. (1995). Carboxymethyl cellulases active and stable at alkaline pH from alkalophilic *Cephalosporium* sp.RYM-202 Biotech.Letters, 17,5, 507-512.

Kierulff, J. V. (1997). Denim bleaching. Textile Horizons. 8, 33-36.

Lachke, A. H. (1988). 1,4-*b* -D-Xylan Xylohydrolase of *Sclerotium rolfsii* Methods in Enzymology, 160, 679-684.

Miller, G. L. (1959). Use of dinitrosalicylic acid reagent for determination of reducing sugar. Anal. Chem., 31, 426-428.

Miller, G. L., Blum, R. Gelnnon, W. E and Burton, A. (1960). Measurement Carboxymethyl cellulase activity; Analytical Biochemistry 2, 127-132.

Peterson, G. C., Screws, G. A., and Quadroon, D. M. (1992). Biopolishing of cellulosic fabric Canadian textile Journal. Oct. 31-35.

Reese, E.T. and Mandels, M. (1963). Enzymatic hydrolysis of cellulose and its derivatives. Methods in Carbohydrate Chemistry (Whistler, L) 3, 139-143, Academic Press, New York, London.

Sadana, J.C., Lachke, A.H. and Patil, R.V., (1984). Endo -(1→ 4) b-D-glucanase from *S.rolfsii.* Purification, substrate specificity and mode of action. Carbohydrate Research 133, 297-312.

Schulein, M. (1997). Enzymatic properties of cellulases from *Humicola insolens* J. Biotechnol. 57, 71-81.

Susumo, Ito (1997). Alkaline cellulases from alkaliphilic *Bacillus* : Enzymatic properties, genetics and application to detergents. Extremophiles, 1, 61-66.

Teather. R.M. and Wood, P.J. (1982) Applied Environmental Microbiology. 43, 777.

Wheals, A. E., Basso, L. C., Denise, M. G., and Amorim, H. V. (1999). Fuel ethanol after 25 years. Trends in Biotechnology. 17, 482-487.

Microbiology and Biotechnology for Sustainable Development (Ed. P.C. Jain),
CBS Publishers & Distributors, New Delhi (2004), pp. 293–299.

B-13

Xylanase Production by Thermophilic Fungi from Soil and Decomposing Organic Matter

Naveen Kango, S.C. Agrawal and P.C. Jain
Department of Applied Microbiology and Biotechnology
Dr. Hari Singh Gour University, Sagar, (M.P.) 470 003.

Abstract

Forty thermophilic fungal forms isolated from soil and naturally decomposing organic matter of varied nature were tested for their ability to produce xylanase on medium containing wheat bran as the sole carbon source. Among these, culture filtrates of thirty three test strains produced a distinct zone of xylan hydrolysis on xylan-agarose plates. The quantitative estimation of xylanase activity showed that Thermomyces lanuginosus strains (# NK-2, NK-25, NK-4, NK-14, NK-26, NK-6, NK-41) produced higher level of xylanase activity while Aspergillus nidulans NK-62, T. lanuginosus NK-33, Malbranchea sp. NK-106, and Emericella nidulans NK-43 showed fairly good amount of xylanase activity.

Key Words: Xylanase, Thermophilic fungi.

INTRODUCTION

Xylans are hemicellulosic heteropolysaccharides of the plant secondary wall consisting of a β-1,4-linked xylo-pyranosyl backbone substituted with 4-O-methyl-D-glucuronic acid, D-glucuronic acid, arabinose and acetate. They form a prominent portion (7-30%) of hemicelluloses of annual, softwood and hardwood plants (Timell, 1967; Gregory *et al.*, 1998). The enzymatic hydrolysis of xylan using microbial xylanases has potential applications in bioconversion of lignocelluloses to sugar, clarifying fruit juices, increasing the nutritional value of silage and fodder (Wong and Saddler, 1992), production and prebleaching of kraft pulp (Paice *et al.*, 1988, Viikari *et al.*, 1994). Owing to increasing biotechnological importance of thermostable xylanases several thermophilic molds have been examined for production of thermostable xylanases (Yoshioka *et al.*, 1981; Yu *et al.*, 1987; Anand and Vithyathil, 1990; Monti *et al.*, 1991; Banerjee *et al.*, 1995; Saraswat and Bisaria, 1997). In the present study we have screened forty thermophilic fungal isolates for production of xylanase on wheat bran using xylan-agarose plate assay method as described by Bernier Jr. *et al.*, (1983). The xylanaolytic activity of these isolates was quantified by measuring release of reducing sugar from xylan.

MATERIALS AND METHODS

Test Organisms: The thermophilic fungal cultures used in this study were isolated from soil samples and naturally decomposing organic matter (Kango *et al.*, 2002).

Enzyme production: For the production of xylanase, commercially available wheat bran was used as substrate. The wheat bran was thoroughly washed to remove starch and oven dried. Erlenmayer flasks (150 ml) containing 50ml Czapeck's salt solution with 2% wheat bran (w/v) were inoculated with mycelial agar discs (diameter 10 mm) cut from the periphery of the seven day old colony of these fungi grown on YpSs agar. The flasks were incubated under stationary condition at 45°C for seven days. The contents were then filtered through Whatmann No. 1 filter paper and the filtrate was used as crude enzyme sample.

Preparation of substrate: One percent Oat spelt xylan (w/v), was dissolved in 200mM sodium acetate buffer (pH 5.0) by continuous stirring for 8 hrs. This suspension was centrifuged at 10,000 rpm for 20 minutes to separate insoluble fraction while the supernatant was used as a source of xylan.

Xylan-agarose plate assay: Xylanolytic activity was detected by radial diffusion of the culture filtrate in xylan bearing agarose gel. Xylan agarose gel was prepared by adding agarose (2% w/v) to xylan solution. 50 ml aliquots of molten xylan-agaorse solution were poured in 12 cm petriplates. Wells of equal diameter (6 mm) were cut on these gels and filled with 75 μl of crude enzyme samples. These gels were incubated for 16 hrs. at 45°C and then stained by 1% solution of congo red to visualize zone of xylan hydrolysis.

Xylanase activity: Xylanase activity was quantified spectrophotometrically by measuring liberation of reducing sugar from xylan solution using 3, 5- dinitrosalicylic acid (Miller, 1959). Suitably diluted enzyme sample was added to 0.5 ml of xylan solution (1% oat spelt xylan in 200 mM sodium acetate buffer, pH:5) and was incubated for 5 minutes at 50°C. The reaction was stopped by adding 3ml of DNS reagent and boiling the tubes for 15 minutes. The tubes were cooled and the absorbance was read at 550 nm. One unit of xylanase was defined as the amount of enzyme that liberated 1μ mol of xylose per min.

RESULTS AND DISCUSSION

The results of xylanolytic activity of forty thermophilic fungal strains as tested by xylan-agarose plate assay are presented in Table 1. Out of forty thermophilic fungal strains thirty-three fungal strains showed xylanase activity in their culture filtrates and produced distinct zones of xylan hydrolyis on xylan-agarose plates. In another set of experiment the xylanolytic activity in the culture filtrates of test fungi was quantified by estimating the amount of reducing sugar liberated from oat spelt xylan and was expressed in units/ml of culture filtrate (Table 2). Among eight strains of *Thermomyces lanuginosus, T. lanuginosus* (NK-2) was found to possess enzyme activity equivalent to 1418 U/ml in its culture filtrate while the culture filtrates of other seven strains of *T. lanuginosus* (# NK-25, NK-4, NK-14, NK-26, NK-6, NK-41, NK-33) showed xylanase activity in the range of 330 U/ml to 979 U/ml. The strain of *Aspergillus nidulans* (NK-62) showed xylanase activity equivalent of 362 U/ml while other test strains of *Aspergillus* including *Emericella nidulans* showed xylanase activity in the range of 4.2 to 102 U/ml. Test strains of *Absidia* sp. (NK-39) and Malbranchea *sulfurea* (NK-91) also showed high xylanase activity.

Table 1: Zone of xylan hydrolysis produced by culture filtrates of thermophilic fungal strains on xylan-agarose plate

S.No.	Description	Isolate No.	Zone of Activity (in mm)	S.No.	Description	Isolate No.	Zone of Activity (in mm)
1.	*Absidia corymbifera*	NK-29	Nil	21.	*Mucor strain-III*	NK-66	Nil
2.	*Absidia strain-I*	NK-7	19	22.	*Myceliophthora strain-I*	NK-1	23
3.	*Absidia strain-II*	NK-11	6	23.	*Myceliophthora strain-II*	NK-12	24
4.	*Absidia strain-III*	NK-24	13	24.	*Myceliophthora strain-III*	NK-15	26
5.	*Absidia strain-IV*	NK-39	23	25.	*Rhizomucor sp.*	NK-3	12
6.	*Absidia strain-V*	NK-48	Nil	26.	*Scytalidium sp.*	NK-10	17
7.	*Aspergillus nidulans*	NK-62	24	27.	*Talaromyces dupontii*	NK-9	19
8.	*Aspergillus strain-I*	NK-20	28	28.	*Thermoascus aurantiacus*	NK-23	23
9.	*Aspergillus strain-II*	NK-86	16	29.	*T. lanuginosus strain-I*	NK-6	17
10.	*Aspergillus strain-III*	NK-30	12	30.	*T. lanuginosus strain-II*	NK-25	12
11.	*Aspergillus terreus*	NK-32	Nil	31.	*T. lanuginosus strain-III*	NK-26	21
12.	*Chaetomium thermophilum*	NK-67	Nil	32.	*T. lanuginosus strain-IV*	NK-33	18
13.	*Emericella nidulans strain-I*	NK-43	22	33.	*T. lanuginosus strain-V*	NK-41	20
14.	*E. nidulans strain-II*	NK-205	16	34.	*T. lanuginosus strain-VI*	NK-2	22
15.	*Humicola insolens*	NK-37	13	35.	*T. lanuginosus strain-VII*	NK-4	24
16.	*Malbranchea sulfurea strain-I*	NK-106	21	36.	*T. lanuginosus strain-VIII*	NK-14	18
17.	*M. sulfurea strain-II*	NK-91	20	37.	*Thielavia albomyces*	NK- 58	Nil
18.	*Mucor pusillus*	NK-17	27	38.	*Thielavia terrestris*	NK-28	14
19.	*Mucor strain-I*	NK-19	13	39.	Unidentified	NK-18	28
20.	*Mucor strain-II*	NK-55	19	40.	Unidentified	NK-51	Nil

A comparision of the data obtained by two methods (Table 1 and 2) showed enormous variation in the size of zone of hydrolysis (Fig. 1) and its corresponding activity in terms of liberation of reducing sugar from xylan eg. Unidentified strain (NK-18) produced a hydrolysis zone of 28 mm on xylan-agarose plate while it was found to possess only 1.5 U/ml of xylanase activity. Similar contrasting result was also seen in case of *T. lanuginosus* (NK-25) having 979 U/ml of xylanase activity while it produced a comparatively smaller zone of hydrolysis. A difference in the xylanase activity as determined by the two methods may be because of certain limitations of the assay methods. As in case of xylan-agarose plate assay, the appearance of zone of activity mainly depends on the diffusibility of the enzyme present in crude culture filtrate while partially degraded substrate may also produce a clear zone of hydrolysis on staining with congo red. On the other hand, xylanase activity as *quantified* by measurement of reducing sugar represents the amount of end product i.e., xylose formed as a result of xylan hydrolysis.

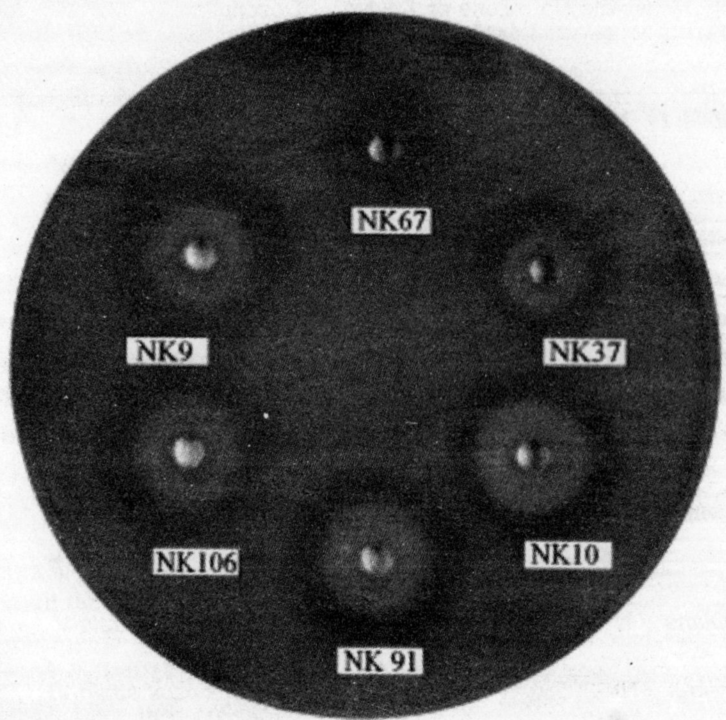

Fig. 1: Zones of xylan hydrolysis formed by radial diffusion of crude enzyme samples on xylan agarose gel. (See colour figure on Plate 2 at page 202)

Several workers have reported high level of xylanase production from *T. lanuginosus*. Kitpreechavanich *et al.*, (1984) found *Humicola lanuginosa* to produce 2050 U/ml xylanase using wheat bran under solid state fermentation while Gomes *et al.*, (1993) have reported of 9168 nKat/ml of xylanase activity when grown on xylan in liquid fermentation. In the present study *T. lanuginosus* (NK-2) was found to produce 1418 U/ml while other strains of the fungi also showed high activity.

Table 2: Xylanase production by thermophilic fungal strains grown on wheat bran at 45°C for seven days

S.No.	Description	Isolate No.	Activity (U/ml)	S.No.	Description	Isolate No.	Activity (U/ml)
1.	*Absidia corymbifera*	NK-29	Nil	21.	*Mucor strain-III*	NK-66	4.2
2.	*Absidia strain-I*	NK-7	1.2	22.	*Myceliophthora strain-I*	NK-1	19.4
3.	*Absidia strain-II*	NK-11	2.18	23.	*Myceliophthora strain-II*	NK-12	35.38
4.	*Absidia strain-III*	NK-24	2.80	24.	*Myceliophthora strain-III*	NK-15	33.3
5.	*Absidia strain-IV*	NK-39	308.0	25.	*Rhizomucor sp.*	NK-3	Nil
6.	*Absidia strain-V*	NK-48	14.8	26.	*Scytalidium sp.*	NK-10	Nil
7.	*Aspergillus nidulans*	NK-62	362.0	27.	*Talaromyces dupontii*	NK-9	54.9
8.	*Aspergillus strain-I*	NK-20	4.2	28.	*Thermoascus aurantiacus*	NK-23	19.2
9.	*Aspergillus strain-II*	NK-86	62.5	29.	*T. lanuginosus strain-I*	NK-6	628.2
10.	*Aspergillus strain-III*	NK-30	43.0	30.	*T. lanuginosus strain-II*	NK-25	979.6
11.	*Aspergillus terreus*	NK-32	35.4	31.	*T. lanuginosus strain-III*	NK-26	786.7
12.	*Chaetomium thermophilum*	NK-67	4.6	32.	*T. lanuginosus strain-IV*	NK-33	330.4
13.	*Emericella nidulans strain-I*	NK-43	102.0	33.	*T. lanuginosus strain-V*	NK-41	553.3
14.	*E. nidulans*	NK-205	41.0	34.	*T. lanuginosus strain-VI*	NK-2	1418.0
15.	*Humicola insolens*	NK-37	4.3	35.	*T. lanuginosus strain-VII*	NK-4	810.
16.	*Malbranchea sulfurea strain-I*	NK-106	268.8	36.	*T. lanuginosus strain-VIII*	NK-14	802
17.	*M. sulfurea strain-II*	NK-91	182.9	37.	*Thielavia albomyces*	NK- 58	Nil
18.	*Mucor pusillus*	NK-17	5.4	38.	*Thielavia terrestris*	NK-28	14.15
19.	*Mucor strain-I*	NK-19	4.2	39.	Unidentified	NK-18	1.5
20.	*Mucor strain-II*	NK-55	33.9	40.	Unidentified	NK-51	Nil

Xylanolytic activity of Thermophilic mucorales has also been reported by Banerjee *et al.* (1995) and Grajek, (1987). In the present study several strains of *Absidia, Mucor* and *Rhizomucor* sp. (NK-3) isolated from decomposing organic matter and soils have been examined for the production of xylanase. Among these *Absidia* sp. (NK- 39) produced higher xylanolytic activity (308 U/ml) while *Mucor* sp.(NK-55) showed xylanolytic activity equivalent to 33 U/ml.

The test strains of *Talaromyces dupontii* (NK-9), *Thermoascus aurantiacus* (NK-23), *Thielavia terrestris* (NK-28) and *Chaetomium thermophile* (NK-67) produced 54.9 U/ml, 19 U/ml, 14 U/ml and 4U/ml of xylanase in their culture filtrates, respectively. Test strains of *Malbranchea* i.e. Malbranchea *sulfurea* (NK-106) and *M. sulfurea* (NK-91) produced 268 U/ml and 182 U/ml of xylanase, respectively. Production of xylanase by *Themoascus aurantiacus, Malbranchea pulchella, Thielavia terrestris, Talaromyces emersonii, Chaetomium thermophile,*

Myceliophthora etc. has been reported earlier by other workers (Tuohy and Coughlan,1992; Matsuo *et al.* 1975; Yu *et al.*,1987; Durand *et al.*,1984, Ganju *et al.*, 1989; Dubey and johri,1987). Test strains of *Aspergillus nidulans* (NK-62), *Emericella nidulans* (NK-205), and *Aspergillus terreus* (NK-32) showed a great variation in xylanase activity in their culture filtrates (362 U/ml, 102 U/ml, 35 U/ml respectively). Strains of *Myceliophthora* sp. produced xylanase in the range of 35-19 U/ml. The results of the present study indicate the common occurrence of xylanolytic system in test thermophilic fungi while the amount of xylanase produced varies enormously among them. A few test strains have been found to be good candidates for xylanase production. However, the level of xylanase activity can be enhanced in these strains for their practical application.

REFERENCES

Gregory, A.C.E., O'connell, A.P. and Bolwell, G.P. (1998) Xylans. In Biotechnology and Genetic Engineering Reviews (Ed. M.P. Tombs) 15, 439-455.

Anand, L. and Vithyathil, P.L. (1990) Production of extracellular xylanase by thermophilic fungus *Humicola lanuginosa* bunce. Indian Journal of Experimental Biology 25, 434-437.

Banerjee, S., Archana, A. and Satyanarayana, T. (1995) Xylanolytic of activity and xylose utilization by thermophilic molds. Folia Microbiol.40, 279-282.

Bernier, Jr. R., Desrochers, M., Jurasek, L.and Paice, M.G. (1983) Isolation and characterization of a xylanase from *Bacillus subtilis*. Appl. Environ. Microbiol., 46, 511-514.

Ganju, R.K., Vithayathil, P.J. and Murthy, S.K. (1989) Purification and Characterization of two xylanases form *Chaetomium thermophile var. coprophile*. Can. J. Microbiol. 35, 836-842.

Dubey, A.K., and Johri, B.N. (1987) Xylanolytic activity of thermophilic *Sporotrichum* sp. and *Myceliophthora thermophilum*, Proc. Ind. Acad. Sci (Plant Sciences) 97, 247-255.

Durand, H., Soucaille, P. and Tiraby, G. (1984) Comparative study of cellulase and hemicellulases from four fungi: Mesophiles *Trichoderma reesei* and *Penicillium* sp. and thermophiles *Thielavia terrestris* and *Sporotrichum cellulophilum*. Enzyme Microb. Technol. 6, 175-180.

Kango, N., Agrawal, S.C. and Jain, P.C. (2002) Isolation of thermophilic fungi from soil and decomposing organic matter.

Kitpreechavanich, V., Hayashi, M. and Nagai, S. (1984) Production of xylan degrading enxymes by thermophilic fungi *Aspergillus fumigatus* and *Humicola lanuginosa*. J. Ferment. Technol. 62; 63-69.

Matsuo, M., Yasui, T. and Kobayashi, T. (1977) Purification adn some properties of B-xylosidase from *Malbranchea pulchella var sulfurea* No. 48, Agric. Biol. Chem. 41, 1593-1599

Miller, G. L. (1959) Use of dinitrosalicylic acid reagent for determination of reducing sugars. Anal Chem., 31, 426-428.

Monti, R., Terenzi, H.F. and Jorge, J.A. (1991) Purification and properties of an extracellular xylanase from thermophilic fungus *Humicola grisea* var. *thermoidea* Canadian Journal of Microbiology 37, 675-681.

Paice, M.G., Bernier, R.Jr. and Jurasek, L. (1988) Viscosity – enhancing bleaching of hardwood kraft pulp with xylanase from a cloned gene. Biotechnol. Bioeng. 32, 235-239.

Saraswat, V. and Bisaria, V.S. (1997) Biosynthesis of xylanolytic and xylan-debranching enzymes in *Melanocarpus albomyces* IIS 68. Journal of Fermentation and Biotechnology 84, 352-357.

Timell, T.E. (1967) Recent progress in the chemistry of wood hemicelluloses. Wood Sci. Technol. 1, 45-70.

Tuohy, M.G. and Coughlan, M.P. (1992) Production of thermostable xylan degrading enzymes by *Talaromyces emersonii*. Biores. Technol. 39, 131-137.

Viikari, L., Kantellinen, A., Sundquist, J. and Linko, M.(1994) Xylanases in bleaching: From an idea to the industry. FEMS Micribiol. Rev. 13, 335-350.

Wong, K.K.Y. and Saddler, J.N. (1992) *Trichoderma* xylanases: Their properties and application. In: Xylans and Xylanases (Visser, J., Beldman, G., Someren, M.A.K. and Voragen, A.G.J., Eds.), pp. 171-186, Elsevier, Amsterdam.

Yoshioka, H, Nagato, N., Chavanich, S., Nilubol, N. and Hayashida, S. 1981 Purification and properties of thermostable xylanase from *Talaromyces byssochlamydoides* YH-50. Agricultural and Biological Chemistry 45, 2425-2432.Microbiology 37, 675-681.

Yu, E.K.C., Tan, L.U.L., Chan, M.K. and Saddler, J.N. (1987) Production of thermostable xylanase by *Thermoascus aurantiacus*. Enzyme and Microb. Technol. 9, 16-24.

Microbiology and Biotechnology for Sustainable Development (Ed. P.C. Jain),
CBS Publishers & Distributors, New Delhi (2004), pp. 300–306.

B-14

Extracellular Production of α-Amylase by some Thermophilic Fungi from Saw Dust and Compost

Sharmeela Singhai and P.C. Jain
Department of Applied microbiology and Biotechnology
Dr. H.S. Gour Vishwavidyalaya, Sagar 470 003, M.P. India.

Abstract

Thirty seven thermophilic fungal strains belonging to 25 species of 14 genera isolated from saw dust and compost were screened for the production of α-amylase during their growth on amylase assay agar medium and in three liquid culture media. Amongst these, 12 strains showed greater activity of α-amylase. Culture filtrates of Malbranchea cinnamonea (T-47) and Talaromyces themophilus (T-46) have been found to possess activity of this enzyme even at a reaction temperature of 70ºC. The cultures of Myceliophthora vellerea (T-15), Myceliophthora sp. (T-64), Sagenomella sp. (T-51) and Thermomyces lanuginosus (T-31) have showed moderate activity of this enzyme at 70ºC.

Key words: Thermophilic fungi, compost, saw dust, α-amylase.

INTRODUCTION

Biopolymers such as cellulose, strach, xylan, lignin etc. are abundant in nature and constitute a major part of living matter. α-amylase is used in the production of maltose syrup from starch, for liquefaction of starch in winery and brewery, wallpaper removing, baby food preparations, laundries etc. (Palmer, 1975; Norman, 1979). Thermostable α-amylase involved in starch conversion technology is of major commercial importance (Forgarty and Kelly, 1979, 1980; Forgarty, 1983). Starch processing provides a range of products with specific composition and properties (Crabb and Mitchinson, 1997). Action of α-amylase on starch results in a rapid loss in its viscosity and reduction in iodine staining power, with the formation of oligosaccharides. The attack of α-amylase on α-1, 4 linkages near the branch points of the branched dextrins allows the formation of α-limit dextrins of few glucose units.

Prolonged action of α-amylase on linear oligosaccharides, results in the formation of maltose and glucose.

In the present investigation thermophilic fungi isolated from saw dust and compost have been tested for the production of starch hydrolyzing enzyme(s) and to know whether they are of any industrial significance.

MATERIALS AND METHODS

(A) Screening of fungi for amylase production using solid media :

Screening of fungi for amylase production was done following the method of Hankin and Anagnostakis (1975). The medium used was having Difco Nutrient Agar plus 2% soluble starch (pH.-6). Twenty ml of sterlized amylase assay medium was poured in Petridishes. The plates were then inoculated with test fungi and incubated at 45°C. After three days incubation radial growth of the colony was measured and the plates were then flooded with Iodine reagent. Iodine reagent was prepared by diluting 1 ml stock iodine solution (6.00 g kI, 600 mg I_2 and 100 ml distilled water) to 100 ml with 0.5 M HCl. The growth of fungal colony and the width of Non-blue zone of enzyme activity around the colony were recorded and relative enzyme activity (REA) of each organism was calculated using following formula:

$$\text{REA} = \frac{\text{Width of Non} - \text{blued zone (mm) around the colony}}{\text{Diameter of fungal colony}}$$

(B) Production of α-amylase in broth culture medium

To study extra cellular α-amylase production test thermophilic fungi were grown in 3 different culture media having following composition:

(1) **Czapek's dox broth :** 30.0 gm. Sucrose, 1.0 gm. KH_2PO_4, 0.5 gm. $MgSO_4.7H_2O$, 0.5 gm KCl, 0.01 gm. $FeSO_4.7H_2O$, 1000 ml Distilled water.

(2) **YpSs broth:** 5.0gm soluble starch, 1.0 gm KH_2PO_4, 0.5 gm. $MgSO_4.7H_2O$,1.0 gm. Yeast Extract, 1000ml Distilled water.

(3) **Glucose asparagine broth:** 2.0 gm. Asparagine, 10.0 gm. Glucose, 1.0 gm. . KH_2PO_4, 0.5 gm. $MgSO_4.7H_2O$, 100μg. Biotin, 5μg. Thiamine, 1000 ml Distilled water, 2ml Microelement solution.

Erlenmeyer flasks of 150 ml capacity containing 40 ml of culture medium were autoclaved for 15 minutes at 20 1bs pressure. The flasks were inoculated with spore suspension (having 2×10^6 spores/ml) of test organisms and then incubated at 45°C for 7 days. After incubation, cell free culture filtrates were obtained by filtering the content of the flasks through Whatman No.1 filter paper. So obtained culture filtrates were used as crude enzyme samples in each case.

Amylase activity in the culture medium was determined following the method of Chrispeel and Varner (1970). The reaction mixture containing 50 μl of enzyme sample, 950 μl of distilled water and 1000 μl of starch solution (150 mg native starch, 600 mg KH_2PO_4 and 200 μmol $CaCl_2$ in 100 ml of distilled water) were mixed simultaneously and then incubated at

45°C for 30 minutes. 1ml Iodine solution was then added to stop the reaction. The sample was then diluted with 9 ml distilled water and absorbance was read at 620nm. With the help of standard curve of starch, amount of hydrolyzed starch was calculated in each case. Amylolytic activity was recorded as the amount of hydrolyzed starch per ml crude enzyme sample (Total enzyme activity).In order to compare amylase production by test strains Relative Enzyme Yield was calculated using following formula:

$$\text{REY} = \frac{\text{Amount of hydrolysed starch (mg) / hr / ml}}{\text{Wet weight of mycelia (g)}}$$

(C) Effect of temperature on α-amylase activity

The cultures of 12 test fungi, which showed greater activity of α-amylase have been selected on the basis of results of previous experiments and were further assayed to study the effect of different temperatures on the activity of α-amylase. The effect of different reaction temperatures (ranging from 15°C-75°C) on α-amylase activity was determined following the method as described earlier.

RESULTS AND DISCUSSION

All the test thermophilic fungi were found to synthesize α-amylase on amylase assay agar medium. Maximum activity of this enzyme was recorded around the growing colonies of *Malbranchea cinnamonea* (T-34) followed by *Talaromyces thermophilus* (T-46), *M. cinnamonea* (T-47), *M. cinnamonea* (T-2), *A. niger* (T-18), *A. terreus* (T-23). Other test strains also produced extracellular amylase around their colonies (Table 1).

Table 1: Amylase Activity of Some Thermophilous Fungi is Recorded after 3 Days Incubation at 45°C

Fungi	Isolate number	REA
Absidia corymbifera	T-28	0.02
A. corymbifera	T-26	0.04
Absidia sp.	T-21	0.01
Absidia sp.	T-68	0.02
Aspergillus fumigatus	T-3	0.06
A. fumigatus	T-17	0.10
**A. fumigatus*	T-22	0.13
A. fumigatus	T-7	0.03
A. flavus	T-27	0..11
A. nidulans	T-11	0.09
**A. nidulans*	T-19	0.08
**A.niger*	T-18	0.18
**A. terreus*	T-23	0.168

(Contd.)

Fungi	Isolate number	REA
**A. terreus*	T-50	0.10
**A. terreus*	T-49	0.11
A. ustus	T-36	0.11
Aspergillus sp.	T-6	0.19
**Corynascus sepedonium*	T-29	0.01
**Corynascus sepedonium*	T-40	0.02
**Emericella nidulans*	T-10	0.10
**Emericella nidulans.*	T-38	0.13
Humicola grisea	T-5	0.02
Humicola sp.	T-61	0.05
**Malbranchea cinnamonea*	T-2	0.216
**M. cinnamonea*	T-34	0.316
**M. cinnamonea*	T-47	0.221
Mucor sp.	T-14	0.04
Myceliophthora thermophila	T-33	0.02
M. vellerea	T-15	0.02
Myceliophthora sp.	T-64	0.06
Penicillium olivicolor	T-4	0.05
**Rhizomucur pusillus*	T-37	0.06
**Sagenomella sp.*	T-51	0.135
**Talaromyces thermophilus*	T-46	0.257
**Thermoascus aurantiacus*	T-44	0.05
Thermoascus sp.	T-1	0.02
**Thermomyces lanuginosus*	T-31	0.11

*Data recorded after five days of incubation.

Effect of media on enzyme production

Fungi were grown in three different media and α- amylase activity in their culture filtrates was determined. The results are recorded in Table-2. Maximum production of amylase was recorded in the cultures of *Malbranchea cinnamonea* (T-47) when grown on YpSs medium followed by Glucose asparagine medium. Czapek's dox medium also favoured production of this enzyme in cultures of this fungus but its activity was recorded very less. Amylase production was noted greater in the cultures of *Absidia* sp. (T-68), 3 strains of *Aspergillus fumigatus* (T-22, T-3 T-17). *A. nidulans* (T-ll), *A. niger* (T-18), *A. ustus* (T-36), *Corynascus sepedonium* (T-29, T-40) *Emericella nidulans* (T-10), *Myceliphthora vellerea* (T-15), *Myceliphthora* sp. (T-64), *Talaromyces thermophilus* (T-46) and *Thermoascus* sp. (T-1) when grown on Glucose asparagine medium.

Table 2: Effect of Culture Medium on the Growth and Production of α-Amylase by Some Thermophilous Fungi at 45°C after 7 days Incubation

Fungi	Isolate	Enzyme Activity								
		Amount of hydrolyzed starch in mg hr^{-1} ml^{-1} crude enzyme sample								
		Medium used								
		YpSs			Czapek's dox			Glucose Asparagine		
		Wet weight (mg)	Enzyme activity	REY*	Wet weight (mg)	Enzyme activity	REY*	Wet weight (mg)	Enzyme activity	REY*
1	2	3	4	5	6	7	8	9	10	11
Absidia corymbifera	T-28	0796	3.92	4.92	0685	3.72	5.43	1479	3.72	2.52
A. Corymbifera	T-26	1002	3.84	3.82	0265	3.84	14.49	1235	3.76	3.04
Absidia sp.	T-21	2003	2.68	1.33	0295	2.68	9.08	3105	2.36	0.76
Absidia sp.	T-68	0552	3.60	6.52	0292	3.20	10.95	1898	4.00	2.10
Aspergillus fumigatus	T-3	0163	3.60	2.20	0563	4.00	7.10	0402	2.80	6.96
A. fumigatus	T-22	0370	4.00	1.08	0403	2.80	6.94	0366	4.40	12.02
A. fumigatus	T-7	0464	0.40	0.86	0632	3.60	5.69	0352	4.00	11.36
A. fumigatus	T-17	0399	4.80	12.03	0406	3.20	7.88	0181	4.80	26.51
A. flavus	T-27	0430	0.80	1.86	0543	0.20	0.36	0426	2.00	4.69
A. nidulans	T-11	0230	3.20	13.91	0299	3.60	12.04	0212	4.00	18.86
A. nidulans	T-19	2008	2.76	1.37	0535	1.28	2.39	2266	2.44	1.07
A.niger	T-18	0278	2.80	10.07	0316	3.60	11.42	0269	4.00	14.86
A. terreus	T-23	0291	3.60	12.37	0703	3.60	5.12	0323	3.60	11.14
A. terreus	T-50	0847	1.52	1.79	0414	3.60	8.69	1271	3.60	2.83
A. terreus	T-49	0363	4.40	12.12	0536	3.04	5.37	0463	4.28	9.24
A. ustus	T-36	0291	2.80	9.62	0275	4.80	17.45	0280	5.20	18.57
Aspergillus sp.	T-6	1963	2.68	1.36	0647	2.68	4.14	2128	2.36	1.10
Corynascus sepedonium	T-29	1348	3.44	2.55	0624	3.36	5.38	1812	3.60	1.98
Corynascus sepedonium	T-40	0664	3.00	4.51	0515	3.20	6.21	2012	5.00	2.48
Emericella nidulans	T-10	1984	2.80	1.49	0090	4.80	53.33	2265	5.20	2.29
Emericella nidulans	T- 38	0464	1.96	4.22	0632	3.76	5.94	0352	6.24	17.72
Humicola grisea	T-5	0982	1.84	1.87	0178	1.84	10.33	0389	4.00	10.28
Humicola sp.	T-61	0480	3.60	7.52	0470	3.60	7.65	0430	3.60	8.37
Malbranchea cinnamonea	T-2	0754	10.00	13.26	0184	2.84	15.43	1552	5.60	3.60
M. cinnamonea	T-34	0604	9.92	16.42	0451	2.52	5.55	1365	7.40	5.42
M. cinnamonea	T-47	1074	9.80	9.12	0231	3.28	14.19	0950	7.60	8.00

(Contd.)

1	2	3	4	5	6	7	8	9	10	11
Mucor sp.	T-14	2002	2.36	1.17	0112	1.96	17.50	0340	3.36	9.88
Myceliophthora thermophila	T-33	0367	3.92	10.4	0098	3.36	34.28	1384	3.28	2.36
M. vellerea	T-15	0679	2.84	4.18	0393	3.16	8.04	1397	4.40	3.14
Myceliopthora sp.	T-64	0650	3.90	6.00	0067	3.36	50.14	0981	4.80	4.89
Penicillium olivicolor	T-4	0653	2.00	3.06	1032	3.36	3.25	0957	2.80	2.92
Rhizomucor pusillus	T-37	0278	3.60	12.94	0316	4.00	12.65	0280	2.80	10.00
Sagenomella sp.	T-51	0706	4.52	6.40	0624	7.92	12.69	1271	1.84	1.44
Talaromyces thermophilus	T-46	0100	4.92	49.20	0314	2.84	9.04	0627	6.28	10.01
Thermoascus aurantiacus	T-44	1109	2.48	2.23	0279	1.88	6.73	1152	2.84	2.46
Thermoascus sp.	T-1	1230	3.20	2.60	1504	3.04	2.02	1752	4.00	2.28
Thermomyces lanuginosus	T-31	0495	3.96	8.00	0636	3.20	5.03	0447	3.52	7.87

$$\text{*REY} = \frac{\text{Amount of hydrolysed starch (mg) / hr / ml}}{\text{Wet weight of mycelia (g)}}$$

Table 3: Effect of Different Temperatures on Activity of α-Amylase

FUNGI	Isolate	Mycelial Dry weight in mg	Amount of hydrolyzed starch in mg hr^{-1} ml^{-1} crude enzyme sample											
			15°C	25 °C	30 °C	35 °C	40 °C	45 °C	50 °C	55 °C	60 °C	65 °C	70 °C	75 °C
Aspergillus nidulans	T-11	0217	0.16	1.00	1.72	2.36	2.48	6.76	6.00	4.44	4.04	0.24	0.00	0.00
Aspergillus niger	T-18	0117	0.36	3.12	3.96	8.80	8.04	7.20	6.40	4.84	4.24	0.64	0.24	0.00
Aspergillus ustus	T-36	0246	0.80	0.92	2.76	4.00	4.40	7.20	6.76	6.64	6.20	1.64	0.20	0.00
Humicola grisea	T-5	0102	0.08	0.20	0.44	2.40	3.20	5.20	1.48	1.44	1.44	0.64	0.00	0.00
Humicola sp.	T-61	0101	0.20	1.20	2.02	4.28	4.56	7.68	5.29	5.16	4.96	1.64	0.96	0.00
Malbranchea cinnamonea	T-47	0204	2.36	6.80	7.40	8.04	8.24	10.00	9.92	9.80	9.60	5.64	5.60	0.00
Myceliophthora thermophila	T-33	0285	0.20	2.02	2.08	2.24	3.56	4.52	3.68	3.16	2.88	0.76	0.48	0.00
Myceliophthora vellerea	T-15	0203	0.20	2.02	2.28	2.48	3.04	5.04	3.60	3.56	3.48	1.72	1.24	0.00
Myceliopthora sp.	T-64	0314	0.12	1.88	2.36	2.76	3.22	5.16	4.88	4.36	4.24	4.20	2.44	0.00
Sagenomella sp.	T-51	0155	0.08	0.60	1.56	2.16	2.64	5.40	4.60	3.96	3.92	2.40	2.32	0.00
Talaromyces thermophilus	T-46	0264	2.36	4.40	6.08	7.00	7.40	10.00	9.80	9.60	9.60	9.40	8.40	0.00
Thermomyces lanuginosus	T-31	0173	0.16	1.20	1.72	3.36	5.04	7.56	7.20	7.04	6.64	4.00	3.24	0.00

Note:

1. Data given in table is a mean of two independent determinations.
2. Cultures grown at 45°C.

Effect of different temperature

Results of effect of different temperatures on the activity of α- amylase in crude culture filtrate of test fungi are recorded in Table 3. Culture filtrates of Aspergillus niger (T-18) indicated optimum amylase activity at 35°C. Maximum activity of α-amylase was noted in the culture filtrates of *Malbranchea cinnamonea* (T-47) and *Talaromyces thermophilus* (T-46) at 45°C. However, only a little decrease in the amylase activity was noted at reaction temperatures ranging from 45°-60°C in case of *Malbranchea cinnamonea* (T-47) and 45°C to 70°C in case of *Talaromyces thermophilus* (T-46). In cultures of *Aspergillus ustus* (T-36) α- amylase activity was recorded with little variation at temperatures ranging from 45°-60°C.

In the present investigation 4 thermophilic fungi, *Malbranchea cinnamonca* (T-47), *Talaromyces thermophilus* (T-46), *Aspergillus ustus* (T-36) and *Thermomyces langinosus* (T-31) have indicated production of α-amylase starch hydrolyzing enzymes greater activity and also their thermostable nature. Activity of α-amylase in cultures grown in different media was found different. This indicates the possibility of improving α-amylase production in these potential strains by manipulation in their cultural conditions.

ACKNOWLEDGEMENTS

Authors are thankful to Head of the Botany Department, Dr. H.S. Gour Vishwavidyalaya, Sagar, for Laboratory facilities. One of the author (S.S.) is also thankful to Director General Health Services, Govt. of India for award of JRF.

REFERENCES

Crabb, W.D. and Mitchinson, C. (1997). Enzyme involved in the processing of starch of sagurs. Trands in Biotechnology 15: 349-352.

Chrispeel, M.J. and Varner, J.E. (1967) Gibberellic acid enhanced synthesis and release of α-amylase and ribonuclease by isolated barley aleuron layers. Plant Physiology. 42: 398-406.

Forgarty, W.M. (1983) Microbial amylases. In : Microbial enzymes and biotechnology, (Ed. Forgarty W.M.) Applied Science pyblishers, London. 1-92.

Forgarty, W. M. and Kelly, C.T. (1979) Starch degrading enzymes of microbial origin. In: Bull AH (ed) Progress in Indstrial Microbiology, Vol 15, Elsevier, Amsterdam, pp. 87-150.

Forgarty, W.M. and Kelly, C.T. (1980) Amylases and Amyloglucosidases and realted glucanases. In Economic Microbiology Microbial enzymes and bioconversions, Vol. 5, (Ed. Rose, A.H.) Academic Press, New York pp. 115-170.

Hankin, L. and Anagnostakis, S.L. (1975). The use of solid media in detection of enzyme production by fungi. Mycologia 97 : 597-607.

Normam, B.E. (1979) The application of polysaccharide degrading enzyme in starch industry. In: Microbial polysaccharides and polysaccharides. (Ed. Berkeley R. C.W., Gooday G.W., Ellwood DC), Academic Press, London, 339-376.

Palmer, T.J. (1975) Glucose syrups in food and drink. Process Biochem. 10 : 19-20.

Peterson, W.H. and Fred, E.B. (1932) Butyl-acetone fermentation of corn meal: interrelation of substrate and products. Ind. Eng. Chem. 24: 237-242.

Microbiology and Biotechnology for Sustainable Development (*Ed.* P.C. Jain),
CBS Publishers & Distributors, New Delhi (2004), pp. 307–313.

B-15

Production of Enzymes by some Keratinolytic Bacteria

P.C. Jain and Shama J.P. Khanam
Department of Applied Microbiology & Biotechnology
Dr. H.S. Gour University Sagar (M.P.)

Abstract

Four strains of bacteria isolated from dropped off feathers using keratin enrichment technique have been tested for their ability to degrade human hair and hen feathers. Two test bacteria i.e. strain CO2 and strain AO1 indicated high keratinolytic properties. They were also found to produce gelatinase and caseinase and caused greater weight loss of feathers than hair. For lipase activity two bacteria i.e. Strain CO1 and strain CO2 have been found positive.

Key Words: Keratinolytic bacteria, keratin, human hair, hen feather

INTRODUCTION

In nature keratin is found in skin and its appendages of man and animals such as horns, hooves, feather, hair, nails etc. Natural keratinic materials contain only a small amount of pure keratin while a large portion of these consist of chemically different cementing materials. Hence, in order to achieve a complete hydrolysis of natural keratinic matter a group of enzymes with varied hydrolytic properties is required, which can be obtained from one organism or different organisms. Amongst prokaryotes only a few bacterial strains are known to produce keratinolytic enzymes (Atalo and Gashe 1993; Cheng *et al.*, 1995; Lin *et al.*, 1992; Takami *et al.*, 1999) while a large number of potential strains could be isolated with desired characteristics. In order to achieve keratinolytic system the prokaryotes may prove better tools. In the present study an attempt has been made to characterize feather degrading capabilities of four bacteria isolated from dropped off feathers by using keratin enrichment technique (Jain, 2000).

MATERIALS AND METHODS

Four strains of bacteria (strain A01, B02, C01 and C02) isolated from dropped off feathers have been tested for their lipolytic, proteolytic and keratinolytic activity. For this the test bacterial strains were grown in a basal medium containing K_2HPO_4 -0.4gm, $MgSO_4.7H_2O$ - 0.05gm; NaCl - 0.01gm; $FeCl_3$ - 0.01gm; glucose - 10.00-gm per liter of distilled water (pH was maintained to 7.5). An aliquot of 75 ml of the basal medium was taken in 150 ml Erlenmeyer flask with natural and defatted hairs and feathers as substrate.

A. Keratin degradation

The keratinic substrate (0.5 gm) was added in each flask and sterilized at 121°C for 15min. The flasks were inoculated with 1ml spore suspension (2 x 10^6 spores/ml) of each test organism and kept for incubation at 28°C and 37°C for 20 days. A set of flasks having 0.5 gm keratin substrates in basal medium were also kept without inoculum and treated as keratin controls.

Keratin decomposing ability of test organisms was determined using the method as described by Jain and Agarwal (1980). From all the flasks the substrates, along with growing bacterial biomass were removed by filtration and dried at 70-80°C for 24 hour. The total dry weight in each case was determined and compared with the substrate in control (Table 1). If the weight of the control + bacterial biomass was found more, bacterium was considered to be non-keratinolytic and the increased weight was attributed to the production of biomass due to utilization of nutrients present in the basal medium and also from the substrate. If the substrate with bacterial biomass weighed less than the control, the bacterium was considered keratinolytic. The weight loss was calculated by subtracting the dry weight of uninoculated keratin substrate. The filtrate was processed further for determination of activity of enzymes and amount of amino acids and proteins.

Net loss of wt. = wt. of keratin in control – (wt.of keratin + bacterial biomass in test flask).

B. Lipase activity

The cultivation fluids thus obtained were tested for their extra-cellular enzyme production by agar well diffusion method. The medium was prepared according to Hankin and Anagnostakis (1975). Sorbitan monolaurate (Tween 20) was used as the lipid substrate. The medium contained per liter: peptone-10gm; NaCl-5gm; $CaCl_2.2H_2O$-0.1gm; agar-20gm, (pH 6). The tween 20 was sterilized separately by autoclaving for 15min at 15 pounds pressure and 1ml of this was added per 100ml of sterile and cooled basal medium. 500µl of cultivation fluid was dispensed in the agar well prepared using cork borer. The inoculated plates were incubated at 28°C and 37°C for 24 hours and were then observed for lipolytic activity in each case. Visible precipitate formed due to formation of crystals of the calcium salt of the lauric acid was considered positive reaction indicating presence of lipolytic enzyme in test culture fluid.

C. Protease (gelatinase) activity

The culture fluids were tested for the two proteases i.e. gelatinase and casinase activity using two different media. For the gelatinase activity Difco nutrient agar medium was prepared according to Hankin and Anagnostakis (1975) to this 0.4% gelatin was added. The pH was maintained to 6.0. An 8% solution of gelatin in water was sterilized separately and added to the nutrient agar at the rate of 5ml per 100ml of medium 500μl of cultivation fluid was dispensed in the agar well and the plates were incubated at 28°C and 37°C for 24 hours. After incubation, complete degradation of gelatin was seen as a clearing in the somewhat opaque agar around the well.

D. Protease (Caseinase) activity

For casinase activity the medium was prepared according to Rajamani and Hilda (1987). The medium contained: skimmed milk - 20g in 200ml distilled water and phosphate buffer - 600ml of 0.5M, pH 7. All the three constituents of medium were autoclaved separately to avoid coagulation and charring of milk due to the presence of buffer salts and later mixed under sterile conditions. 500μl of cultivation fluid was dispensed in the well bored in milk agar medium and incubated at 28°C and 37°C for 24 hour. Zone of proteolysis was observed after flooding the plates with 5% TCA for 10min.

E. Keratinase activity

Keratin degradation by bacterial strains was also confirmed according to Wainwright (1982) using keratin azure. This technique involved use of keratin azure; a commercially available keratin substrate dyed with Ramazol Brilliant Blue R. The dye is covalently linked to the substrate and release of the blue color is a measure of keratin degradation.

Substrate, keratin azure was weighed 0.010g in sterile screw cap tubes and inoculated with 5 ml spore suspension of each test organism. One tube containing sterile distilled water and keratin azure was run as keratin control. All the tubes were incubated at 37°C. Development of blue color in each tube was measured at 595 nm up to 12 days at an interval of 3 days to determine the rate of keratin degradation by test bacteria.

RESULT AND DISCUSSION

The results of keratin degrading capabilities of test bacterial strains are given in Table-1.Bacterial strain A01 caused maximum degradation of defatted human hair at both the test temperatures i.e. 28°C and 37°C. A total loss in weight of defatted human hair was found to be 32% and 37% at 28°C and 37°C respectively. However, this bacterium caused only 2-6% loss in the weight of natural hair. The degradation of defatted feathers was found to be 24 and 26% at 28°C and 37°C temperatures respectively. Bacterial strain B02 responded well when grown at 28°C causing 14-17 and 18-22% weight loss in human hair and hen feathers, respectively. Bacterial strain CO1 and CO2 caused 32 and 35% weight loss in defatted feathers at 37°C respectively. While at 28°C temperature they caused a total of 38% loss in defatted feathers.

These strains also showed better activity on natural feathers at 28°C. The results presented in table1, indicates that, using strain CO1 and CO2 maximum keratinolysis can be achieved at the test range of temperatures between 28°C to 37°C.

Table 1: Degradation of hair and feathers by four strains of bacteria at different temperatures

Test Bacteria	Weight loss in percentage*							
	28°C				37°C			
	Hair		Feather		Hair		Feather	
	Natural	Defatted	Natural	Defatted	Natural	Defatted	Natural	Defatted
Strain A01	32	2	21	24	6	37	20	26
Strain B02	14	17	22	18	8	15	6	-
Strain C01	14	26	29	38	2	-	26	32
Strain C02	2	4	32	38	18	16	14	35

*incubation of 20 days.

Lipase Activity

Bacterial strains CO1 and CO2 showed lipolytic activity in the extra cellular fractions when grown on natural and defatted human hair and hen feather. While activity of this enzyme, was not detected in cultures of other test bacteria i.e. AO1 and BO2 (Table 2).

Table 2: Lipase production by bacteria in Keratin rich media at 24 hrs of incubation

Test Bacteria	Zone of enzyme activity*							
	28°C				37°C			
	Hair		Feather		Hair		Feather	
	Natural	Defatted	Natural	Defatted	Natural	Defatted	Natural	Defatted
Strain A01	-	-	-	-	-	-	-	-
Strain B02	-	-	-	-	-	-	-	-
Strain C01	20	20	16	20	21	22	24	22
Strain C02	15	20	15	15	16	14	16	13

*Including the diameter of well i.e. 10mm

Gelatinase Activity

Gelatinase activity was noted in extra cellular fractions of all the test bacteria when grown on natural and defatted human hair and hen feather (Table 3). A zone of gelatinase activity was found to be in the range of 24 to 38 mm.

Caseinase Activity

Caseinase activity was noted in the culture fluid of all the test bacteria when grown on natural and defatted human hair and hen feather (Table 4).

Table 3: Gelatinase production by bacteria in keratin rich media at 24 hours of incubation.

Test Bacteria	Zone of enzyme activity*							
	28°C				37°C			
	Hair		Feather		Hair		Feather	
	Natural	Defatted	Natural	Defatted	Natural	Defatted	Natural	Defatted
Strain A01	26	30	30	30	30	38	35	30
Strain B01	24	38	38	30	24	30	30	28
Strain C01	38	24	30	38	24	30	30	31
Strain C02	30	30	28	30	30	30	27	26

*Including the diameter of well i.e. 10mm.

Table 4: Caseinase production by bacteria in keratin rich media at 24 hours of incubation.

Test Bacteria	Zone of enzyme activity*							
	28°C				37°C			
	Hair		Feather		Hair		Feather	
	Natural	Defatted	Natural	Defatted	Natural	Defatted	Natural	Defatted
Strain A01	24	24	30	24	30	38	30	24
Strain B01	20	18	18	20	16	19	20	20
Strain C01	16	16	24	18	18	18	24	14
Strain C02	24	14	18	18	24	24	12	20

*Including the diameter of well i.e. 10mm.

Keratinase activity

Keratinase activity was noted, using keratin azure as substrate and the results are given in Table 5. Strain AO1 caused degradation of 7.891mg keratin azure in 12 days while strain BO1 caused degradation of only 2.116 mg of keratin azure. Test strain CO1 and strain CO2 caused degradation of 4.766 and 4.752 mg keratin azure, respectively in 12 days (Fig. 1).

For degradation of feather keratin three strains of bacteria have showed remarkable activity causing 21 to 38 per cent weight loss when tested at 37°C. The keratin degrading ability and production of enzyme keratinase by test bacteria has also been confirmed by another set of experiment in which, we have used keratin azure as substrate. It is interesting to note that the test bacteria, also showed good activity of gelatinase and caeinase. This showed that the test strain of bacteria possess a wide range of proteases which may help

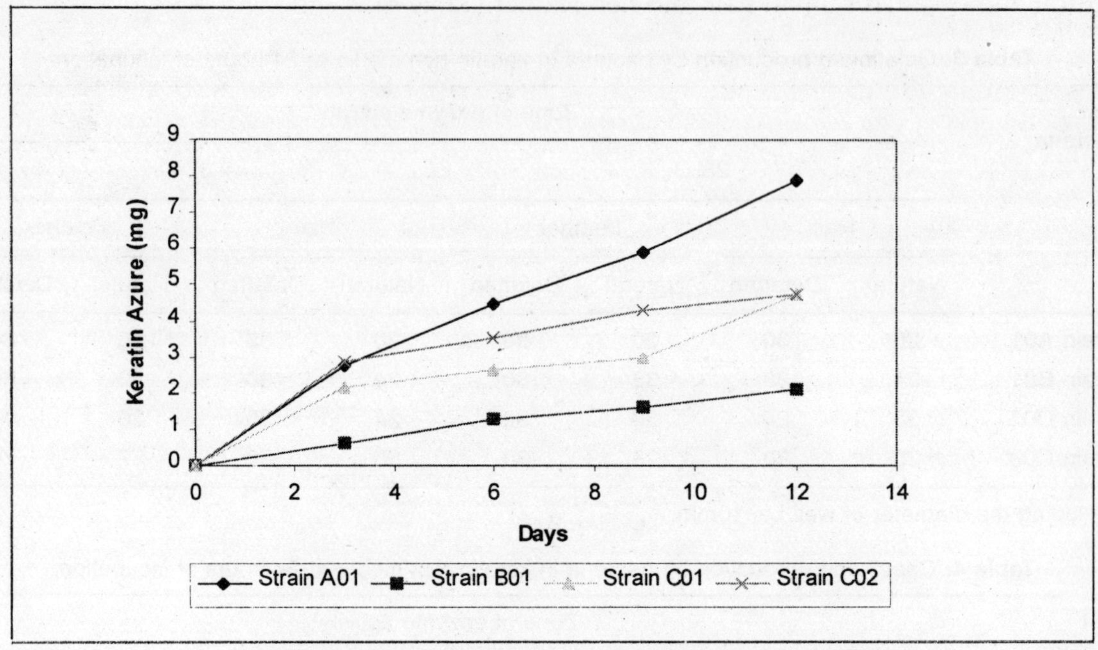

Fig. 1. Keratinase Activity

them in complete degradation of keratin in nature while their potential can be exploited for the biotransformation of keratin waste to protein and amino acids. In the present study only two strains (i.e. strain CO1 and strain CO2) showed lipase activity. Lipase production by present test strains of bacteria is significant from the point of view of degradation of natural keratinic matter. The results of present study are sufficient to trigger an interest to search some more promising strains of bacteria from naturally decomposing keratin materials.

Table 5: Keratinase activity

Test Bacteria	Degradation of Keratin azure(mg)*			
	3 days	6 days	9days	12 days
Strain A01	2.750	4.464	5.932	7.891
Strain B01	0.619	1.296	1.612	2.116
Strain C01	2.145	2.664	2.995	4.766
Strain C02	2.894	3.528	4.320	4.752

* Initial inoculum strength 10^7 spores/ Tube

ACKNOWLEDGEMENT

Authors are thankful to the Head Department of Applied Microbiology and Biotechnology. Dr. H.S. Gour Vishwavidyalaya, Sagar for laboratory facilities and senior author (PCJ) is thankful to U.G.C., New Delhi for grant of minor Research project.

REFERENCES

Atalo, K., and Gashe, B.A. (1993). Protease production by a thermophilic *Bacillus* species (P-001A) which degrades various kinds of fibrous proteins. *Biotechnol. Lett. 15*: 1151-1156.

Cheng, S.W., Hu, H.M., Shen, S.W., Takagi, H., Asano, A. and Tsai, Y.C. (1995). Production and characterization of keratinase of a feather - degrading *Bacillus licheniformis* PWD-1. *Biosci. Biotechnol. Biochem.* 59 : 2239-2243.

Hankin, L. and Anagnostakis, S.L. (1975). The use of solid media for detection of enzyme production by fungi. Mycologia. Vol. LXVII, No. 3 : 597-607.

Jain, P.C. and Agrawal, S.C. (1980). A note of keratin decomposing capability of some fungi. *Trans. Mycol. Soc. Japan, 21* : 513-517.

Jain, P.C. (2000). Enumeration and characterization of keratinolytic bacteria from dropped off feathers. 40th Annual conference of microbiologists of India, Bhubneswar. (Abst. GMM-88). 22-24 Jan. 2000.

Lin., X., Lee, C.G., Gasale, E.S., and Shih, J.C.H. (1992). Purification and characterisation of a keratinase from a feather degrading *Bacillus licheniformis* strain. *Appl. Environ. Microbiol.* 58 : 3271-3275.

Rajamani, S. and Hilda, A. (1987). Plate assay to screen fungi for proteolytic activity. *Curr. Sci. 56 :* 1179-1181.

Takami, H., Nogi, Y. and Horikoshi, K. (1999). Reidentification of the keratinase -producing facultatively alkaliphilic *Bacillus* sp. AH-101 as *Bacillu halodurans. Extremophiles*, *3* : 293-296.

Wainwright, M. (1982). A new method for determining the microbial degradation of keratin in soils. *Experientia. 38* : 243-244.

Microbiology and Biotechnology for Sustainable Development (Ed. P.C. Jain),
CBS Publishers & Distributors, New Delhi (2004), pp. 314–325.

B-16

An Improved Method for the Preparation of Spheroplast from *Escherichia coli*

Manoj Kumar, S.C. Agrawal*, R.K. Upreti**
*Biomembrane Division, Industrial Toxicology Research Center, M.G. Marg, Lucknow (UP), * Department of Applied Microbiology and Biotechnology, Dr.H.S.Gour University, Sagar (MP).*

Abstract

A lysozyme-osmotic shock method is described for spheroplast preparation from variously grown Escherichia coli cells. Use of glucose rather than sucrose showed efficient spheroplasting. This procedure found to be equally effective for all stages of growth in minimal as well as rich medium and from early exponential phase to the late stationary phase cells. Resultant spheroplast may be suitably used for the subsequent localization and fractionation of various macromolecules, without affecting their biological activity.

Keywords: Spheroplast, *E.coli*, Lysozyme, subcellular fractionation, membrane.

INTRODUCTION

Anatomically, *Escherichia coli* cell has very simple organization. The outer envelope is composed of three distinct layers viz.cell wall, peptidoglycan and cytoplasmic membrane. The cell envelope encloses the protoplasm comprising of cytoplasm, cytoplasmic granules and nucleic acids (DNA and RNA). In addition to these essential components, some strains of *E.coli* possess additional structures like capsules, flagella, S–layer, fimbriae etc. To obtain various components of *E.coli* cells in pure form and to carry out functional analysis, the subcellular fractionation is essentially required. Many techniques like rupturing of cell either by freezing and thawing, grinding with abrasive, extrusion under mechanical pressure or exposure to high frequency sound waves are not recommended for this purpose due to possible intermixing of constituents of anatomical structures of cells. Further more, these drastic methods of cell disruption may cause extensive damage to various polymer

** for correspondence: E-mail: upretirk@rediffmail.com

constituents, resulting in the loss of their biological activity (Osborn *et al.*, 1972). One of the most important approaches for subcellular fractionation is by converting cells to spheroplast followed by controlled lysis to various fractions (Birdsell and Cota–Robles, 1967; Miura and Mizushima, 1969; Weiss and Fraser, 1973; Witholt *et al.*, 1976). The lysozyme treatment is the choice of approach used for converting cells to spheroplast. Spheroplasts of Gram–negative bacteria are also used in variety of investigations like release of enzymes, accumulation of metabolites (Zhu *et al.*, 1999), purification of enzyme (Davidson and Kumar, 1989) and assay of biological activity of viral nucleic acid.

Variety of techniques have been utilized to render Gram–negative bacteria susceptible to lysis by lysozyme, but they have usually been tailored for particular cell or for the study of specific function. Procedures developed for certain bacteria have been proven less effective for other bacteria. This may be due to the difference in structure of envelope among bacteria and variation in role of various factors, like metallic ions in maintaining cell wall integrity among them. Besides that lysozyme sensitivity varies within species. It also varies in strains with the culture age, growth phase, medium composition and cultivation conditions. Therefore to obtain the most efficient sub cellular fractions, which could render variously grown cells completely susceptible to lysozyme for a particular strain, it is necessary to standardize the sub cellular fractionation procedure.

The present paper describes a procedure, for the preparation of spheroplast from *E. coli* cells grown under different conditions, including stationary as well as exponential growth phase.

MATERIALS AND METHODS

Chemicals

Lysozyme (egg white, Crystalline), Agarose, Proteinase K, BSA, EDTA, pNPP was purchased from Sigma, USA. All other chemicals used were procured from Qualigens, E.Merck, and Sigma–Aldrich. Microbiological media were purchased from Hi–media, India.

Organism and cultivation conditions

Three strains of *Escherichia coli* (*E.coli PCRO 1687, E.coli* B37, *E.coli* DH5 α) were used. Organisms were grown in nutrient broth or basal mineral media. Nutrient broth (NB) contained (g/liter); peptone 2.0, beef extract 3.0; NaCl, 5.0 (pH 7.0$\pm$4). The Basal mineral medium (pH 7.0$\pm$0.2) contained 2.0 gram of NH_4Cl, 6.0 gram of Na_2HPO_4, 3.0 gram of KH_2PO_4, 0.026 gram of Na_2SO_4, 0.021gram of $MgCl_2$, a trace of $FeCl_3$ per liter. Carbon source, 0.5% Glucose (filter sterilized) was added after autoclaving the salts. Bacteria were cultured at 30 °C with shaking (200 $\pm$ 10 rpm) in one liter Erlenmeyer flasks, each containing 400 ml of medium. To solidify, 2% agar was added as and when required in each medium. Cultures were maintained on nutrient agar slant, and glycerol stock at–40 °C. Majority of the experiments were confined to *E.coli* PCRO1687.But final protocol was verified with all strains. Typically, each measurement was carried out in three replicate samples and repeated at least twice.

Growth studies

Cultures were started with over–night nutrient broth grown culture broth. Growth was measured at timed intervals by turbidimetry at 610 nm in a Baush and Lomb spectronic–21 instrument. Viability testing was done, by counting colony–forming units (C.F.U.) at timed intervals. For that, serial ten–fold dilutions of sample were plated on nutrient agar, which were incubated at 37°C for 24 hours and then colonies were counted.

Spheroplast Formation

Lysozyme sensitivity depends upon bacterial strain, growth phase of cells, cell densities, lysozyme concentration and buffer system etc. (Birdsell and Cota–Robles, 1967). In order to render *E.coli* cells, more sensitive to lysozyme, the effect of these variables in lysozyme sensitivity was investigated. Cells in various densities were suspended in buffer containing different concentrations of Tris–HCl (pH 8.0), EDTA, osmotic stabilizer and lysozyme. Beside the composition and concentration of suspension buffer, the time sequence of additions to the cell suspension was also analyzed.

In a series of experiments, to prepare Spheroplasts, cultures were harvested by centrifugation and suspended in Tris–HCl (pH 8.0), sucrose (pH 8.0) and EDTA (pH 7.6) in a manner resulting suspension contained 5 to 20 mg (dry weight) of cells/ml in 10–200 mM Tris–HCl (pH 8.0), 0.25–2.0 mM EDTA (pH 7.6) and 0.1–1.0 M sucrose (pH 8.0) (SET suspension). Egg white Lysozyme (E.C.3.2.1.17) was added to SET suspension to final concentration of 10–100 μg / ml and after which the cells were exposed to mild osmotic shock by two fold dilution in water to trigger lysozyme penetration to membrane. Mg^{2+} was added to the final concentration of 5–20 mM to stabilize the spheroplasts. They could then be concentrated by centrifugation and suspended in dilute buffer containing no osmotic stabilizers. Experiment were also carried out to assess osmotic sensitivity of spheroplast by chelating Mg^{2+} with the addition of equimolar concentration of EDTA.The efficiency of glucose (Zhu *et al.*, 1999), Glycine and NaCl separately and in combination to adjust osmotic strength instead of sucrose was also evaluated.

Cell lysis (osmotic sensitivity) was measured according to Witholt *et al.* (1976) in all cases to determine lysozyme sensitivity. Briefly, five minutes after the addition of lysozyme, portions of suspension were diluted ten fold in water and OD was recorded at 399 nm. The OD observed two minutes after dilutions was corrected for the dilutions, which occurred when lysozyme, EDTA or water was added to the cells. The lysozyme sensitivity was expressed as the percent decrease in the OD five minutes after treatment compared to before the lysozyme treatment. All lysozyme sensitivities were repeated to obtain an average value of four separate determinations.

The effect of lysozyme on the conversion of rod–shaped cells to sphere one was further confirmed under phase contrast microscope. Furthermore taking the advantage of inability of spheroplast in growing on solid media, comparisons of C.F.U of control cells (with out Lysozyme treatment) and experimental cells (with Lysozyme treatment) on basal mineral media–agar was also taken as criteria for Lysozyme effect. Results were presented in %production of spheroplast in comparison to respective controls.

Sub–cellular fractionation

Sub cellular fractionation was carried out according to Kumar and Upreti (2000).Briefly the spheroplasts were collected by centrifugation at 15,000 x g for 15 minutes at 4°C and the resulting supernatant obtained was termed as the periplasmic fluid consisting of periplasmic proteins and peptidoglycan residues. The spheroplasts were then suspended in Tris–HCl buffer. Cells were disrupted by four-30 seconds bursts of Vibronic Ultrasonic Processor and centrifuged at 3000 x g for 10 minutes at 4°C to remove debris and unbroken cells. Resulting supernatant consisting of total membrane and cytoplasmic fractions was centrifuged at 50,000 rpm for 150 minutes at 4°C .The pellet consisting of both outer and inner membrane envelop, designated as crude membrane fraction. This was washed twice and resuspended in buffer. The final supernatant obtained was termed as cytoplasmic fraction. Routinely, the $Ca^{2+}Mg^{2+}$ ATPase was used as marker of crude membrane fraction; alkaline phosphtase marker for periplasmic fluid while hexokinase was used as marker of cytoplasmic fraction. Beside that, lipid: protein ratio was also taken as marker of purity of membrane fractions. The typical membrane preparation contains average 25–30% lipids and 55–65%proteins.

Biochemical estimations

Alkaline phosphatase was determined according to Weiser (1962). Ca^{2+} -Mg^{2+} -ATPase and Hexokinase assays were carried out according to the procedures described by Hidalgo *et al.* (1983) and Datta *et al.* (1969), respectively. Enzyme units were defined as micromoles of product formed per minute under the assay conditions. Specific activity was defined as units/mg protein. Total protein was estimated according to the method of Lowry *et al.* (1957) using bovine serum albumin as standard. Total hexoses were estimated by anthrone reagent method of Roe (1955) after hydrolysis of sample in 1.5 N H_2SO_4 at 100°C for 6 h using glucose as standard.

Statistical analysis

The results were expressed as mean ± S.D. Comparisons were made with appropriate control employing student 't'–test. Differences were considered significant at p 0.05.

RESULTS

It is evident from Fig. 1a and b that when the concentration of Tris–HCl was lower than 50mM and no EDTA was present in the suspension medium, the lysozyme sensitivity of cells harvested at different time intervals during the incubation decreased from about 30–45 % in exponential growth phase to about 15–25 % after they had entered the stationary phase. The lysozyme sensitivity increased somewhat after 15 to 20 hours of incubation. The cells remained viable during the entire incubation time, indicating that decreased lysozyme sensitivity in the stationary phase was not related to change in cell viability. The similar results were obtained in mineral media but the lysozyme sensitivity was averaged between 25–35% and never exceeded that. Increasing the concentration of lysozyme did not improve the formation of spheroplasts particularly in stationary phase cells at this concentration of Tris–HCl.

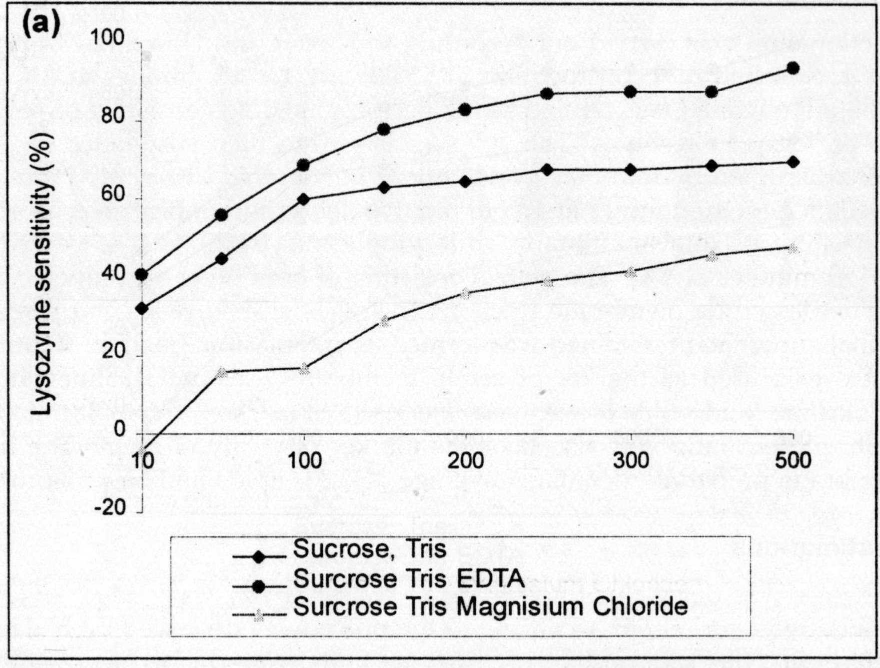

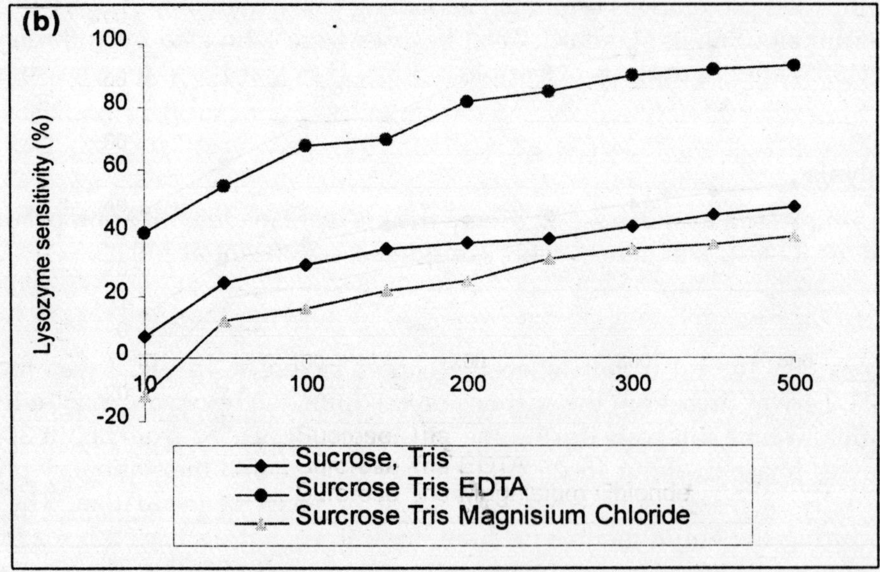

Fig. 1a and b. Sensitivity of lysozyme as a function of suspension buffer. (a) Exponential phase cells. (b) stationary phase cells. Sucrose final concentration was 0.5M. If used, concentration of EDTA, and $MgCl_2$ was 0.5 mM and 10mM, respectively (prior to addition of lysozyme). Cell density 10 mg/ml (dry weight); Lysozyme 50 μg/ml.

When the cells were suspended in a buffer containing variable concentration of Tris–HCl buffer and sucrose, most cells remain resistant to lysozyme, especially at lower Tris–HCl concentrations. The addition of 10–mM Mg^{2+} to buffer further increased the resistance of stationary phase cells to lysozyme. The negative lysozyme sensitivity was monitored at low Tris–HCl concentration in presence of Mg^{2+}.

When EDTA was present in the suspension buffer, cells rendered osmotically sensitive efficiently, provided the concentration of Tris–HCl exceeded 50 mM. Significant spheroplasting was observed at Tris–HCl concentration ranging from 100 to 300mM and EDTA concentrations ranging from 0.25–0.50mM. Similar results were obtained when osmotic sensitivity was determined by ten-fold dilution in 10 mM EDTA instead of water. Results shows that exponential cells differed from stationary phase cells with respect to their susceptibility to lysozyme. However, when no EDTA was present, exponential phase cells were still susceptible to lysozyme. In the presence of 10 mM Mg^{2+} about 30–40 % of cells became osmotically sensitive at Tris–concentration above 100 mM. Stationary as well as exponential phase cells are sensitive to lysozyme if the suspension buffer contains EDTA and a high concentration of Tris–HCl. Lysozyme treatment rendered about 85–90 % in SET–suspended exponential phase cells osmotically sensitive as well the case for stationary phase cells.

Use of glucose rather than sucrose showed efficient lysozyme sensitivity in stationary phase and exponential phase cells (Fig. 2). The sensitivity of lysozyme increased when glucose was used instead of sucrose. Both stationary phase as well exponential phase cells showed approximately 5% more sensitivity than SET buffer, irrespective of the media used. The cells remained fully viable under all the above growth condition. Glycine, NaCl alone and in combination found to be effective but not as good as glucose.

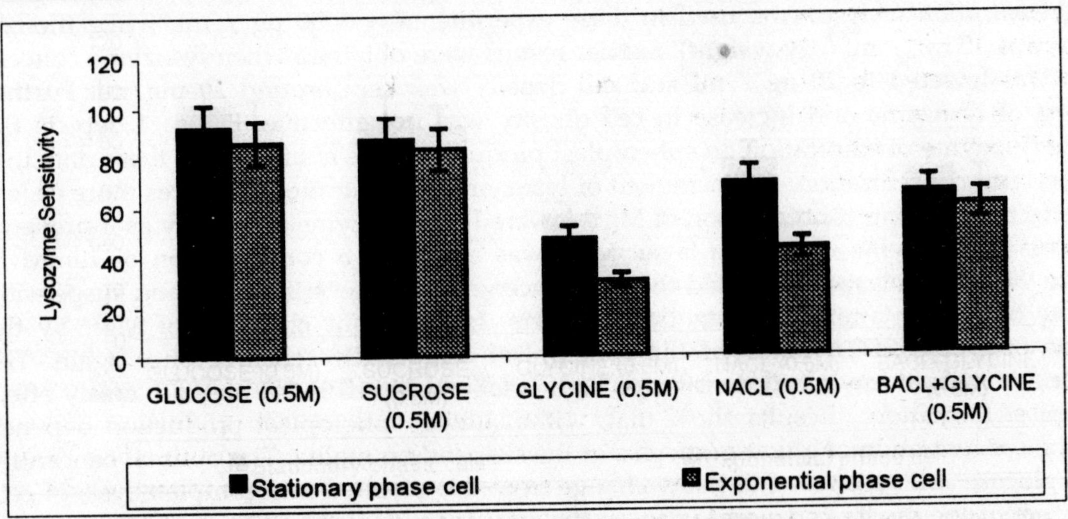

Fig. 2. Effect of various osmotic-stabilizer on lysozyme sensitivity. The suspension buffer contains 250mM Tris-HCl ,0.5 mM EDTA and) 0.5 M osmotic stabilizer. In case of combination, both are taken 0.25 M.

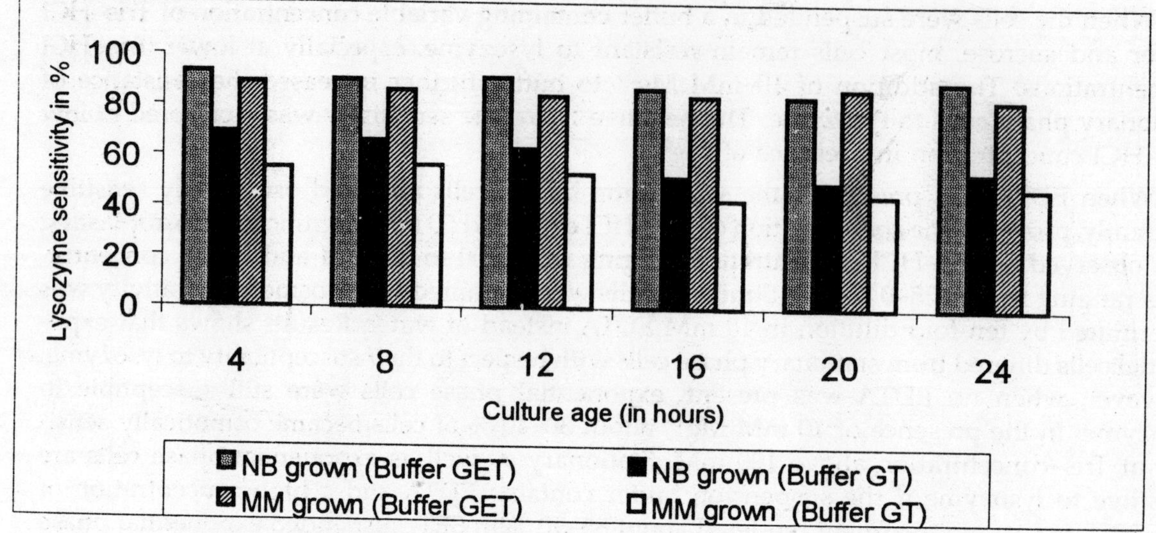

Fig. 3. Sensitivity of *E.coli PCRO 1687* to lysozyme as a function of culture age. Suspension buffer (GET buffer) contain 250mM Tris-HCL, 0.5M Glucose and 5mM EDTA. Cells were grown in nutrient broth (NB) and basal mineral media (MM), separately and taken at density of 10 mg/ml(dry weight). Lysozyme was used at 50μg/ml concentration .For comparison lysozyme treatment was given in buffer containing 250 mM of Tris –HCl and 0.5M of glucose (GE buffer).

The effectiveness of SET and GET (glucose, EDTA, Tris) lysozyme treatment was tested as a function of culture age and as a function of the minimal nutritional supplement. *E. coli* was fully sensitive to lysozyme, regardless to culture age and media composition (Fig. 3). The concentration of lysozyme used in these experiments was 50 μg / ml, while the cell density was 10 mg / ml (dry weight). Similar results were obtained when lysozyme concentration was lowered to 20 μg / ml and cell density was kept around 20 mg/ml. Further lowering of lysozyme and increase in cell density was not effective. Figure 4 depicts the effect of lysozyme concentration on spheroplast production. It is evident from these data that after a certain concentration, the increment of lysozyme concentration produces more or less same effect. Increasing concentration of Mg^{2+} lowered the lysozyme sensitivity as it prevents the access of lysozyme to murein layer. Mg^{2+} was added to a concentration of 10mM to stabilize the spheroplasts; they could then be concentrated by centrifugation and suspension in dilute buffer containing no osmotic stabilizers. Interestingly, chelation of Mg^{2+} by the addition of excess EDTA rendered the spheroplast osmotically sensitive once again. The clumping of cells at lower cell density (or high lysozyme / cell ratio) may adversely affect spheroplast formation. Results show that, within limits, spheroplast production depends upon the concentration of glucose/sucrose in the suspending media. The optimal concentration of glucose /sucrose was 0.5M; any change from this resulted into complete lysis of cell. The nature of the media had no bearing on the effectiveness of the SET and GET lysozyme treatment. When the mineral media was used, the sensitivity of resulting stationary phase cells remained constant at about 90 %. Figure 5 demonstrates the typical pattern of osmotic lysis of *E.coli* after lysozyme treatment in GET buffer. Rod shaped cells, which change to spheroplast, have been converted to sphere, as seen by phase contrast microscopy (Figure not shown). There was a good relationship between the spheroplast formation and inability to grow on solid medium, as significant concentration dependent decrease in C.F.U. after lysozyme treatment was evident (Data not shown). The present protocol was found effective for all three strains studied, as all showed more or less same results.

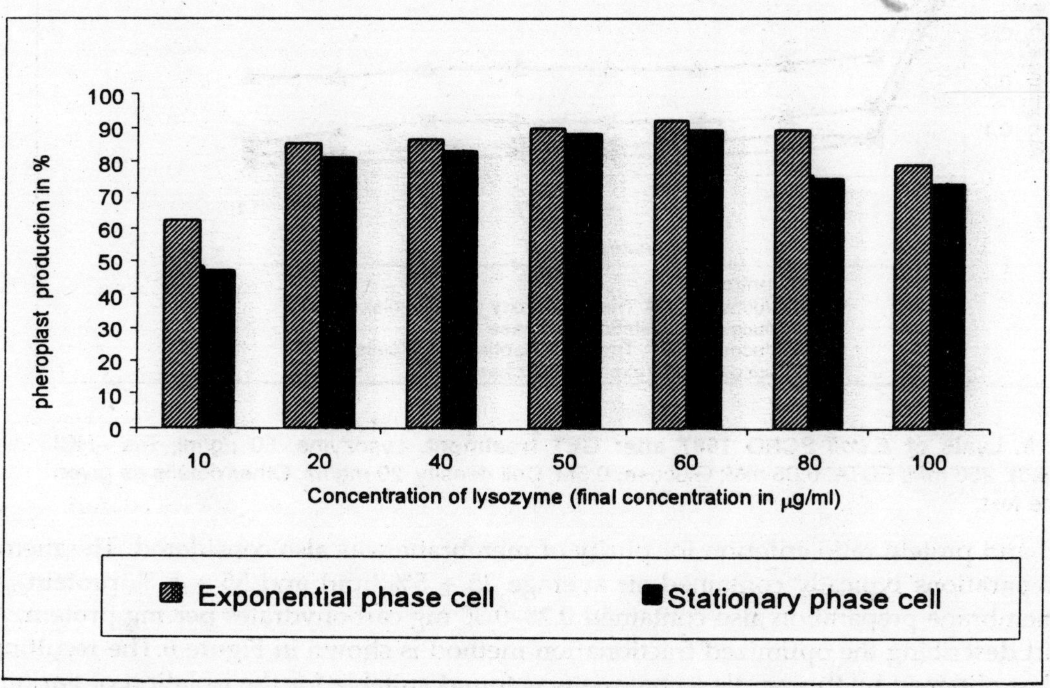

Fig. 4. Effect of lysozyme concentration on spheroplast production. Spheroplast production was measured by c.f.u. on agar plate and microscopically

Spheroplasts prepared from cells of various growth phases with GET lysozyme treatment were ruptured by sonication. The resulting sub cellular fraction was collected. Table 1 shows the percent recovery of enzyme markers in different sub cellular fractions. Approximately 85 % recovery of marker enzymes was noticed in all fractions.

Table 1: Distribution of marker enzyme activity in different cell fractions

Cell fraction	% Total recovery		
	Ca^{2+} -Mg^{2+} -ATPase	Alkaline phosphatase	Hexokinase
Periplasm	9.1±0.6	84.5±7.6	10.9±0.1
Cytoplasm	2.4±0.2	9.8±0.4	84.8±5.4
Membrane fraction	86.5±5.9	6.7±0.2	5.3±0.2

Values are mean ± S. D. from five different preparations.

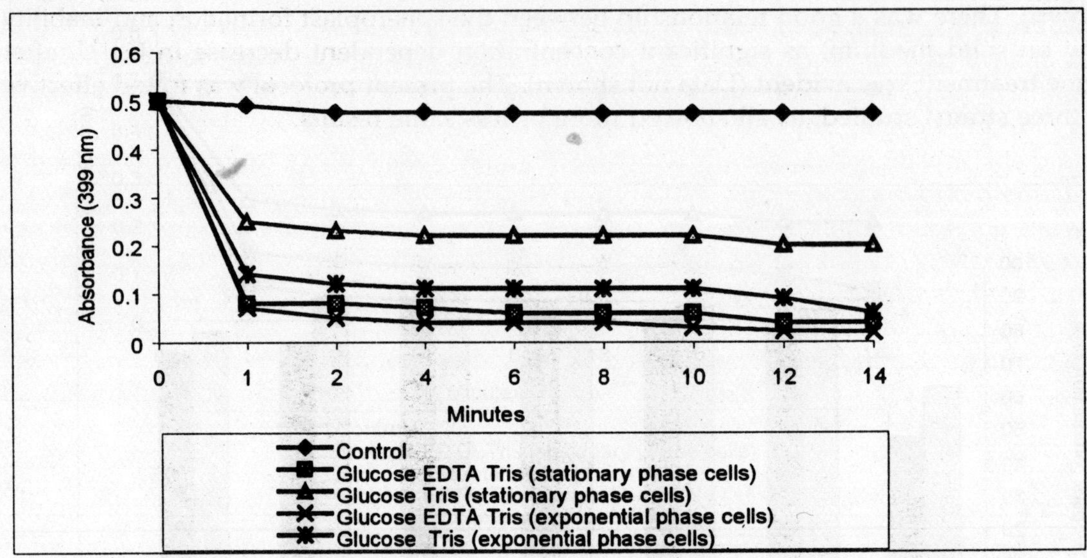

Fig. 5. Lysis of *E.coli* PCRO 1687 after GET treatment. Lysozyme, 50 μg/ml; Tris –HCl (pH8.0), 250 mM; EDTA, 0.05 mM; Glucose, 0.5M; Cell density, 20 mg/ml. Other details as given in the text.

Lipid and protein ratio criterion for purity of membrane was also considered. The membrane preparations typically contained an average 25 ± 5% lipid and 55 ± 5 % protein. A typical membrane preparation also contained 0.25–0.30 mg carbohydrates per mg protein. A flow chart describing the optimized fractionation method is shown in Figure 6.The resulting spheroplast obtained by this gentle technique was found suitable for the isolation of various bioactive proteins, DNA, RNA etc (Data not shown).

DISCUSSION

The envelope of stationary–phase *E. coli* differs from that of exponentially phase with respect to several characteristics (Deutscher *et al.*, 1974; Pagan and Mackey, 2000) including protein composition (Chai and Foulds, 1977) and phospho-lipids (Berger *et al.,* 1980). Therefore, most of the procedure applied for fractionation of one phase (log phase) may not employ to other phase (e.g., stationary phase). Further more, cell grown in minimum mineral media, devoid of supplementation with small amount of rich media, has been reported to be very poor for spheroplast formation, even in case of exponential phase cells, in comparison to the cells grown in rich media. Link and co–workers (1997) have shown the differences in protein composition of cytoplasm, periplasm and membrane in *E. coli* grown in rich media and minimum medium. Even various envelope proteins of *E. coli* may lose by mutation without affecting the vital function of cell. A variety of techniques have been utilized to render Gram–negative bacteria susceptible to lysis by Lysozyme. Several conditions must be met before lysozyme can penetrate the outer membrane of cells. All of these alter, either structurally or chemically, the outer membrane exposing the rigid layer to enzymatic degradation. A mild osmotic shock is essential to drive lysozyme through the outer membrane because lysozyme fails to penetrate through the outer membrane, particularly of stationary phase cells, to significant extent when it is simply added to such cells. Thus cells are exposed to lysozyme and diluted two fold with water, the resulting mild shock allows lysozyme to penetrate through the outer membrane. Moreover, destabilization of outer membrane is required to permit the lysozyme during osmotic shock. Thus, Tris–HCl was used at concentration of 100–300 mM with EDTA. Mg^{2+} was avoided at time of osmotic shock, since EDTA facilitates while Mg^{2+} prevents the access of lysozyme to the murein layer. Evidences shows that divalent cations have an important role in maintenance the cell wall integrity. EDTA treatment of *E. coli* results in to the release of cell lipopolysaccharide. Since Lysozyme penetrates the outer membrane very efficiently following a mild shock in presence of EDTA, only small amounts of lysozyme are necessary to produce spheroplast.

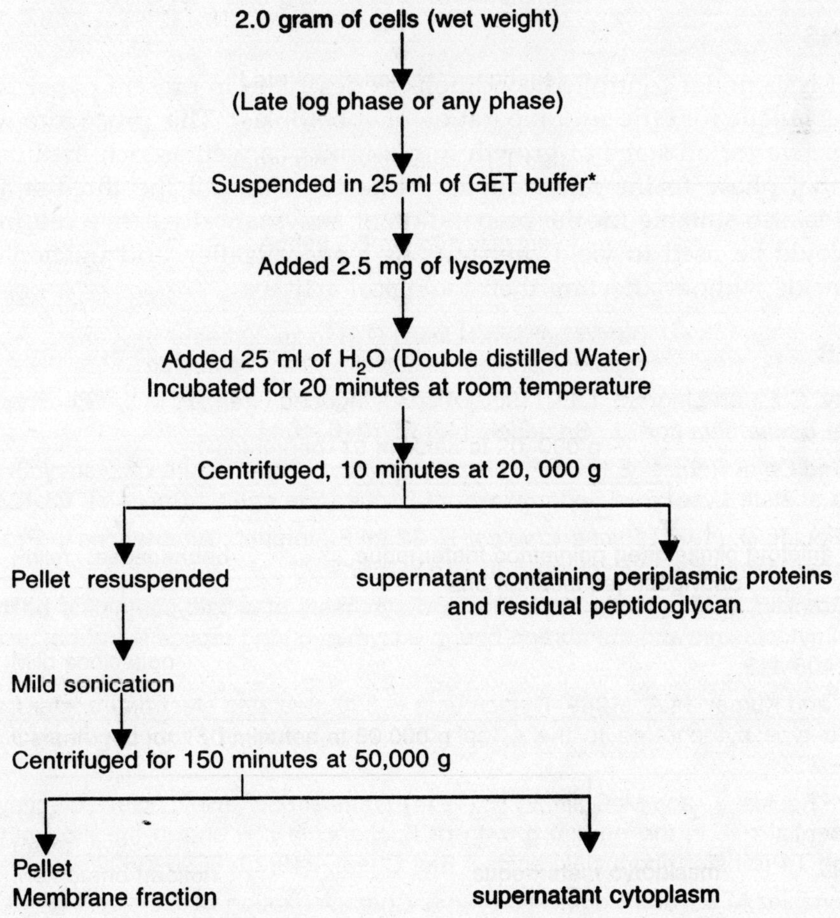

Fig. 6. Flow chart for optimal fractionation of *E.coli* (*Final concentration of Glucose 0.5M, EDTA 0.5mM (pH 7.6) and 0.25 M Tris –HCl (pH 8.0))

Use of glucose rather than sucrose allowed efficient fractionation of the cells. It could be due to small exclusion size of the outer membrane porin of bacterium, which restricts the easy diffusion of sucrose (Ishii and Taijii, 1988; Zhu *et al.*, 1999). In case of the sub cellular fractionation of bacteria, the lysozyme treatment is normally used for the conversion of cells to spheroplast. This procedure has proven effective with all stages of growth in minimal as well as in rich media, from the early exponential to the late stationary phase. This procedure of Lysozyme treatment with the use of Tris–HCl, EDTA, and Glucose worked equally well with unwashed and washed cells, over a period of at least 12 hours following harvesting, provided the cells are stored in 200 mM Tris–HCl (pH 8.0) containing 1mM $MgCl_2$ to prevent autolysis. Findings revealed the spheroplast resulting from this procedure are an excellent source for subsequent fractionation. In present study a few enzyme markers have been investigated, however the distribution of their activities in various fractions resembles broadly the distribution pattern reported in the literature for *E. coli.*

CONCLUSIONS

The method of lysis under controlled conditions as described in present paper is a comparatively gentle technique for efficient preparation of spheroplast. This procedure was found to be equally effective for all stage of growth in minimum as well as rich medium, and from early exponential phase to the late stationary phase, in the all the three strains studied. Besides that it is also suitable for the preparation of enzymatically active cell free extract of bacteria and could be used to yield preparations for localization and fractionation of proteins, nucleic acids without affecting their biological activity.

REFERENCES

Berger, E., Carty, C.E., and Ingram, L.O. (1980) Alcohol induced changes in the Phospholipid molecular species of *Escherchia coli.* J. Bacteriol. 142(3): 1040–1044.

Birdsell, D.C., and Cota–Robles, E.H. (1967) Production and ultrastructure of Lysozyme and Ethylene diamine tetra acetate Lysozyme Spheroplasts of *Escherichia coli.* J Bacteriol. 93:427–437.

Chai, T.J. and Foulds, J. (1977) *Escherichia coli* K–12 tol F Mutants : Alternations in Protein composition of the outer Membrane. J.Bacteriol.130: 781–786.

Datta, A. and Franklin, R.M., (1969) Structure and synthesis of a lipid-containing bacteriophage (ii) Alterations in cytoplasmic and membrane-bound enzymes during replication of bacteriophage PM2. Virology, 39:408-418.

Davidson, V.L., and Kumar, M.A. (1989) Cytochrome c–550 mediates electron transfer from inducible periplasmic c–type cytochrome to the cytoplasmic membrane of *Paracoccus denitrificans.*FEBS Lett.245:271–273.

Deutscher, M.P., Foulds, J., and McClain, W.H. (1974) Transfer ribonucleic acid nucleotidyl–transferase plays an essential role in the normal growth of *Escherichia coli* and in the biosynthesis of some bacteriophage T4 transfer ribonucleic acids.J Biol Chem. 249(20):6696–6699.

Hidalgo, C., Gonzalez,M.E., and Logos, R. (1983) Characterization of Ca^{2+} or Mg^{2+}–ATPase of the transverse tubule membranes isolated from rabbit skeletal muscle. J. Biol. Chem. 258: 1397–13945.

Ishii, J. and Taiji, N. (1988) Size of diffusion pore of *Alkaligenes faecalis.*Antimicrob.Agents.Chemother. 32:378–384.

Kumar, M. and Upreti, R.K. (2000) Impact of lead stress and adaptation in *E.coli.* Ecotox Envir Saf.47: 246–252.

Link, A.J., Robison, K. Church, G.M. (1997) Comparing the predicted and encoded in the genome of *E.Coli.* Electro phoresis. 18 : 1259–1313.

Lowry, O.H., Rosebrough, N.J., Farr, A.L., and Randall. R.J. (1957) Protein measurement with folin phenol reagent. J. Biol. Chem. 193: 265–275.

Miura, T., and Mizushima, S. (1969) Separation and properties of outer and cytoplasmic membranes in *Escherichia coli.*Biochim Biophys Acta.193(2):268–276.

Osborn, M.J., Gander, J.E., Parisi, E., and Carson, J. (1972) Mechinism of assembly of the outer membrane of *Salmonella typhimurium.* Isolation and characterization of cytoplasmic and outer membrane.J Biol Chem. 247(12): 3962–3972.

Pagan, P. and Macky, B. (2000) Relationship between membrane damage and cell death in pressure–treated *Escherichia coli* cells:Differences between exponential–and sationary–phase cells and variation among strains.Appl. Environ.Microbiol. 66: 2829–2834

Roe, J.H. (1955) The determination of sugar in blood and spinal fluid with anthrone reagent. J. Biol. Chem. 212: 335–343.

Weiser, M. M., (1973) Intestinal epithelial cell surface membrane glycoprotein synthesis. J. Biol. Chem., 348: 2536-2540.

Weiss, R.L., and Fraser,D. (1973) Surface structure of intact cells and spheroplast of *Pseudomonas aeruginosa*.J.Bacteriol.113: 963–968.

Witholt, B., Boekhout, M. Brock, Kingma, van Heerikhuizen and de Leij, L.(1976) An efficient and reproduciable procedure for the formation of spheroplast from variously grown *Escherichia coli.*Anal Biochem.74:160–170.

Zhu, Z. Sun, D. and Davidson, V.L. (1999) Localization of periplasmic redox proteins from *Alkaligens faecalis* by a modified general method for fractionating Gram–negative Bacteria.J.Bacteriol. 181:6540–6542.

Microbiology and Biotechnology for Sustainable Development (Ed. P.C. Jain),
CBS Publishers & Distributors, New Delhi (2004), pp. 326–333.

B-17

Characterization of Yeasts from Deteriorating Milk Based Sweets

P. K. Jain, Sarita Gupta, Avni Patel and P.C. Jain
Department of Applied Microbiology and Biotechnology
Dr. H.S. Gour Vishwavidyalaya, Sagar 470003 (M.P.)

Abstract

During a survey of spoilage microorganisms from deteriorating khoa and chhena based sweets, a total of 38 strains of different yeasts have been isolated from 25 sweet samples. These strains have been identified and tested for the assimilation, fermentation and oxidative fermentation of 11 sugars and for the production of intracellular oil, using standard methods. Almost all test strains (>95%) utilized lactose but none of these produced acid from lactose oxidation or fermentation. Most strains (>90%) produced acid from dextrose under both aerobic and anaerobic conditions. Twenty five strains produced acid from sucrose under aerobic condition while only 19 strains were found to be positive for fermentation of sucrose. Two strains of test yeasts (i.e., isolate No. 7 and 14) indicated greater production of oil in their cells while others have also found positive for oil production but with lesser amounts. In the present communication, the possible role of different yeast strains have been discussed in relation to spoilage of milk based sweets during their storage.

Key words: Yeast, milk, sweets, oxidative fermentation.

INTRODUCTION

Yeasts are known to occur in a variety of substrates depending on their nutritional behaviour (Lodder, 1970; Von Arx *et al.*, 1977). Assimilation and fermentative properties of yeasts are significant from the point of view of utilization of a variety of carbohydrate substrates in nature and also in bringing a undesirable change in the product thus making them unusable.

Khoa and chhena based sweets are rich source of carbohydrates and proteins and considered to be delicious food. These are often used on festive occassions all over India. Depending upon the water content of the product, a variety of microorganisms particularly bacteria and yeasts are expected to play important role in spoilage phenomenon of Indian sweets during storage. The fermentative properties of yeasts and their intracellular products may be the major cause for development of odour in them.(Jacob, 1996). Keeping above point in mind, present study was performed to investigate the assimilation, fermentation and oxidation of 11 different sugars by yeasts and production of intracellular oil in their cells.

MATERIALS AND METHODS

In the present study a total of 38 isolates of different yeast genera have been tested for their properties of assimilation and fermentation of 11 sugars by using methods as described by Loddar and Kreger-Van-Rij (1952) and for the production of intracellular oil (SCO) by them. The methods used are as follows :

Assimilation of carbon Source

To study the assimilation of carbohydrates, yeast nitrogen base (Himedia) 6.7 gm/100 ml distilled water (solution A)and carbohydrate solution containing carbohydrate 5 gm/1000 ml distilled water (solution B) were prepared and sterlized separately by filtration. Carbohydrate assimilation medium was then prepared by mixing 0.5 ml of solution A and 4.5 ml of solution B in a presterilized culture tube. Medium was then inoculated with a loopful suspension of test yeast isolates. The tubes were incubated at 28°C and were observed after 7 days for the growth of inoculated yeast in them.

Fermentation of sugars

To study the fermentation of sugars by isolated yeast strains oxidation/fermentation basal medium of following composition was used :

Tryptone	-	2.0 g
NaCl	-	5.0 g
Dipotassium phosphate	-	0.3 g
Bromothymol blue	-	0.08 g
Distilled water	-	1000 ml

To this composition 1.0 % carbohydrate was added as a carbon source. A 10 ml aliquot of this medium was dispensed in culture tubes and then sterlized by autoclaving. The tubes were inoculated by spore suspension of test yeast strain. One set of the inoculated tubes was kept as such to observe oxidative fermentation of sugar while in other set of culture tubes the medium was overlaid by *2.0 ml* of sterlized mineral oil to test their capability to ferment sugar anaerobically. All the tubes were then incubated at 28°C for 96 hours. After incubation the tubes were observed for a change in colour of the medium as caused by fermentation of sugar associated with a change in pH. A change in colour of the medium was recorded as positive result.

Production of oil

To observe the precense of oil within yeast cells an intracellular lipid staining technique of Burdon as followed by Venkateswaran *et al.,* (1992) was used. For this, staining solution containing 0.3% Sudan black-B in 70% ethyl alcohol was used to stain intracellular lipids. For visualizing oil globules inside the cells, the smear of each yeast isolate was heat fixed, flooded with sudan black-B solution and allowed to react for about 10-12 hours. The excess stain was drained off and the smear was rinsed with xylene and blot dried. After this it was counter stained with 0.5% saffranin for 5-10 seconds. The slide was rinsed with water and observed under microscope for presence of oil globules in the cells.

RESULTS AND DISCUSSION

The property of assimilation of different sugars has been used to differentiate species and strains of a given taxon because this property is closely related to the fermentation of sugars. All fermentable sugars are generally assimilated, however, reverse of this may not always be true.

In the present study, almost all the isolated yeast strains assimilated sucrose, sorbitol and mannose while about 90% test strains assimilated other sugars also (Table 1). Morphologically

Table 1: Assimilation of Sugars by Yeasts associated with Indian Sweets

Organism	Isolate No.	Sugars Used*										
		Lac	Suc	Dex	Fru	Mat	Sor	Mal	Xyl	Gal	Raf	Man
1	2	3	4	5	6	7	8	9	10	11	12	13
Saccharomyces	1, 3, 34, 36	+	+	+	+	+	+	+	+	+	+	+
Saccharomyces	6	+	+	+	+	+	+	+	d	d	+	+
Saccharomyces	9	W+	+	+	+	+	+	+	W+	+	-	+
Saccharomyces	15, 31	+	+	+	+	+	+	-	-	+	+	+
Saccharomyces	19	+	+	+	+	+	+	+	-	+	+	+
Saccharomyces	22	W+	+	+	+	+	+	W+	W+	+	+	+
Saccharomyces	24	-	+	-	-	+	+	-	-	+	+	+
Torulopsis	23, 30	+	+	+	+	+	+	+	-	+	+	+
Torulopsis	28	+	+	+	+	+	+	+	+	+	+	+
Schizosaccharomyces	8	+	+	+	+	+	+	+	+	+	+	+
Schizosaccharomyces	26	+	+	+	+	+	+	+	-	+	+	+
Candida –	2,10,13, 25	+	+	+	+	+	+	+	+	+	+	+
Candida	16	+	+	+	+	+	+	+	-	+	+	+
Candida	35	+	+	+	+	+	+	+	+	-	+	+
Pichia	5	+	+	+	+	+	+	+	+	+	+	+

(Contd.)

1	2	3	4	5	6	7	8	9	10	11	12	13
Pichia	17, 18, 32	+	+	+	+	+	+	+	-	+	+	+
Pichia	21	w+	+	+	+	+	+	+	-	+	+	+
Brettanomyces	4	+	+	+	+	+	+	+	+	+	+	+
Hansenula	29	+	+	+	+	+	+	+	-	+	+	+
Trichosporon	11	+	+	+	+	-	+	+	+	+	+	+
Unknown	7	+	+	+	+	+	+	+	+	+	+	+
Unknown	14,33, 37, 38	+	+	+	+	+	+	+	+	+	+	+
Unknown	12	+	+	+	+	+	+	+	+	+	w+	+
Unknown	20	w+	+	+	+	+	+	+	w+	+	+	+
Unknown	27	+	+	+	+	+	+	+	-	+	+	+

* Sugars Used: Lac, Lactose; Suc, Sucrose; Dex, Dextrose; Fru, Fructose; Mat, Mannitol; Sor, Sorbitol; Mal, Maltose; Xyl, Xylose; Gal, Galactose; Raf, Rafinose; Man, Mannose d, doubtful; w+, weak positive.

similar isolates of *Saccharomyces* have been found to be different for assimilation of lactose, dextrose, maltose, xylose and raffinose. Similarly the isolates of *Torulopsis* and *Schizosaccharomyces* responded differently for assimilation of xylose. Other test strains of *Candida* and *Pichia* were also found different in their assimilative properties for certain sugars. Properties relating to fermentation of sugars by any given taxon is considered to be a stable character and hence the isolated strains have also been tested for their fermentative properties. The data given in Table 2 indicate the oxidative fermentation of 11 sugars by isolated yeasts. Amongst the test strains none was found to produce acid from lactose while only one isolate of *Saccharomyces* (Isolate No. 31) and *Schizosaccharomyces* (Isolate No. 26) have been found positive for production of acid from mannose. Other isolates of test yeasts have also responded differently for oxidative fermentation of test sugars.

Anaerobic fermentation of sugars is another criterion for the differentiation of given taxa. The anaerobic fermentative properties of test yeasts are given in Table 3. It is interesting to note that a few isolates of *Saccharomyces* (i.e. Isolate No. 3,9, 36) failed to ferment sucrose. On the other hand one isolate of *Candida* (Isolate No. 16) was found to ferment mannitol and sorbitol anaerobically while all other isolates failed to ferment these sugars anaerobically.

Intracellular lipid production by yeasts particularly those occuring in food products is important since the fatty acids present in their cells may change the product quality during their growth under storage and may reduce the shelf life of the product concerned (Moretan, 1988). In the present study, almost all the yeast isolates were found to synthesize lipids in their cells/pseudomycelium (Table 4).

It could be concluded that assimilatory and fermentative properties of the isolated yeasts and their lipid production potential might be playing some role in the deterioration of khoa and chhena based sweets.

Table 2: Oxidative fermentation of Sugars by Yeasts associated with Indian Sweets

Organism	Isolate No.	Sugars Used*										
		Lac	Suc	Dex	Fru	Mat	Sor	Mal	Xyl	Gal	Raf	Man
Saccharomyces	1	-	+	+	+	-	-	+	+	+	+	-
Saccharomyces	3	-	-	+	+	-	-	-	-	-	-	-
Saccharomyces	6	-	+	+	+	-	-	-	-	+	+	-
Saccharomyces	9	-	-	+	+	-	-	-	-	+	-	-
Saccharomyces	15	-	+	+	+	-	-	-	-	-	-	-
Saccharomyces	19, 22	-	+	+	+	-	-	+	-	+	-	-
Saccharomyces	24	-	+	+	+	-	-	+	-	-	-	-
Saccharomyces	31	-	+	+	+	-	-	-	-	-	-	+
Saccharomyces	34	-	+	+	+	-	-	-	-	-	-	-
Saccharomyces	36	-	+	+	+	-	-	+	-	-	-	-
Torulopsis	23	-	-	+	+	-	+	-	-	-	-	-
Torulopsis	28	-	+	+	+	-	-	-	-	-	-	-
Torulopsis	30	-	-	+	+	-	-	-	-	-	-	-
Schizosaccharomyces	8	-	-	+	+	-	-	+	-	+	-	-
Schizosaccharomyces	26	-	+	+	+	-	+	+	-	-	+	+
Candida	2	-	-	+	+	-	-	+	+	-	-	-
Candida	10	-	-	+	+	-	+	+	+	+	+	-
Candida	13	-	-	+	+	-	-	-	+	+	-	-
Candida	16	-	+	+	+	+	+	+	+	+	-	-
Candida	25	-	+	+	+	-	-	+	-	-	-	-
Candida	35	-	+	+	+	+	-	-	-	-	-	-
Pichia	5	-	+	+	+	-	-	+	-	-	+	-
Pichia	17, 21	-	-	+	+	-	-	-	-	+	-	-
Pichia	18	-	-	+	+	-	-	+	-	+	-	-
Pichia	32	-	+	+	+	-	-	-	-	-	-	-
Brettanomyces	4	-	+	+	+	-	-	+	-	+	-	-
Hansenula	29	-	-	+	+	-	-	-	-	-	-	-
Trichosporon	11	-	+	+	+	-	-	-	-	+	+	-
Unknown	7	-	+	+	+	-	-	+	+	+	+	-
Unknown	12	-	-	-	-	-	-	-	+	+	-	-
Unknown	14, 20, 38	-	+	+	+	-	-	-	-	-	-	-

* Sugars Used: Lac, Lactose; Suc, Sucrose; Dex, Dextrose; Fru, Fructose; Mat, Mannitol; Sor, Sorbitol; Mal, Maltose; Xyl, Xylose; Gal, Galactose; Raf, Rafinose; Man, Mannose

Table 3: Fermentation of Sugars by Yeasts associated with Indian Sweets

Organism	Isolate No.	Sugars Used*										
		Lac	Suc	Dex	Fru	Mat	Sor	Mal	Xyl	Gal	Raf	Man
Saccharomyces	1, 19	-	+	+	+	-	-	+	+	+	-	-
Saccharomyces	3	-	-	+	-	-	-	-	-	-	-	-
Saccharomyces	6, 24	-	+	+	+	-	-	+	-	-	-	-
Saccharomyces	9	-	-	+	-	-	-	-	-	+	-	-
Saccharomyces	15, 31, 34	-	+	+	+	-	-	-	-	--	-	-
Saccharomyces	22	-	+	+	+	-	-	+	+	+	-	+
Saccharomyces	36	-	-	+	+	-	-	+	-	-	-	-
Torulopsis	23, 28, 30	-	-	+	+	-	-	-	-	-	-	-
Schizosaccharomyces	8	-	-	+	+	-	-	+	-	+	-	-
Schizosaccharomyces	26	-	+	+	+	-	-	+	-	+	+	-
Candida	2	-	-	-	-	-	-	+	-	-	-	-
Candida	10	-	+	+	-	-	-	-	-	-	-	-
Candida	13	-	+	+	+	-	-	+	+	+	+	-
Candida	16	-	+	+	+	+	+	+	+	+	-	+
Candida	25	-	+	+	+	-	-	+	+	+	-	-
Candida	35	-	-	+	+	-	-	-	-	-	-	+
Pichia	5	-	+	+	+	-	-	-	-	-	-	-
Pichia	17, 18, 21	-	-	+	+	-	-	-	-	+	-	-
Pichia	32	-	+	+	+	-	-	-	-	-	-	+
Brettanomyces	4	-	+	+	+	-	-	+	+	+	-	-
Hansenula	29	-	+	+	+	-	-	-	-	-	-	-
Trichosporon	11	-	+	+	+	-	-	-	-	-	+	-
Unknown	7	-	+	+	-	-	-	+	-	+	-	-
Unknown	12	-	-	+	-	-	-	+	-	-	-	+
*Unknown***	14, 27, 37	-	-	-	-	-	-	-	-	-	-	-
Unknown	20, 33	-	-	+	+	-	-	-	-	-	-	-
Unknown	38	-	-	+	+	-	-	+	-	-	-	-

* Sugars Used*:* Lac, Lactose; Suc, Sucrose; Dex, Dextrose; Fru, Fructose; Mat, Mannitol; Sor, Sorbitol; Mal, Maltose; Xyl, Xylose; Gal, Galactose; Raf, Rafinose; Man, Mannose

** Only partial fermentation of all sugars shown by Isolate 14, 27, 37.

In order to increase shelf life of the products, both yeast and bacterial growth should be prevented on the finished product. The possibility of using bacteriocins for this purpose is of immense value (Klaenchammer 1988, 1993; Daba et. al. 1991) and hence further investigations on these lines are required to yield desirable results.

Table 4: Presence of Intracellular oil globules in cells

Organism	Isolate No.	Oil globules in cells*	Organism	Isolate No.	Oil globules in cells*
Saccharomyces	1	+++	*Candida*	16	++
Saccharomyces	3	++	*Candida*	25	++
Saccharomyces	6	++	*Candida*	35	+++
Saccharomyces	9	++	*Pichia*	5	+++
Saccharomyces	15	+	*Pichia*	17	+++
Saccharomyces	19	++	*Pichia*	21	+
Saccharomyces	22	+	*Pichia*	18	+++
Saccharomyces	24	+++	*Pichia*	32	++
Saccharomyces	31	+++	*Brettanomyces*	4	+
Saccharomyces	34	+++	*Trichosporon*	11	++
Saccharomyces	36	++	*Unknown*	7	++++
Torulopsis	28	+	*Unknown*	12	+
Torulopsis	30	+++	*Unknown*	14	++++
Schizosaccharomyces	8	+++	*Unknown*	27	+
Schizosaccharomyces	26	++	*Unknown*	33	++
Candida	2	++	*Unknown*	37	++
Candida	13	+++	*Unknown*	38	+++

*Presence of intracellular oil globules in cells :- + Poor, ++ Fair, +++ Good, ++++ Excellent

ACKNOWLEDGEMENT

Authors are thankful to Prof. S.C. Agrawal, Head, Department of Applied Microbiology and Biotechnology, for providing laboratory facilities and encouragement.

REFERENCES

Daba, H.S., Pandian, J.F., Gossolin, R.E., Huang, S.J., and Lacroix, C. (1991). Detection and activity of a bacteriocin produced by *Leuconostoc mesenteroides.* Appl. Environ. Microbiol. 57:3450-3455.

Jacob, Z.(1996). Yeast lipid biotechnology. In, Advances in Applied Microbiology. Vol. 39. Academic Press. Inc. p.185-213.

Klaenchammer, T.R. (1988). Bacteriocins of lactic acid bacteria. Biochemec. 70:337-349.

Klaenchammer, T.R. (1993). Genetics of bacteriocins produced by lactic acid bacteria. FEMS Microbiol Rev. 12:39-87.

Lodder, J. and Kreger-Van-Rij, N.J.W. (1952) The Yeasts. A Taxonomic Study, Interscience North Holland Publishing Company, Amsterdam Publishers, Inc. New York. pp. 713.

Lodder, J. (1970) The Yeast, A Texonomic Study. North Holland Publishing Company, Amsterdam, pp.1385.

Moreton, R.S. (1988). Physiology of lipid accumulating yeasts. In, Single Cell Oil (*Ed.* Moreton R.S.) Harlow Longman Scientific and Technical press, pp. 1-32.

Venkateswaran, G., Shashi, K. and Joseph, R. (1992). Influence of nitrogen status and mutation on the fatty acid profile of *Rhodotorula gracilis.*, Current Science 62 (8): pp. 580-582.

Von Arx J. A., Rodrigues de Miranda, L., Smith, M. and Yarrow, D. (1977). The Genera of Yeast and Yeast Like Fungi, Centraalbureau Voor Schimmelcultures, Baarn, The Netherlands, pp. 42.

Microbiology and Biotechnology for Sustainable Development (Ed. P.C. Jain),
CBS Publishers & Distributors, New Delhi (2004), pp. 334–342.

B-18

Oxidation and Fermentative Properties of some Bacteria Associated with Spices

Amita Shrivastava and P.C. Jain*
Department of Botany, Dr. H.S. Gour Vishwavidyalaya, Sagar-470003 M.P.
**Deptt of Applied Microbiology & Biotechnology, Dr. H.S. Gour Vishwavidyalaya, Sagar 470003 M.P.*

Abstract

Indian spices are widely used in perfumery and cosmetics, medicines and food preparations. Hence examination of microbial contaminants associated with them is important from commercial and health point of views. Contaminating microorganisms may spoil them by utilization of active ingredients present in spices or may cause toxicity of various nature. A survey of storage fungi from six spices was conducted and fungi were isolated using standard methods. During enumeration of fungal contaminants a few samples yielded some bacteria. These bacteria were isolated, purified and tested for their oxidative and fermentative properties using API CH-50 strips (Bio-Merieux Sa, France). The tests were conducted as per the instructions of the manufacturer of API CH-50 strips. This test allows the study of production of acid by fermentation and oxidation of 49 carbohydrates.

In the present investigation almost all the test bacteria utilized and assimilated L-arabinose, ribose, D-xylose, D-fructose, D-arabitol and gluconate. However, test bacteria differ greatly in their ability to produce acid by oxidation and fermentation of different carbohydrates. The results are discussed in relation to their medical and commercial importance.

Key words: Spices, bacteria, oxidation, fermentation, sugars.

INTRODUCTION

The spices are herbs and their products which are commonly used to develop flavour and taste in various foods. Similar to other organic materials the association of microorganism with them is natural and constant. In a survey, a number of fungi have been isolated from six spices (Shrivastava and Jain 1992; 1993). During isolation of fungi some strains of bacteria have also been collected.

The spices are being used world wide in perfumery and cosmetics, medicines, in food preparations and food preservation etc. Some of the spices are used in the form of crude powder and hence the consumers are consuming the associated microflora also, which may effect the health of consumers adversely and hence the isolated bacterial strains have been tested for their assimilatory and fermentative properties of 49 carbohydrates using API 50 CH test Strips (Bio-Merieux Sa, France).

MATERIALS AND METHODS

In the present study carbohydrate metabolism of 7 bacterial strains have been studied by using API 50 CH testing system (Bio-Merieu Sa, France) The details of the materials and methods are as follows:

PREPARATION OF INOCULUM

Seven strains of bacteria i.e., M-1, M-2, M-3, M-5, M-6, M-7 and M-9 were isolated from spices (Shrivastava, 1993) and were used in the present study. The test strains were grown on nutrient agar medium (Peptone, 5.0g; NaCl, 5.0g; Beef extract, 3.0g in 1000 ml distilled water) for 48 hours at 37°$\pm$1°C and spore suspension was prepared in Hugh and Leifson's fermentation medium which contained Peptone, 2.0g; NaCl, 5.0g; K_2HPO_4, 0.3g; Neutral red, 0.025g as pH indicator in 1000 ml distilled water. So prepared bacterial suspension was used as inoculum to study production of acid by oxidative fermentation and assimilation of 49 carbohydrates by test bacteria.

API 50 CH TEST STRIPS

It consists of 50 microtubes each containing an anaerobic zone (the tube portion) for the study of fermentation, and an aerobic zone (the cupule portion), for the study of oxidation and assimilation.

PREPARATION OF THE STRIP

Complete strip is made up of 5 small strips (No. 1 to 5), each containing 10 numbered tubes. The strips are incubated in a honey combed incubation tray, which serves as a support and individual incubator. The lid protects it from contaminants in the air assuring the humid atmosphere necessary to avoid dehydration of strips during the incubation period. In the honey combed base tray, about 10.00 ml of distilled water was dispended to maintain humidity during incubation period. The API 50 CH test strips were then placed in the tray. Bacterial suspension was then filled in each tube with the help of sterile Pasteur pipette. The tubes were completely filled following the instructions of the manufacturer. After inoculation the tray was covered with the lid and incubated at 37°$\pm$1°C. These were observed after 48 hours for change of colour in cupule tubes indicating oxidative fermentation of sugars and for the growth of test bacteria as a result of assimilation of sugar.

RESULTS AND DISCUSSION

The results of carbohydrate metabolism of 49 sugars by 7 test bacterial strains (i.e., M-1, M-2, M-3, M-5, M-6, M-7 and M-9) are presented in Table 1 and 2. The details of assimilation and oxidative fermentation of different carbohydrates by test bacteria are as follows:

Table 1: Assimilation of different Carbohydrates by some spice contaminating bacteria.

Tube No.	Carbo-hydrate	Incubation time (hours) at 37ºC																				
		Strain M-1			Strain M-2			Strain M-3			Strain M-5			Strain-6			Strain M-7			Strain M-9		
		6	24	48	6	24	48	6	24	48	6	24	48	6	24	48	6	24	48	6	24	48
1	2	3	4	5	6	7	8	9	10	11	12	13	14	15	16	17	18	19	20	21	22	23
0	Control	-	-	-	-	-	-	-	-	-	-	-	-	-	-	-	-	-	-	-	-	-
1	Glycerol	-	+	+	-	+	+	-	+	+	-	-	-	-	+	+	-	+	+	-	+	+
2	Erythritol	-	-	+	-	-	+	-	+	+	-	-	-	-	-	+	-	-	+	-	+	+
3	D-Arabinose	-	-	-	-	-	-	-	-	+	-	-	-	-	-	+	-	-	-	-	-	-
4	L-Arabinose	-	-	+	-	-	+	-	+	+	-	-	+	-	-	+	-	-	+	-	-	+
5	Ribose	-	+	+	-	+	+	-	+	+	-	+	+	-	-	+	-	-	+	-	+	+
6	D-Xylose	-	+	+	-	+	+	-	+	+	-	+	+	+	+	+	-	-	+	-	-	+
7	L-Xylose	-	+	+	-	-	-	-	-	-	-	-	+	-	-	-	-	-	-	-	-	-
8	Adonitol	-	+	+	-	-	-	-	-	-	-	-	-	+	+	+	-	-	-	-	-	+
9	β-menthyl-xyloside	-	-	-	-	-	-	-	+	+	-	+	+	+	+	+	-	-	-	-	-	-
10	Galactose	-	-	-	-	+	+	-	+	+	-	-	+	+	+	+	-	-	+	-	+	+
11	D-Glucose	-	-	+	-	+	+	-	+	+	-	-	-	+	+	+	-	+	+	-	-	-
12	D-Fructose	-	-	+	-	+	+	-	+	+	-	+	+	+	+	+	-	-	+	-	+	+
13	D-Mannose	-	-	-	-	+	+	-	+	+	-	+	+	+	+	+	-	-	+	-	+	+
14	L-Sorbose	-	-	-	-	-	-	-	-	-	-	-	-	-	-	-	-	-	-	-	-	-
15	Rhamnose	-	+	+	-	-	-	-	-	-	-	+	+	+	+	+	-	-	-	-	-	-
16	Dulcitol	-	+	+	-	-	-	-	-	-	-	+	+	-	-	-	-	-	-	-	-	-
17	Inositol	-	+	+	-	+	+	-	-	+	-	-	+	+	+	+	-	-	-	-	+	+
18	Mannitol	-	+	+	-	+	+	-	+	+	-	+	+	+	+	+	-	-	-	-	+	+
19	Sorbitol	-	+	+	-	+	+	-	+	+	-	-	+	+	+	+	-	-	-	-	+	+
20	α-Methyl-D-mannoside	-	-	+	-	+	-	-	-	-	-	-	-	-	-	-	-	-	-	-	-	-
21	α-Methyl-D-glucoside	-	-	+	-	+	-	-	-	-	-	-	-	-	-	-	-	-	-	-	-	-
22	N-Acetyl glucosamine	-	-	+	-	+	+	-	+	+	-	-	-	+	+	+	-	-	+	-	-	+
23	Amygdaline	-	-	+	-	+	+	-	+	+	-	+	+	-	-	-	-	-	-	-	-	+
24	Arbutine	-	-	+	-	+	+	-	+	+	-	-	-	-	-	-	-	-	-	-	-	-

(Contd.)

1	2	3	4	5	6	7	8	9	10	11	12	13	14	15	16	17	18	19	20	21	22	23
25	Esculine	-	-	+	-	+	-	-	-	+	-	-	-	-	-	-	-	-	-	-	+	+
26	Salicine	-	-	+	-	-	+	-	+	+	-	-	+	-	-	-	-	-	-	-	-	-
27	Cellobiose	-	-	+	-	+	+	-	+	+	-	+	+	-	+	+	-	-	-	-	-	+
28	Maltose	-	-	+	-	+	+	-	+	+	-	+	+	-	+	+	-	-	-	-	+	+
29	Lactose	-	-	+	-	+	+	-	+	+	-	-	-	-	-	-	-	-	-	-	-	-
30	Melibiose	-	-	+	-	+	+	-	+	+	-	-	-	-	-	-	-	-	-	-	-	-
31	Saccharose	-	-	+	-	+	+	-	+	+	-	-	-	-	+	+	-	-	-	-	+	+
32	Trehalose	-	-	+	-	+	+	-	+	+	-	+	+	-	+	+	-	-	-	-	-	+
33	Insuline	-	-	-	-	-	-	-	-		-	-	+	-	-	-	-	-	-	-	-	-
34'	Melezitose	-	-	-	-	-	-	-	-	+	-	+	+	-	-	-	-	-	-	-	-	-
35	D-Raffinose	-	-	-	-	-	+	-	+	+	-	+	+	-	-	-	-	-	-	-	-	-
36	Amldon	-	-	+	-	+	+	-	+	+	-	-	-	-	-	+	-	-	-	-	+	+
37	Glycogene	-	-	-	-	-	+	-	+	+	-	+	+	-	-	-	-	-	-	-	-	-
38	Xylitol	-	-	-	-	-	-	-	-	-	-	-	-	-	-	+	-		-	-	+	+
39	β-Gentiniose	-	-	+	-	+	+		+	+	-	+	+	-	-	-	-	-	-	-	-	-
40	D-Turanose	-	-	+	-	+	+	-	+	+	-	-	-	-	-	-	-	-	-	-	-	-
41	D-Lyxose	-	-	+	-		+	-	-	-	-	-	-	-	-	+	-	-	-	-	-	-
42	D-Tagetose	-	-	+	-	-	-	-	-	-	-	-	-	-	-	-	-	+	+	-	-	-
43	D-Fucose	-	-	+	-	-	-	-	-	-	-	-	-	-	-	-	-	+	+	-	-	-
44	L-Fucose	-	-	+	-	-	+	-	+	+	-	-	-	-	-	+	-	+	+	-	-	-
45	D-Arabitol	-	-	+	-	-	+	-	+	+	-	+	+	-	-	+	-	-	+	-	+	+
46	L-Arabitol	-	-	-	-	-	+	-	+	+	-	-	+	-	-	+	-	-	+	-	-	+
47	Gluconate	-	+	+	-	+	+	-	+	+	-	+	+	-	-	+	-	+	+	-	+	+
48	2-Ceto-gluconate	-	+	+	-	-	-	-	+	+	-	-	+	-	-	+	-	+	+	-	-	-
49	5-Ceto-gluconate	-	+	+	-	-	-	-	+	+	-	-	-	-	-	+	-	+	+	-	-	-

+, Assimilation of carbohydrates; -, No visible growth

Fermentation of carbohydrates

The results of the acid production by metabolism of different sugars are given in Table 2. D-glucose fermentation was noted in almost all the test bacteria after 6 and 24 hours of incubation at 37°C. However, the colour produced in the medium by the production of acids was found depleting in some cases when the incubation period was increased to 48 hours. All the test bacteria except strain M-9 also caused acid production in 24 hours of incubation by fermentation of D-fucose. However, strain M-9 indicated acid production by D-fucose only after 48 hours. Strain M-1 was found to ferment only 7 carbohydrates out of 49 tested by API 50 CH test strip. Strain M-6 was found to ferment maximum number of carbohydrates, i.e., 29 out of 49 tested. Strain M-2, M-3, M-5, M-7 and M-9 were found to ferment 10, 22, 17, 7 and 23 carbohydrates, respectively. Strain M-2 was found to produce acid by the metabolism of glucose quickly as pink colour was observed both in tube and cupule portion after 6 hours incubation period while fermentation of ribose, D-fructose, salicine and D-fucose to acids was observed after an incubation of 24 hours. Acid production by the metabolism of D-xylose, and L-arabitol by this strain was recorded after 48 hours incubation period in both anaerobic and aerobic zone of the tubes. Acid production by this strain as a result of metabolism of D-mannose and amldon was also noted but only in tube portion. Strain M-3 was found to ferment maximum number of sugars under test. It was found to ferment 22 carbohydrates, i.e., glycerol, L-arabinose, ribose, D-xylose, galactose, D-glucose, D-fructose, D-mannose, mannitol, sorbitol, N-acetyl glucosamine, cellobiose, maltose, lactose, melibiose, saccharose, trehalose, D-raffinose, amldon, glycogen, D-fucose and D-arabitol in both cupule and tube portion after 24 hours incubation period. Acid production by the metabolism of amygdaline was noted in cupule portion thus indicating oxidation of this carbohydrate by strain M-3.

Table 2: Metabolism of different Carbohydrate and Production of Acid* by some Spice Contaminating Bacteria.

Tube No.	Carbo-hydrate	Incubation time (hours) at 37°C																				
		Strain M-1			Strain M-2			Strain M-3			Strain M-5			Strain-6			Strain M-7			Strain M-9		
		6	24	48	6	24	48	6	24	48	6	24	48	6	24	48	6	24	48	6	24	48
1	2	3	4	5	6	7	8	9	10	11	12	13	14	15	16	17	18	19	20	21	22	23
0	Control																					
1	Glycerol								CT			CT			CT			CT			CT	T
2	Erythritol																					T
3	D-Arabinose															T						
4	L-Arabinose								CT				CT									
5	Ribose					CT	CT		CT							CT				CT	T	T
6	D-Xvlose		T	CT		T	CT		CT	CT		CT	CT			CT		CT			C	CT
7	L-Xylose																					
8	Adonitol														T	T						
9	β-menthyl-xyloside																					
10	Galactose								CT						CT			CT				
11	D-Glucose		CT	C	CT	T			CT		T	CT	T		CT		C	CT		T	CT	T
12	D-Fructose					CT			CT	T					CT			CT		T	CT	T
13	D-Mannose								CT	CT	T	CT	CT		CT			CT		T	CT	T
14	L-Sorbose																			T	T	T
15	Rhamnose											CT	T		CT							

(Contd.)

1	2	3	4	5	6	7	8	9	10	11	12	13	14	15	16	17	18	19	20	21	22	23
16	Dulcitol											CT	T									
17	Inositol														T	T					CT	T
18	Mannitol			CT	T				CT			CT	CT		CT					CT	CT	T
19	Sorbitol				CT				CT						CT						CT	T
20	α-Methyl-D-mannoside																					
21	α-Methyl-D-glucoside																					
22	N-Acetyl glucosamine								CT		T	CT		T	T					CT	T	
23	Amygdaline										C		T									
24	Arbutine										T					T		T	C	CT	T	
25	Esculine																					
26	Salicine										T					T				T	T	
27	Cellobiose								CT	CT		CT										
28	Maltose								CT	CT	T	CT	T	T	CT					T	CT	T
29	Lactose								CT	CT			T	T	T							
30	Melibiose								CT			CT	T							T		
31	Saccharose								CT						C		C			T	T	T
32	Trehalose								CT		T	CT			T		C			T	T	T
33	Insuline									CT					T							
34	Melezitose																					
35	D-Raffinose								T													
36	Amidon						T		CT							T						T
37	Glycogene								CT			T										
38	Xylitol								C							CT						T
39	β-Gentiniose			T												T						
40	D-Turanose																					
41	D-Lyxose					C	T									CT						
42	D-Tagetose																					
43	D-Fucose		CT	CT		CT	CT		CT	CT		CT	CT		CT	CT		CT	CT			CT
44	L-Fucose															CT						
45	D-Arabitol								T						T	T						
46	L-Arabitol						CT		C						C	T					T	
47	Gluconate		T											C	C						T	T
48	2-Ceto-gluconate																					
49	5-Ceto-gluconate																					

* Production acid, C – in Cupule, T – in Tube, CT – in both Cupule and Tube.

Strain M-5 was found to produce acid by the metabolism of 17 different carbohydrates. It was found to ferment 4 sugars i.e., amygdaline, arbutine, salicine and glycogen only in tube portion. While acid production by metabolism of other 13 carbohydrates was noted both in tube and cupule. Acid production by fermentation of arbutine and salicine was recorded after 6 hours, while fermentation of amygdaline and glycogen was noted after 24 hours. It is interesting that initially this bacterium produce acid from D-glucose, D-mannose, N-acetyl glucosamine, maltose and trehalose in anaerobic zone but later indicated the production of acid(s) in both the zones i.e., aerobic and anaerobic (Table 2).

The strain M-6 was found to produce acid by metabolism of 30 sugars. However, production of acid by metabolism of D-xylose, adonitol, inositol, N-acetyl glucosamine, arbutine, salicine, cellobiose, trehalose, amldon, B-gentiobiose and L-arabitol was noted in anaerobic zone of the inoculated tube with this test strain.

Fermentation of erythritol, galactose, salicine, melibiose, saccharose, trehalose, amldon, xylitol, gluconate, 5-ceto-gluconate was observed in anaerobic zone when the strips were inoculated with strain M-9. In addition to these this bacterium also produced acids by metabolism of 13 other carbohydrates.

Assimilation of carbohydrates

A perusal of the data indicates that almost all the bacteria utilized and assimilated L-arabinose, ribose, D-xylose, D-fructose, D-arabitol and gluconate (Table 1). Almost all test bacterial strains except strain M-3 utilized L-arabinose very slowly as indicated by the appearance of bacterial growth in the test cupule after 48 hours of incubation. Bacterial strain M-7 utilized only 18 carbohydrates out of 49 tested. Bacterial strain M-1 was found most efficient for utilization of different test carbohydrates as sole carbon source. It was found to assimilate 38 carbohydrates out of 49 tested (Table 1). Next to this, strain M-3 showed its efficiency to utilize 37 carbohydrates as sole carbon source. Other test strains of bacteria, i.e., M-2, M-5, M-6 and M-9 were found to assimilate 33, 27, 30 and 24 different carbohydrates, respectively. Utilization of D-arabinose was recorded by strain M-3 and strain M-6 only. Utilization of inuline as sole source of carbon was recorded by test strain M-1 and M-5, while melezitose was utilized and assimilated by strain M-3 and M-5. Assimilation of D-tagetose and D-fucose was recorded by strain M-1 and M-7. Amongst the test strains of bacteria, strain M-6 was found to posses high metabolic potential as it utilized and assimilated most of the sugars within 6 hours of incubation and produced visible turbidity in the test cupules.

In some of the cases the test organisms indicated acid production during early incubation i.e., 6-24 hours but no positive reaction for acid was noted when observations were made after 48 hours. Depletion of the acids in late incubation may be (i.e. 48 hours) due to the metabolism of acids to the acetoin (acetyl methylacarbinol) by the bacteria. This compound does not produce acid reactions. Most of the bacteria produced acid both in cupule and tube portion. Thus indicating both the oxidative and partial fermentative metabolism of different carbohydrates to acids. However, such organisms do not come in the category of obligate anaerobes. In fact, most genera of aerobic bacteria have been reported to have the capacity to oxidize and ferment carbohydrates (Cheesbrough, 1984). But these bacteria indicate very slow production of acid, hence, requiring a long incubation period. In addition to this the fermentative organisms also have the capacity to utilize carbohydrates both in the presence of oxygen and in absence of the oxygen.

For test organisms, as being inhabitants of spices, it is quite possible that these may get entry into human digestive system through various food items in which the spices are used to develop taste and flavour. However, their role in the development of enteric diseases in human beings is a subject of investigation. In the present study spice contaminating strains of bacteria were found capable to produce acids by the oxidation and/or fermentation of various carbohydrates thus their role in imparting gastric disorders can be assumed.

Species have been regarded as food preservatives and anti-oxidant (Zaika *et al.*, 1978). In addition to this a number of spices have also been found effective in retarding rancidity during frozen storage of group pork and beef, and pork sausage (Dubois and Tressler, 1934; Atkinson *et al.*, 1947; Chipault *et al.*, 1956). The spices are also known for antimicrobial properties (Corran and Edgar, 1933; Fabian *et al.*, 1939; Webb and Tanner, 1945; Dold and Knapp, 1948; Bullerman, 1974; Beuchat, 1976). Above studies suggested that the spices constitute one or more antimicrobial substances in them. Association of bacterial contaminants with spices, hence, indicates the presence of some resistance factors in spice contaminating micro-organism, which support the survival of these micro-organism on spices.

It is a common observation that the intake of spicy food generally cause more gas and acid production in human beings, whether these health disorders are by the chemical constituents of spices or by the micro-organism which are associated with them is a subject of investigation. Some investigations on spices suggest that the spices have some common component, which induce the fermentative activity of the micro-organisms such as *Pediococcus cerevisiae* (Zaika *et al.*, 1978; Zaika and Kissinger, 1984), some Micrococci (Salzer *et al.*, 1977) and yeast (Corran and Edgar, 1933; Wright *et al.*, 1954). However, at this juncture it is difficult to conclude, whether, spices alone can cause the gastric disorders in human beings by inhibiting or stimulating the activities of enteric microflora which help the digestion process or the spice associated micro-organisms in the presence of spices, are producing health disorders by the production of acids and gases of varied nature.

ACKNOWLEDGEMENT

The authors are thankful to Head Department of Botany, Dr. H.S. Gour Vishwavidyalaya, Sagar for laboratory facilities and Prof. S.C. Agrawal for encouragement. Senior author (AS) is thankful to Directorate General Health Service, New Delhi, for award of JRF.

REFERENCES

Atkinson, I., Cecil, S. R. and Woodroof, J.G. (1947). Extending keeping quality of frozen pork sausage. *Food Ind.* 19: 1198.

Beuchat, L.R. (1976). Sensitivity of *Vibrio parahaemolyticus* to spices and organic acids. *J. Food Sci.*, 41: 899.

Bullerman, L.B. (1974). Inhibition of Aflatoxin production by cinnamon. *J. Food Sci.*, 39: 1163-1165.

Cheesbrough, Monica (1984). Medical Laboratory Manual for Tropical Countries Vol. II: Microbiology. Butterworth and Co. (Publisher) Ltd. Kent, U.K.

Chipault, J.R., Mizuno, G.R. and Lundberg, W.O. (1956). The antioxidant properties of spices in foods. *Food Technol.,* 10: 209.

Corran, J.W. and Edger. S.H. (1933). Preservative action of spices and related compounds against yeast fermentation. *J. Soc. Chem. Ind.,* 52: 149-152 I.

Dold, H. and Knapp, A. (1948). The antibacterial action of spices. *Z. Hyg. Infektionskrankh,* 128 : 696 (*Chem. Absr.*, 47: 9419a (1953).

Dubois, C.W. and Tressler, D.K. (1934). Seasonings, their effect on maintenance of quality in storage of frozen ground pork and beff. *Proc. Inst. Food Technol.*, 202 (*Chem. Absr.,* 38: 6410).

Fabian F.W., Krehl, C.F. and Little, N.W. (1939). The role of spices in pickled food spoilage. *Food Res,* 4: 269.

Salzer, U.J., Broker, V., Klie, H.F. and Liepe, H.U. (1977). Wirkung von pfefler and pfefferinhaltss toffen aufdie mikroflora von. Wurstwaren. *Fleischwirtschaft.* 57 : 2011.

Shrivastava, Amita and Jain, P.C. (1992). Seed mycoflora of some spices. *J. Fd. Sci. Technol.,* 29(4): 228-230.

Shrivastava, Amita and Jain P.C. (1993). Biochemical characteristics of some Bacteria isolated from Indian Spices. Proc. 80th Ind. Sc., Cong Goa, part IV (Late Abstracts), Sec. Botany Abstract No. 45, p. 121.

Webb A.H. and Tanner, F.W. (1945). Effect of spices and flavouring materials on growth of yeasts. *Food Res.,* 10: 273.

Wright, W. J., Bice C.W. and Fogelberg, J.M. (1954). The effect of spices on yeast fermentation. *Cereal Chem.,* 31: 100.

Zaika, L.L. and Kissinger, J.C. (1984): Fermentation enhancement by spices: Identification of active component. *J. Food Sci.,* 49: 5-9.

Zaika, L.L., Zell, T.E., Palumbo, S.A. and Smith, J.L., (1978). Effect of spices and salt on fermentation of Lebanon bologna-type sausage. *J. Food Sci.,* 43: 186-190.

Microbiology and Biotechnology for Sustainable Development (Ed. P.C. Jain)
CBS Publishers & Distributors, New Delhi (2004), pp. 343–346.

B-19

Field Evaluation of Chloramphenicol as an Agriculture Fungicide against Betelvine *Phytophthora* Diseases

J.P. Chaurasia
Plant Pathology Laboratory, Department of Botany,
Dr. H.S. Gour Vishwavidyalaya, Sagar (MP) 470 003 India

Abstract

Field evaluation of chloramphenicol was conducted for the control of devastating foot rot and leaf rot of Piper betel caused by Phytophthora parasitica var. piperina.

As foliar spray in the field all the concentrations of this antibiotic showed remarkable fungitoxic effect even at very low concentration and reduced lesion development effectively. 500ppm concentration appeared to be highly fungitoxic to the test pathogen with 100% control of disease under field condition. The concentration of chloramphenicol used did not change quality, colour, aroma, and taste of the betel leaves. Interestingly, the net profit and yield also increased by the application of this fungicide @ 500 ppm concentration (150 gm/ha.).

This is the first report of using the chloramphenicol against foot rot and leaf rot diseases of Piper betle.

Key Words: Field evaluation, Antibiotic, *Piper betel, Phytophthora parasitica* var. *piperina*, Foot rot and Leaf rot diseases.

INTRODUCTION

Betel vine (*Piper betel* L.) is a well-known aromatic medicinal cash crop of India with approximate turn over of about 1,64,500 crores rupees per year. It provides livelihood to millions of families engaged in its cultivation and trade. It is exported to several countries and is a valuable foreign exchange earner. It has got immense ethnic, religious, social, medicinal, industrial and economic importance.

Foot rot and leaf rot caused by fungus *Phytophthora parasitica* var. *piperina* happens to be the most severe and devastating disease in all the betel vine growing areas. It causes 40 to 100% loss when the attack is of severe nature. Under these circumstances the cultivators are forced to change over to other profession for their livelihood. Hence, management of betel vine *Phytophthora* disease has been the subject of immense and active research interest.

Normally, betel vine crop is a money crop and successful cultivation yield give very large returns. Looking to the magnitude of the disease problems various workers have made very sincere efforts and used chemical based fungicides and pesticides for its management (Tiwari, 1968; Vyas and Chaurasia, 1976; Madhadevan, 1982; Shrivastava, 1985; Chaurasia, 1995, 1996, 1998, 1999, 2001). Since, chemical based fungicides are possessing mammalian and phytotoxicity, there seems a need of some alternative biological compound to control *Phytophthora* diseases of this crop.

In the present investigation Chloramphenicol has been used as an alternative agriculture fungicide for its practical application to control *Phytophthora* diseases of betel vine.

MATERIAL AND METHODS

Chloramphenicol is water soluble substance produced by *Streptomyces venzualae*. Chemically it is a Nitrobenzene derivative of dichloracetic acid. It is broad spectrum antibiotic used for treating plant pathogenic bacteria but its activity against the fungus *Phytophthora parasitica* var. *piperina* has not been investigated.

A field trial of chloramphanicol was conducted during March 2001 (Tilli Village Sagar) against foot rot and leaf rot diseases. Six concentrations (50,100,250,500,1000 and 2000 ppm) of this antibiotic were prepared and evaluated against the lesion development under field condition using foliar spray. For each concentration a separate plot was used. Drug was sprayed once on the crop. The control plot was sprayed with water. The development of lesion was recorded in control and treated plants separately, every 24 hours upto 6 days, the percent efficacy over control was calculated at 24 hours interval upto 144 hours of sprays.

Field trial of test antibiotic was conducted in local Bareja (a plot of field with diffused sunlight) on naturally growing crop for which a test plot and a control plot were taken side by side.

RESULTS AND DISCUSSION

All the tested concentrations of chloramphenicol were found effective in the reduction of disease severity. Data regarding the fungitoxicity of chloramphenicol in terms of percentage efficacy of disease control are presented in Table 1. About 41%, 53% and 76% reduction in leaf rot infection was observed at 50, 100 and 250 ppm concentration, respectively. A complete control of leaf rot development was observed at 500 ppm concentration of this antibiotic. Kachhwaha (1993) has also reported inhibitory effect of chloramphenicol on development of fruit rot of Alubukhara and Grape caused by *Coniella granati* and *Geotrichum candidum*.

Chloramphenicol inhibits protein synthesis by binding to the 50S ribosomal subunit and blocking the peptide transferase of the amino acid from S-RNA to ribosome (Malik, 1972). It may also have a direct inhibitory effect on peptidyl transferase and termination. It increases the uptake of transport of organic molecules in host plants (Crowdy *et al.*, 1950). Chaurasia (1995) has reported antifungal activity and possible mode of action of chloramphenicol against *Phytophthora parasitica* var. *piperina.* It has been found to be non-mutagenic, non-carcinogenic and non-phytotoxic when applied at a rate of 500-ppm concentration. According to Thirumalachar (1973) and Thirumalachar *et al.*, (1973) it may stimulate the growth of the host plant. Chloramphenicol inhibit nucleic acids metabolism of *Phytophthora parasitica* var. *piperina.* It may effect the expansion of cotyledons of *Piper betle* in light and in the presence of kinetin. It has been observed that this antibiotic increases the host resistance against the disease-causing organism (Chaurasia, 1995). Further, its foliar spray in the field at a concentration of 500 ppm did not change quality, colour aroma and taste of betel leaves.

Table 1: Effect of Chloramphenicol on the Leaf rot (lesions) development of Betel vine caused by *Phytophthora parasitica* var. *piperina* under field conditions

Observation time (Hours)	Diameter of rotten (lesions) area (mm) of treated plant Concentration (ppm) treated							Percent Efficacy over control Concentration (ppm) treated					
	Control	50	100	250	500	1000	2000	50	100	250	500	1000	2000
24	12.0	6.0	0.0	0.0	0.0	0.0	0.0	50.0	100	100	100	100	100
48	14.0	8.0	6.0	0.0	0.0	0.0	0.0	42.8	57.1	100	100	100	100
72	19.0	10.0	8.0	6.0	0.0	0.0	0.0	47.3	57.8	68.4	100	100	100
96	24.0	12.0	10.0	7.0	0.0	0.0	0.0	50.0	58.3	70.8	100	100	100
120	30.0	18.0	13.0	8.0	0.0	0.0	0.0	40.0	56.6	73.3	100	100	100
144	43.0	25.0	20.0	10.0	0.0	0.0	0.0	41.8	53.4	76.7	100	100	100

Each datum given in Table is an average of three replicates.

The use of antibiotics as agricultural fungicides for the control of plant diseases is gaining attention of many farmers may be because of their biological origin. It is the first report on use of chloramphenicol as a field fungicide for the control of *Piper betle* diseases caused by fungus *Phytophthora parasitica* var. *piperina.* It is water-soluble and hence its translocation all over the plant body is quite rapid. The application of chloramphenicol is not only a cheap alternative for betel vine diseases but also helps in maintaining the crop yield.

Further work on the use of chloramphenicol as agriculture fungicide is required to broaden its application on other crops particularly those affected by bacterial and fungal pathogens.

ACKNOWLDGEMENT

Author is grateful to Prof. K. M. Vyas, Head Department of Botany, Dr. A. S. Mishra, Reader, Department of Botany and Hari Sankar Chaurasia, Dr. H.S. Gour Vishwavidyalaya, Sagar (M.P.) 470 003 India, for providing necessary Laboratory and Field facilities.

REFERENCE

Chaurasia, S.C.(1976). Studies on foot rot and leaf rot diseases of pan (*Piper betle* L.) with special reference to pathogenesis and control measures. Ph.D. Thesis, University of Sagar.

Chaurasia, J.P. (1995). Studies on the management of Betel vine *Phytophthora* diseases in Sagar Division. Ph.D. Thesis, University of Sagar.

Chaurasia, J.P. (1996). Effect of hepar sulph. on betel vine *Phytophthora* diseases. Madhya Bharti Jouranl 36 A-40B, PP, 65-71.

Chaurasia, J.P. (1998). Management of Betel vine *Phytophthora* disease by homoeodrugs : A novel approach, (Abs) XIII M.P. Young Scientist Congress, Gwalior, P. 24-25.

Chaurasia, J.P. (1997). In vitro evaluation of some homeopâthic drugs against betel vine *Phytophthora* disease, Indian Phytopath. 50(4) : 542-547.

Chaurasia, J.P. (2001). Betel vine cultivation and management of diseases. Scientific Publishers (India) Jodhpur, PP 359.

Crowdy, S.H., J.F. Grove, H.G. Hemming and K.C. Robinson (1950). The translocation of antibiotics in higher plants. II The movement of griesofluvin in broad-bean and tomato, J. Exp. Bot. 7, 42-64.

Kachhawaha, M.(1993).Studies on the plant growth regulatory activities of certain antibiotics, Ph.D. Thesis, Univ. of Sagar.

Madhavan, A. (1982). Biochemical aspects of plant disease resistance part-I Performed inhibitory substances prohibition, to day and tomorrows printers and publishers, New Delhi.

Malik, V.S. (1972). Chloramphenicol Adv. Appl. Microbial. 15, 297-336.

Rendi, R. and Ochoa, S. (1962). Action of chloramphenicol, J. Biol. Chem., 237:3711.

Shrivastava, A. (1985). Studies on the efficacy of certain antibiotic against betel vine *Phytophthora*, Ph.D. Thesis University of Sagar.

Thirumalachar, M.J. (1973). Antibiotics in crop protection. Presidential Address 60th (Diamond Jubilee) Session Indian Science Congress, Chandigarh.

Thirumalachar, M.J., Govindu, H.C. and Yaraguntaiah, R.C. (1973). Chemotherapeutic control of tomato leaf curl virus disease. Indian Phytopath. 26;323-332.

Tiwari D.P. (1968). Studies on foot and leaf rot diseases of *Piper betel* L. with special reference to microbiology and measures of control. Ph.D. Thesis, University of Sagar.

Vyas K.M. and Chaurasia, S.C. (1976). Efficacy of certain antibiotics against betel vine *Phytophthora*, Phytophthora News Letter 7:28.

Microbiology and Biotechnology for Sustainable Development (*Ed.* P.C. Jain),
CBS Publishers & Distributors, New Delhi (2004), pp. 347–353.

B-20

Effect of Aflatoxin-B_1 on Seed Germination and Mitotic Cell Division

Kiran Jain, S.K. Yadav, S.C. Agrawal* and P.C. Jain*
Department of Botany, Dr. H.S. Gour Vishwavidyalaya,
Sagar-470003 M.P.
**Department of Applied Microbiology and Biotechnology,*
Dr. H.S. Gour Vishwavidyalaya, Sagar M.P.

Abstract

The term aflatoxins refers to the group of bisfuranocoumarin metabolites biosynthesized by Aspergillus flavus group of fungi. Amongst these, Aflatoxins B_1 has been reported to possess high toxicity and proved to be hepatotoxic, carcinogenic, teratogenic and mutagenic for animals and poults. Whether, these toxic metabolites are affecting germination of seeds and seedling vigour in wheat and gram and mitotic cell division in cells of Allium cepa roots have been studied choosing Aflatoxin B_1 as test fungal metabolite. Experiments have been conducted separately for each study. The data obtained were analyzed statistically and are expressed as mean±SE together with 't' test for mitotic index (MI) and as percentage for chromosomal abnormalities.

Lower concentrations of Aflatoxin B_1 (upto 2.5 ppm) have not been found effective against seed germination in wheat but reduced seedling vigour. Aflatoxin B_1 inhibited cell division process. The results of present investigations are discussed in terms of their immediate and also delayed effect of different concentration of this toxin on MI value.

Key words: Aflatoxin B_1, Mitotic cell Division, Seed, Germination.

INTRODUCTION

The mycotoxins that are of certain significance include aflatoxins, citrinine, sterigmatocystin, ochratoxin, patulin and penicillic acid. Amongst these, aflatoxins are widely distributed and have variously been reported from a variety of agricultural products, used as food and feed (Wyllie and Morehouse, 1977, 1978). The term aflatoxins normally refers to the group of bisfuranocoumarin metabolites biosynthesized by *Aspergillus flavus* group of fungi, the major members are designated as B_1, B_2, G_1, and G_2 (Hartley *et al.*, 1963).

In some dairy cattle aflatoxin B_1 and B_2 are partially metabolized to aflatoxin M_1 and M_2 respectively. Another aflatoxins, i.e. Aflatoxin P_1 is the principal urinary metabolite of aflatoxin B_1, but it has not been recorded in mould cultures (Dalezios *et al.*, 1971).

A number of reviews that appeared on the aflatoxins and their toxicity in animals and poultry established that aflatoxins are hepatotoxins, carcinogens, teratogens and mutagens (Goldblatt, 1969; Ciegler *et al.*, 1971; Mirocha and Christensen, 1976, Wyllie and Morehouse, 1977, 1978). The most well known effect of the mycotoxic fungi on the plant system is the inhibition of seed germination of some crop plants and oil seeds resulting in chlorotic and albino effect in leaves during early stages of plant growth (Christensen and Kaufmann, 1965, 1969; Neergaard, 1977; Joffe, 1969; Kang, 1970; Mehan and Chohan, 1974a). 'Aflaroot' disease syndrome in groundnut is the most severe effect of aflatoxin in plant system (Mehan and Chohan, 1974 b). Culture filtrates of *A.flavus* have been found mitodepressive (Mito-inhibitory) in root meristem of *Allium cepa* (Kiran, 1992). The present study was planned to characterize whether the mitodepressive effect of culture filtrates is due to aflatoxin B_1 or due to some other fungal metabolites.

MATERIAL AND METHODS

Effect of different concentrations of aflatoxin B_1 on seed germination and mitotic cell division was studied.The details of materials and methods are as follows:

(1) Preparation of Test Samples

For the present study standard aflatoxin B_1 sample was obtained from the sigma chemical company, U.S.A. As the methanol is one of the best solvent for this toxin , 1 mg sample of aflatoxin was first dissolved in 1 ml methanol to prepare its solution equivalent to 10^3 ppm. The volume of 1ml methanol solution was then raised to 100ml by adding 99 ml sterilized distilled water to prepare a stock solution of 10 ppm of aflatoxin B_1. Other concentrations were prepared by using sterilized distilled water. By diluting the stock solution with appropriate amount of water, finally 0.05, 0.10, 0.50, 1.00, 2.50, 5.00, and 10.00 ppm concentrations of aflatoxin B_1 were prepared.

(2) Effect of Aflatoxin B_1 on Seed Germination and Seedling Vigour

Effect of five different concentrations of aflatoxin B_1 (i.e. 0.50, 1.00, 2.50, 5.00 and 10.00 ppm) on seed germination and seedling vigour of two crop plants was tested. For this, *Triticum vulgare* (wheat) and *Cicer arietinum* (gram) seeds were used. Seeds were surface sterilized by using 0.1% mercuric chloride solution and for the treatment of aflatoxin B_1, sterlized seeds were soaked in different concentrations of this toxin separately for 24 hour. After the treatment, seeds were placed aseptically in sterilized Petridishes lined with three layers of moistened filter paper for germination. For control, the surface sterilized seeds were soaked for 24 hour in sterilized distilled water. The Petridishes were then incubated at 28 °C for 3 days in seed germinator. After 3 days incubation, number of germinated seeds, root and shoot length of germinated seeds were noted. Emergence of radical was taken as criteria for seed germination.

The data were analyzed statistically and are expressed as percent germination and per-cent inhibition/stimulation over control.

(3) Effect of Aflatoxin B_1 on Mitotic Cell Division

Effect of six different concentrations of aflatoxin B_1 (i.e., 0.05, 0.10, 0.50, 1.00, 5.00 and 10.00 ppm) was tested on the dividing cells of *Allium cepa* root meristem at room temperature. For this, *Allium cepa* bulbs were pregerminated in sterilized tap water to get fresh crop of roots. The two sets of bulbs were made, roots of the first set were given 12 and 24 hour treatment of different concentrations of aflatoxin B_1. In the second set, roots were given 12 and 24 hour treatment of different concentration of aflatoxin B_1 and then were kept in distilled sterilized water for 36 hour to observe any recovery of the effect of aflatoxin B_1. Fixation of roots after 12 and 24 hours treatment in first set and at an interval of 12 hour during 36 hour recovery period were made using acetic alcohol (1:3). Roots after each interval, i.e., 12, 24, 36, 48 and 60 hours from the bulbs kept as controls, were also obtained and were then fixed in acetic alcohol.

The roots in each case ware examined to note the extent of cell division process and chromosomal abnormalities. For this root squashes were made in 2% aceto-orcein following the method as described by Sharma and Sharma (1965). The data obtained were analyzed statistically and are expressed as mean±standard error together with 't' significance tests for mitotic index (MI) and as percentage for chromosomal abnormalities.

RESULT AND DISCUSSION

(A) Effect of Aflatoxin B_1 on Seed Germination and Seedling Vigour

The results of the effect of different concentrations of aflatoxin B_1 on seed germination and seeding vigour of two crop plants, i.e, *Cicer arietinum* and *Triticum vulgare* were analyzed and are described in the following text :

(i) *Cicer arietinum* (Gram)

Results of the effect of aflatoxin B_1 on seed germination and seedling vigour of gram are presented in Table 1. Pregermination treatment of 0.5, 5.0 and 10.0 ppm concentrations of aflatoxin B_1 showed on effect on seed germination in gram seeds. The percentage of germina-tion in above treated seeds was found almost equal to those observed in control seeds. However, 1.0 and 2.5 ppm concentrations of aflatoxin B_1 caused 2.0% loss in seed germina-tion. An inhibition in the root growth was noted in all the seedlings developed from the seeds treated with the test concentrations of aflatoxin B_1. The maximum inhibition, i.e., 28.24 per cent was observed in the seeds treated with 1.0 ppm concentration of this toxin. Other concentrations of aflatoxin B_1, i.e., 0.5, 2.5, 5.0 and 10.0 ppm caused 9.78, 9.73, 1.59, and 24.35 per cent inhibition in the root length, respectively.

Stimulation in shoot length was noted in the seedlings developed from the seeds treated with 0.5, 1.0, 2.5 and 5.0 ppm concentrations of aflatoxin B_1 while 10.0 ppm concentration of this toxin showed inhibitory effect on shoot growth in gram seedlings.

Though both inhibitory and stimulatory effects of aflatoxin B_1 were noted on the root and shoot growth in some seedlings developed from the treated seeds but in almost all the cases total length of the seedling was found less in treated samples than controls thus, affecting the seedling vigour in all the treated seeds.

Table 1: Effect of different concentrations of aflatoxin B_1 on seed germination and root and shoot length in *Cicer arietinum* (Gram).

Concentration used	Seed germination (%)	Root length (Cm)	Shoot length (Cm)
Control	17.00±0.00	10.02±0.57	0.71±0.09
0.5 ppm	17.00±0.00 (0.00)	9.04±0.46 (-9.78)	1.08±0.09 (+52.11)
1.0 ppm	16.66±0.06 (-2.00)	7.19±0.37 (-28.24)	1.24±0.17 (+74.64)
2.5 ppm	16.66±0.06 (-2.00)	9.05±0.46(-9.73)	1.26±0.19 (+77.46)
5.0 ppm	17.00±0.00 (0.00)	9.86±0.45 (-1.59)	1.05±0.12 (+ 47.88)
10.0 ppm	17.00±0.00 (0.00)	7.58±0.59(-24.35)	0.84±0.11 (-18.30)

Values in parenthesis are representing percent positive/negative effect over control.

(ii) *Triticum vulagare* (Wheat)

The results of the effect of different concentrations of aflatoxin B_1 on the seed germination and seedling vigour of wheat are presented in Table 2. Three concentrations of aflatoxin B_1, i.e., 0.5, 1.0, and 2.5 ppm have been found ineffective on germination in wheat seeds but higher concentrations of this toxin i.e., 5.0 and 10.0 ppm caused inhibition in the seed germination in this crop. Maximum inhibition (i.e., 10.17 per cent) of seed germination was noted in samples treated with 10.0ppm concentration of aflatoxin B_1 (Table 2). Effect of this toxin on the root growth in wheat seedlings was similar to those observed in gram seedlings. In this case all the concentrations of aflatoxin B_1 reduced root length in the seedlings developed from the treated seeds. 10.0 ppm concentration caused maximum inhibition i.e., 71.01 per cent in the root length.

Table 2: Effect of different concentrations of aflatoxin B_1 on seed germination and root and shoot length in *Triticum vulgare* (wheat).

Concentration used	Seed germination (%)	Root length (Cm)	Shoot length (Cm)
Control	19.66±0.06	6.28±0.17	2.90±0.12
0.5 ppm	19.66±0.06(0.00)	4.83±0.07(-23.08)	3.33±0.13(+14.82)
1.0 ppm	19.66±0.06(0.00)	3.57±0.15(-43.15)	2.10±0.16(-27.58)
2.5 ppm	19.66±0.06(0.00)	4.72±0.10(-24.84)	1.00±0.05(-65.51)
5.0 ppm	18.66±0.06(-5.08)	2.89±0.24(-53.98)	2.22±0.14(-23.44)
10.0 ppm	17.66±0.12(-10.17)	1.82±0.14(-71.01)	1.20±0.13(-58.62)

Values in parenthesis are representing percent positive/negative effect over control.

The shoot growth was also found decreased in most of the seedlings developed from the treated seeds except those treated with 0. 5 ppm concentration. However, in almost all the seedlings developed from the treated seeds, the total length of the seedlings was found less when compared with controls. In general, all the concentrations of aflatoxin B_1 reduced seedling vigour in wheat crop also.

(B) Effect of Aflatoxin B_1 on Mitotic Cell Division

The data on the effect of different concentrations of aflatoxin B_1 on root meristem of *Allium cepa* were analysed in terms of the following parameters:

(a) Mitotic index (MI) - comparison between treated and control and 't' significance test.

(b) Induced mitotic abnormalities - any abnormality in the dividing cells at chromosomal level.

The details of the effect of different concentrations of aflatoxin B_1 on the mitotic cell division after 12 and 24 hours treatment and during 36 hour recovery are recorded in Table 3. Data indicate that almost all the concentrations of aflatoxin B_1 inhibit cell division process in root meristam of *Allium cepa*. Further, this effect increases with the increase in recovery period. No chromosomal abnormalities were reported in the samples treated with different concentrations of Aflatoxin B_1.

Table 3: Analysis of the data on the effect of Aflatoxin B_1 on Mitotic Index (MI) in *Allium cepa* root.

		10 ppm Mean±SE	5 ppm Mean±SE	1 ppm Mean±SE	0.5 ppm Mean±SE	0.1 ppm Mean±SE	0.05 ppm Mean±SE	Control Mean±SE
12 hour Treatment		2.12±0.40 (2.05)	1.72±0.22 (2.75)	1.82±0.16 (2.67)	2.36±0.16 (2.01)	2.37±0.14 (2.00)	2.66±0.26 (1.58)	4.01±0.80
Recovery	R_1	2.49±0.17 (2.21)	1.04±0.07 (3.87)	1.51±0.17 (3.11)	3.00±0.16 (1.04)	1.84±0.18 (1.19)	2.36±0.06 (1.98)	3.75±0.54
	R_2	1.17±0.24 (2.09)	0.50±0.03 (3.13)	1.02±0.17 (2.35)	2.60±0.07 (0.21)	1.82±0.21 (1.25)	1.61±0.14 (1.55)	2.76±0.72
	R_3	0.14±0.12 (8.30)	0.32±0.08 (8.25)	0.75±0.36 (4.17)	2.16±0.03 (1.74)	2.45±0.20 (0.52)	1.36±0.18 (3.96)	2.63±0.27
24 hour Treatment		0.00±0.00 (6.94)	0.00±0.00 (6.94)	0.10±0.08 (6.63)	0.29±0.17 (10.48)	2.00±0.24 (2.91)	3.59±0.41 (0.23)	3.75±0.54
Recovery	R_1	0.00±0.00 (3.83)	0.00±0.00 (3.83)	0.02±0.01 (3.80)	0.05±0.03 (3.76)	0.66±0.24 (2.76)	0.48±0.35 (2.85)	2.76±0.72
	R_2	0.00±0.00 (9.74)	0.00±0.00 (9.74)	0.00±0.00 (9.74)	0.04±0.02 (9.59)	0.06±0.03 (9.51)	0.08±0.02 (9.44)	2.63±0.27
	R_3	0.00±0.00 (22.60)	0.00±0.00 (22.60)	0.00±0.00 (22.60)	0.00±0.00 (22.60)	0.00±0.00 (22.60)	0.00±0.00 (22.60)	2.26±0.10

Notes: (1) Table 't' value at 8 degree of freedom and 0.05 probability is 2.3.

(2) Calculated 't' values are given in parenthesis.

(3) Recovery after treatment-R_1, 12hour; R_2, 24hour; R_3, 36hour.

Alfatoxion B_1 ($C_{17}H_{12}O_6$) is a toxin,which was found associated with various deleterious effects on human and animal system (Wyllie and Morehouse, 1977, 1978). In the present study effect of different concentrations of the toxin was studied on seed germination and seedling vigour of two crop plants. The data indicate that 1.0 and 2.5 ppm concentration of aflatoxin B_1 affected the seed germination in *Cicer arietium* (gram), while all other test concentration of this toxin did not show any effect on seed germination. However, when wheat seeds were given pregermination treatment of 5.0 and 10.0 ppm concentrations of this toxin, 5.08 and 10.17 per cent seed failed to germinate, respectively, in comparison to control. In both the crops, almost all the test concentration were found to produce some inhibitory effect on the seedling growth and reduced seedling vigour beside, the stimulatory effect of some concentration of this toxin on root or shoot length in the seedlings of the test crops.

Aspergillus flavus which is a well know storage fungus, producing aflatoxin, has also been reported as a pathogen causing aflaroot disease syndrom in grundnut sedling. The cause of this disease is found to be aflatoxin (Chohan and Gupta, 1968, Kang, 1970). According to Rana (1971) the aflatoxins inhibit the growth of coleoptile by disorganizing the process of cell division dependent on nucleic acid multiplication. Adverse effect of aflatoxins on seed germination was also reported by Schoental and White (1975).

Besides their role in causing loss in germinability in seeds of some crop plants,aflatoxin are also reported to cause chlorosis of leaves by checking the synthesis of chlorophyll by restricting the growth-hormone induced synthesis of RNA, DNA, and proteins in the leaves (Durbin, 1959; Joffe, 1969).

In the present study all the test concentrations (i.e., 0.05, 0.10, 0.05, 1.0, 5.0 and 10.0 ppm) of aflatoxin B_1 inhibited the cell division process in the samples given 12 and 24 hour treatment (Table 3). In addition to the inhibitory or mitodepressive activity of this toxin in the treated sample, present study also confirms the delay effect of this toxin on the root meristem cells of *Allium cepa* as indicated by the increasing repressive effect of this toxin in treated sample during 36 hour of recovery. Kihlman (1966) reported that most mito-deperessive substances perhaps disturb the internal mileu of the sensitive cells in such a manner that their biosynthetic pathways get disturbed. Consequently many cells fail to complete their division cycle and may even get damaged or destroyed.

In the present study, the mito-depressive (mitoinhibitory) effect of aflatoxin B_1 was found persistent even after the treatment i.e. during recovery. In most of the cases, the inhibitory effect was increased with the increase in the recovery period. However, a sudden decrease in mito-inhibitory effect was noted at 10.0 ppm concentration as compared to its lower concentration (i.e. 5.0 ppm). This indicates that the lower concentrations of this toxin are mito-inhibitory and the higher ones are mito-promotary during 12 hour of treatment (Table 3). While studying the effect of aflatoxin on mitotic index, Bilgrami *et al.* (1986) reported a gradual decline in relative division rate (RDR) in root meristematic cells of *Allium cepa* in the concentration range of 10^1 to $8x10^2$ ppb. They also recorded a sudden increase in the RDR at about 1000 ppb which continued to rise steeply surpassing even the control level and thus reported that higher concentrations of this toxin are mito-promotary. The mito-promotary activity of higher concentrations of this toxin in plant system is of normal type or leading to any abnormality in the sensitive cells is a subject of further enquiry.

ACKNOWLEDGEMENT

The authors are thankful to Head, Department of Botany, Dr. H.S. Gour Vishwavidyalaya, Sagar for providing laboratory facilities and encouragements.

REFERENCES

Bilgrami, K.S., Sinha, S.P. and Ranjan, K.S. (1986). Effect of af1atoxin B_1 on mitotic index. *Curr. Sci.*, 21: 1092-1094.

Chohan, J.S. and Gupta, V.K. (1968). *Indian J. Agric. Sci.*, 33 : 561.

Christensen, C.M. and Kaufmann, H.H. (1965). Deterioration of stored grain by fungi. *Ann. Rev. Phytopath.*, 3 : 69-84.

Christensen, C.M. and Kaufmann, H.H. (1969). Grain Storage : The Role of Fungi in Quality Loss. University of Minnesota Press, Minneapolis.

Ciegler, A., Detroy, R.W. and Lillehoj, E.B. (1971). Patulin, Penicillic acid and other carcinogenic lactones. In : "Microbial Toxins", Vol. 6, (Ed. A.Ciegler, S. Kadis and S.J. Ajl), Academic Press New York, p. 409-434.

Dalezios, J., Woga, G.N. and Weinreb, S.M. (1971). Aflatoxin P_1 : A new aflatoxin metabolite in monkeys, *Science*, 171 : 584-585.

Durbin, R.D. (1959). *Dis. Rep.*, 43 : 922.

Goldblatt, L.A. (1969). Aflatoxin, Scientific Background, Control and Implications. Academic Press, New York and London.

Hartley, R.D., Nerbitt, B.F. and O'kelly, J. (1963). Toxic metabolites of *Aspergillus flavus. Nature* (London), 198 : 1056-1058.

Joffe, A.Z. (1969). Aflatoxin produced by 1629 isolates of *Aspergillus flavus* from groundnut kernels and soils of Israel. *Nature*, 221 : 492.

Kang, M.S. (1970). Pathogenesis in groundnut (*Arachis hypogaea* L.) by *Aspergillus flavus* Link ex Fries. Ph.D. Thesis, Punjab Agricultural University, Ludhiana.

Kihlman, B.A. (1966). Action of Chemicals on dividing cells, Prentice Hall, pp. 200.

Kiran, J. (1992). "Mycotoxin contamination in Food and Feed with special reference to their cytogenetic effect on plant system". Ph.D. Thesis, Dr. H.S. Gour Vishwavidyalaya, Sagar.

Mehan, V.K. and Chohan, J.S. (1974a). Effect of temperature on growth and aflatoxin production by isolates of *Aspergillus flavus. Indian Phytopath.* 27 : 168-170.

Mehan, V.K. and Chohan, J.S. (1974b). Virulence of aflatoxigenic and non toxigenic isolates of *Aspergillus flavus* Link ex Fr. on groundnut seedlings. *Phytopath. Med.*, 8 : 108-109.

Mirocha, C.J. and Christensen, C.M. (1976). Mycotoxins and the fungi that produce them. *The American Phytopathological Society*, 3 : 110-123.

Neergaard, P. (1977). "Seed Pathology", The MacMillan Press Ltd., London and Basingstoke.

Rana, B.M. (1971). M.Sc. Thesis, Punjab Agric. Univ., Ludhiana.

Schoental, R. and White, A.F. (1975). *Nature*, 205, 57.

Sharma, A.K. and Sharma, A. (1965). Chromosome Technique Theory and Practice. *Butterworth*, London.

Wyllie, T.D. and Morehouse, L.G. (1977). Mycotoxic Fungi, Mucotoxins, Mycotoxicoses. An Encyclopedic Hand Book, Mycotoxic Fungi and Chemistry of Mycotoxins - Vol. I, Marcel Dekker, Inc., New York.

Wyllie, T.D. and Morehouse, L.G. (1978). Mycotoxic Fungi, Mucotoxins, Mycotoxicoses. Vol. II, Marcel Dekker, Inc., New York.

Microbiology and Biotechnology for Sustainable Development (Ed. P.C. Jain),
CBS Publishers & Distributors, New Delhi (2004), pp. 354–357.

B-21

Incidence of *Candidiasis* in Leukoplakia Cases in Cancer Suspected Patients

Sudhir K. Jain, Archana Shrivastav and S.C. Agrawal*
Department of Applied Microbiology, Cancer Hospital & Research Institute,
Gwalior 474 009 India
** Department of Applied Microbiology & Biotechnology*
Dr. H.S. Gaur University, Sagar 470 003, India

Abstract

An investigation conducted on seven randomly selected cases of oral leukoplakia revealed that majorities of them (71.3%) were positive for Candida albicans; the remaining two revealed the presence of Mucor sp. and Aspergillus fumigatus, respectively. The data presented in the results emphasize the significance of cultural examination of cancer patients particularly those of leukoplakia for detection of bacterial and fungal infections associated with cancer necessitating proper treatment of all maladies. It is evident that during the present study the antifungal treatment showed a marked improvement in leukoplakia cases.

Key words : *Candidiasis*, Cancer patient, Leukoplakia

INTRODUCTION

Fungal infections are a serious and increasingly frequent problem in patients with cancer (Arendrof and Walker, 1980; Menier-Carpenter *et al*,1981; Horn *et al*,1985; Kwon-Chung and Bennett,1992; Deccan,1997). Leukoplakia has been described as a clinical term(WHO,1978). Pindborg *et al* (1988) mentioned the condition in the form of a white patch more than 5 mm in diameter, which could not be removed on rubbing. King (1964) described its microscopic lesions as epithelial atrophy or hyperplasia. Renstrup (1958) observed that the commonest site of leukoplakia was the buccal gingival gutter and in 1970 he recorded that leukoplakia was sometimes associated with *Candida* infection. Waldron and Shafer (1975) examined 3256 cases of oral leukoplakia and found that the highest incidence of epithelial alterations, ranging from dysplasia to carcinoma *in situ* was seen in leukoplakia of the floor of the mouth. Pindborg *et al.* (1988) studied 248 patients with oral leukoplakia for one to ten years, only 4.4% of which developed epidermoid carcinoma. Most of these leukoplakias were of the speckled type. They divided leukoplakia into two types; speckled and homogenous. Over 60% of the speckled ones were record to have superimposed infection of *Candida albicans* (Vanbreuseghem, 1970; Renstrup, 1970; Body, 1984; Horn *et al*, 1985; Douglas, 1995).

Einhorn and Warsell (1967) recorded the occurrence of oral carcinoma in patients suffering from leukoplakia of the oral mucosa. Rosai (1996) summarized the controversial state in which the etiology of leukoplakia stands today, and thus the urgency of this investigation was realized prompting us to undertake the present study.

MATERIALS AND METHODS

The present study was carried out at Cancer Hospital and Research Institute, Gwalior (India). During the course of routine examination of patients suspected of suffering from precancerous or cancerous conditions, only seven of the large number of leukoplakia cases, were randomly selected for microbiological screening. Swabs in triplicate were collected with the aid of a blunt sterile scalpel (so that superficial mucosa could be scraped). Which were then subjected to the microbiological examination on their delivery in the laboratory.

The culture examination was conducted on routine media i.e. Sabouraud's dextrose agar medium containing chloramphenicol (0.5 mg/ ml) with and without actidione (Chloroheximide 0.5 mg/ml). The tubes were incubated at 37° ± 1°C for seven days and the types of fungi were recorded. The positive cultures were identified on the basis of mycelial structure, conidia or budding cells and sporulation by standard procedures (Kwon-Chung and Bennett,1992). *Candida* species were identified, in addition, by standard tests (Kwon-Chung and Bennett,1992). Those cases in which no growth appeared till a period of seven days was declared as negative and wherever possible a second sample from the same patient were obtained for repeat examination to confirm the negative findings.

RESULTS AND DISCUSSION

A view of Table 1 reveals that out of seven samples tested for the presence of etiologic agents, five (71.3%) of them yielded the pure growth of *Candida albicans*, each strain of which produced chlamydospores on chlamydospore agar. One of the remaining two samples was positive for *Mucor* sp and the other showed *Aspergillus fumigatus.* The former has been reported to cause mucormycosis and the role of latter as pathogen causing mucobuccal infections has been well established (Kwon-Chung and Bennett, 1992). The isolation of pathogenic fungi from all seven cases with predominance of *Candida* infections was considered noteworthy. Histopathological examination conducted in a few specimens revealed the presence of yeast like cells.

The follow up of these cases was done up to a period of three months after a continued treatment of all these cases with antifungal agents. The treatment included simultaneous use of local and generalized antifungal agents. After recovery, no recurrence was reported in any of the cases described herein.

Table 1: Incidence of *Candidiasis* in leukoplakia cases

S.No.	Age	Sex	Site	Size of Lesions	KOH preparation	Fungal morphology	Isolated Fungi
1	32	Male	Oral	6mm	Budding cells & hyphae with branching	Budding cells & Pseudo-hyphae with branching	*Candida albicans*
2	30	Male	Oral	4mm	Branching hyphae, Coenocytic	Fast growing, gray fluffy colour unbranched sporangiophore, globose sporangia, spores variable in size and shape, mostly ellipsoidal	*Mucor sp.*
3	37	Male	Oral	5mm	Budding cells & Pseudohyphae with branching	Budding cells & Pseudo-hyphae with branching	*Candida albicans*
4	23	Male	Oral	5mm	Hyphal form	Colony first white then become greenish blue colour, powdery mycelium branched, septate, conidio-phore short and smooth, flask shaped vesicle, single seriate sterigmata, vesicle upper half fertile, rough walled globose conidia	*Aspergillus fumigatus*
5	61	Male	Oral	7mm	Budding cells & Pseudohyphae with branching	Budding cells & Pseudo-hyphae with branching	*Candida albicans*
6	48	Male	Oral	6mm	Budding cells & Pseudohyphae with branching	Budding cells & Pseudo-hyphae with branching	*Candida albicans*
7	52	Male	Oral	7mm	Budding cells & Pseudohyphae with branching	Budding cells & Pseudo-hyphae with branching	*Candida albicans*

The results embodied in the Table 1 confirm the findings of Pindborg *et al.,* (1988), Renstrup (1970) and Vidas *et al.,* (1988), who recorded the presence of *Candida albicans* in varying proportions of patients suffering from leukoplakia. They however, failed to establish the role played by *Candida* organisms in the patients suffering from leukoplakia i.e. whether this organism existed as a real causative agent of the disease or was acting as a secondary superimposed invader. Any way, the results of the treatment were encouraging and the organisms failed to establish or reappear at the site after an antifungal treatment carried out as per schedule. A large number of patients (71.3%) positive for *Candida albicans* were suggestive of a vital role of pathogenicity played by these organisms in leukoplakia. Whether these organisms were responsible for causing disease or were acting as opportunistic pathogens in the event of disease being originated by non-infectious causes has yet to be determined. However, the antifungal treatment has yielded encouraging results and it suggested to carry out cultural examination of all cases of leukoplakia and those found positive for the presence of pathogenic fungus, ought to be treated with proper antifungal drugs.

REFERENCES

Arendrof, T.M .and Walker, D.M. (1980). The prevalence and intra oral distribution of *Candida albicans* in man. *Arch Oral Bio* 25: 1-10.

Body, G.P. (1984). *Candidias*is in Cancer patients. *American Journal of Medicine* 77: 13-19.

Deacon, J.W. (1997).*Modern Mycology* III edn, Blackwell Science Ltd.

Douglas, L.J. (1995) Adhesion-receptor interactions in the attachment of *Candida albicans* to host epithelial cells. *Canadian Journal of Botany* 73 : S1147-1153.

Einhorn, J. and Warsell, J. (1967). Incidence of oral carcinoma in patients with leukoplakia of the oral mucosa. *Cancer.* 20 : 2189-2193.

Horn, R., Wang ,B, Kiehn, J.E and Armstrong, D. (1985) Fungemia in a Cancer Hospital : Changing frequency, earlier onset and result of therapy. *Review of Infectious Diseases* 7: 646-655.

King, O.H. (1964) Intraoral leukoplakia? *Cancer* 17: 131-136

Kwon-Chung K. J. and Bennett, J.E. (1992).*Medical Mycology*, Lea Febiger, Philadelphia.

Mennier-Carpenter, F., Kiehn ,T.E. and Armstrong, D. (1981). Fungimia in the immune compromised host : changing patterns, antigenemia, high mortality. *American Journal of Medicine* 71 : 363-370.

Pindborg, J.J., Jolst, O., Renstrup, G. and Roed-Peterson, B. (1988) Studies in oral leukoplakia : A preliminary report on the period prevalence of malignant transformation in leukoplakia based on a follow-up study of 248 patients. *Journal of American Dental Association* 76 : 767-771.

Renstrup, G.(1958) Leukoplakia of the oral cavity : A clinical and histopathologic study. *Acta Odontol. Scand* 16 : 99-111.

Renstrup, G.(1970). Occurrence of *Candida* in oral leukoplakias, *Acta Pathology and Microbiology.* Scand 78 : 421-424.

Rosai Juan (1996). *Ackerman's Surgical Pathology* vol (1), VII edn, The Mosby-Year Book Inc, St. Lousis; 223-255.

Vanbreuseghem, R. (1970). Post mortem mycological investigation of 100 cancerous patients. *Mykosen* 13 : 337-350.

Vidas, I.O., Temmerk, P. and Palaversic, M.(1988) *Candida albicans* in leukoplakia lesions of the oral Mucosa. *Acta Stomatol Croat* 22 (4) : 311-317.

Waldron, C.A. and Shafer, W.G. (1975) Leukoplakia revisited : A clinico pathologic study of 3256 oral leukoplakia. *Cancer* 36 : 1386-1392.

WHO (1978). Collaborating centre for oral precancerous lesions: Definition of leukoplakia and related lesions - aid to studies on oral precancer. *Oral Surgery*; 46 : 518-539.

Microbiology and Biotechnology for Sustainable Development (Ed. P.C. Jain),
CBS Publishers & Distributors, New Delhi (2004), pp. 358–364.

B-22

Isolation of some Keratinophilic Fungi from Soils of District Chhindwara, M.P.

S. Qureshi[1], M.K. Rai[2] and S.C. Agrawal[3]
[1]*Department of Botany, Danielson College, Chhindwara-480001, M.P.*
[2]*Department of Biotechnology, Amravati University, Amravati-444602, M.S.*
[3] *Department of Applied Microbiology and Biotechnology,*
Dr. H.S. Gour University, Sagar 470003, M.P.

Abstract

A great variety of geophilic keratinophilic fungi were found to be present in 109 samples out of a total of 200 soil samples collected from different localities of Chhindwara. The percentage occurrence of total keratinophilic fungi was 54.50. Mixed growth of keratinophilic fungi was recorded in 4.5% of the soil samples. A total of 14 species of 9 genera were recovered. These include Chrysosporium tropicum (22%), Microsporum gypseum (16.50%), C. indicum (10.50%), Trichophyton terrestre (6%), T. rubrum (2.5%), Histoplasma capsulatum (1%) and Gleocladium catenulatum, Malbranchea species, Aphanoascus species, Verticillium negrescens and Myrothecium roridum (0.5% each).

Key words: Isolation, Keratinophilic, Soils, Fungi, Chhindwara

INTRODUCTION

Generally keratinophilic fungi are a potential danger to man and animals. They are saprophytes widely distributed in the soil, and are directly linked both with the incidence of disease (Rippon, 1982) and with the process of decomposition (Rose, 1980). Our knowledge about distribution of keratinophilic fungi in India is limited. The first report of a dermatophyte in soils of India was made by Dey and Kakoti (1955) who isolated *Microsporum gypseum* from the vicinity of an animal house in Dibrugarh, Assam state. After this various reports were published (Randhawa *et al.*, 1959; Puri, 1961; Randhawa and Sandhu, 1965; Garg, 1966; Padhye *et al.*, 1967; Kushwaha and Agrawal, 1976a, 1976b; Jain and Agrawal, 1977; Sur and Ghosh 1980; Kushwaha, 1980a, 1983; Verma *et al.*, 1982; Deshmukh and Agrawal, 1983, 1998;

Jain, 1983, 1996, 2000; Jain *et al.*, 1985; Kushwaha and Shrivastava, 1989; Jain *et al.*, 1993; and Deshmukh *et al*, 2000).

The present investigation envisages exploring these fungi in Chhindwara soils.

MATERIALS AND METHODS

Soil samples were collected from sites rich in keratinic material as human and animal remains. Research demonstrated that the keratinophilic fungi differ in their substrate preference for colonization (Rai and Qureshi, 1994). Therefore, sites were selected for collection of soil samples on the basis of various keratinic material. The soil samples were recovered from superficial layer of soil (not exceeding 5 cm in depth). In every sample sterile spatula was used as means for taking the sample. These samples were brought to the lab in sterilized polythene bags.

Thickly populated areas of Chhindwara, viz., 'Chhoti Bazar' and 'Azad Chowk area' were found to be highly contaminated. The soils of these places were rich in keratinic matter of human beings of all age groups. Human and animal activity of all kind defined these areas.

Hair, nails, horn, feathers of pigeon and peacock were used as keratin baits. After rinsing in sterilized water the baits were dried, cut into small pieces (2-3 cm) and were sterilized at 15 lb pressure for 15 min. in an autoclave. Keratin baits were scattered over the soil samples in the Petridishes. The plates were incubated at 28°± 2°C for a period of 6-8 weeks.

Isolations were carried out by direct transfer of fungal growth from the baits to Sabouraud dextrose agar (dextrose 40g, peptone 10g, agar agar 15g, distilled water 1000 ml) supplemented with cycloheximide (0.5mg/ml). In case of more than one species found on the bait, the mixed culture was suspended in sterile normal saline and streaked on plates containing SDA medium for purification.

RESULTS AND DISCUSSION

The over all occurrence of keratinophilic fungi was 54.50%. There was mixed growth of keratinophilic species in 4.5% of the soil samples. *Chrysosporium tropicum* showed the highest prevalence (22%.), followed by *Microsporum gypseum* (16.50%) and *C. indicum* (10.50%). The species *Trichophyton terrestre* was recovered by 6% followed by *T. rubrum* (2.5%). Two unidentified species of *Trichophyton* showed very low prevalence, i.e, 0.5% and 1%. Very low occurrence was exhibited by remaining 6 isolates , i.e., *H. capsulatum* (1%), *G. catenulatum*, *Malbranchea* species, *Aphanoascus* species, *V. nigrescens* and *M. roridum* (0.5% each) (Table 1 and 2). The result supports the previous studies (Randhawa and Sandhu, 1965; Jain *et al.*, 1985 and Williamson and Iyer, 1992) indicating *Chrysosporium* species as the commonest keratinophilic fungi. *Microsporum* and *Trichophyton* were the second most common keratinophilic fungi in the Chhindwara soil.

The above results provide information on the nature of the keratinophilic fungal flora of soils of Chhindwara and its regional distribution. *C. tropicum* is known to be the dominant species all over the world (Randhawa and Sandhu, 1965: Garg, 1966; Padhye *et al.*, 1966; Alteras and Evolceanu, 1969: Ajello and Padhye, 1974; Van Oorschot, 1980; Sur and Ghosh,

1980; Abdel Fattah *et al.*, 1982: Verma *et al.*,1982). The occurrence of *M. gypsem* and *C. indicum* followed by *Trichophyton* also agrees well with the findings of several workers (Randhawa and Sandhu, 1965; Jain *et al.*, 1985; and Williamson and Iyer, 1992). The *Trichophyton* species showed low prevalence in the soil of Chhindwara district.

Table 1: Prevalence of Keratinophilic fungi in soils of various habitats of Chhindwara District

Habitat	No. of samples examined	No. of samples positive
School and College	65	31
Densely populated	60	33
Garden and Park	20	11
Hospital and Nursing home	10	08
Different unusual places	45	26
Total No. of samples	200	109

Table 2: Percentage Occurrence of Keratinophilic Fungi

S.No.	Keratinophilic Fungi	No. of Positive Samples	% Occurrence
1	*Chrysosporium tropicum*	44	22
2	*Microsporum gypseum*	23	16.5
3	*Chrysosporium indicum*	21	10.5
4	*Trichophyton terrestre*	12	06
5	*T. rubrum*	05	2.5
6	*T. simii*	01	0.5
7	*Trichophyton Species I*	01	0.5
8	*Trichophyton Species II*	02	01
9	*Histoplasma capsulatum*	02	01
10	*Aphanoascus sp.*	01	0.5
11	*Gleocladium catenulatum*	01	0.5
12	*Myrothesium roridum*	01	0.5
13	*Verticillium negrescens*	01	0.5
14	*Malbranchea* sp.	01	0.5
	Total No. of samples	200	

It was noted that the keratinophilic fungi differ in their substrate preference for colonization. Horn was found to be the most suitable bait for isolation of keratinophilic fungi of Chhindwara region (Table III). In the present investigation, hair was also proved to be a suitable bait for isolation of keratinophilic fungi, which confirmed the previous findings (Kalpan *et al.*, 1958; Marples, 1967; English and Southern, 1967; Knudtson and Robertstand, 1970; Gugnani *et al.*, 1971, 1975; Okafor and Gugnani, 1981). This indicates the suitability of hair as keratin bait for other keratinophilic fungi, viz, *Aphanoascus* species, *V. negrescens, M. roridum* and *H. capsulatum*. Nail was also found as good bait and showed healthy fungal growth. *Chrysosporium* and *Microsporum* grew well on nails. Pigeon and peacock feathers exhibited poor mycelial growth but found to be very suitable baits for isolation of various species of *Chrysosporium* (Table 3).

Table 3: Keratinophilic Fungi Isolated on different Keratin Bait

S.No	Keratin baits	Keratinophilic fungi														Total No of isolates
		Ct	Mg	Ci	Tt	Tr	Ts	TI	TII	Hc	Gc	Vn	As	Mr	Ma	
1	Horn	11	7	4	6	2	-	-	-	-	1	-	-	-	-	31
2	Hair	6	7	7	2	1	-	-	1	1	-	1	1	1	-	28
3	Nail	7	8	2	1	-	-	1	1	-	-	-	-	-	1	214
	Pigeon feather	11	1	3	2	1	1	-	-	-	-	-	-	-	-	195
	Peacock Feather	9	-	5	1	1	-	-	-	1	-	-	-	-	-	17
	Total isolates	44	23	21	12	5	1	1	2	2	1	1	1	1	1	116

Ct = *Chrysosporium tropicum*
Mg = *Microsporum gypseum*
Ci = *C. indicum*
Tt = *Trichophyton terrestre*
Tr = *Trichophyton rubrum*
Ts = *T. simii*
TI = *Trichophyton Species I*
TII = *Trichophyton Species II*
Ma = *Malbranchea spp.*
Mr = *Myrothecium roridum*
Hc = *Histoplasma capsulatum*
Gc = *Gliocladium catenulatum*
Vn = *Verticillium negrescens*
As = *Aphanoascus sp.*

From the soil samples of school and college *Chrysosporium* was isolated as the dominant fungus followed by *Microsporum* and *Trichophyton*. Latha *et al.*, (1992) also reported the occurrence of keratinophilic fungi on the school playgrounds. The presence of *Malbranchea* species was also an important point. There are various reports of keratinophilic strains of *Malbranchea* species from different soil samples of the world (Orr and Kuehn, 1972; Hubalek and Balat, 1974; Ajello and Padhye, 1974 and Jain and Agrawal, 1979). *Chrysosporium* was also recovered from thickly populated areas. On the contrary, *Trichophyton* exhibited poor colonization in populated areas. Soil samples from market, parks and garden showed abundance of *Chrysosporium* followed by *Microsporum* and *Trichophyton*. Nursing home areas and hospital campus exhibited rich population of *Chrysosporium* and *Trichophyton*, whereas *Microsporum* was absent in these regions. Soil samples from poultry and animal farms also exhibited rich keratinophilic fungal flora. It supports the previous findings (Jain, 1983). Soil samples from cultivated fields were poor in colonization of *Chrysosporium*. It also agrees well with the previous studies (Nigam and Kushwaha, 1990).

ACKNOWLEDGEMENTS

We are thankful to Prof. S.A. Brown, Principal, Danielson College, Chhindwara, M.P. for providing laboratory facilities. S.Q. thanks the Council of Scientific and Industrial Research, New Delhi for the award of Senior Research Fellowship during the tenure of which this work was carried out. We thank to Dr P. C. Jain, Reader, Dr H S Gour Vishwa Vidhyalaya, Sagar, M.P. for critically going through the manuscript. We thank Ms Sarika Shende, research fellow, Department of Biotechnology, Amravati University, Amravati for help in typesetting.

REFERENCES

Abdel-Fattah, H.M., Moubasher, A.H., Maghazy, S.M. (1982). Keratinolytic fungi in Egyptian soils. *Mycopathologia* 79, 49-53.

Ajello, L. and Padhye, A.A. (1974). Keratinophilic fungi of the Galapagos islands. *Mykosen,* 17, 239-243.

Alteras, I. and Evolceanu, R. (1969). A ten yars survey of Romanian soil screening for keratinophilic fungi (1958-1967). *Mycopathol Mycol. Appl.* 38, 151-159.

Deshmukh, S.K. and Agrawal, S.C. (1983). Prevalence of dermatophytes and other keratinophilic fungi in soils of Madhya Pradesh (India). *Mykosen*, 26, 574-577.

Deshmukh, S.K. and Agrawal, S.C. (1998). Biology of keratinophilic fungi and related dermatophytes. In: *Microbes: for health, wealth and sustainable environment (Ed.* Ajit Varma). Malhotra Publishing House, New Delhi, India pp 253-272.

Deshmukh, S.K., Agrawal , S.C. and Jain, P.C. (2000). Isolation of dermatophytes and other keratinophilic fungi from soils of Mysore (India). *Mycoses*, 43, 55-57.

Dey, N.C. and Kakoti, L.M. (1955). *Microsporum gypseum* in India. *J. Indian Med. Assoc.*, 25, 160-164.

English, M.P. and Southern, H.N. (1967). *Trichophyton persicolor* infection in population of small wild animals. *Sabouraudia*, 5, 302-309.

Garg, A.K. (1966). Isolation of dermatophytes and other keratinophilic fungi from soil in India. *Sabouraudia* 4, 259-264.

Gugnani, H.C., Randhawa, H.S. and Shrivastava, J.B. (1971). Isolation of dermatophytes and other Keratinophilic fungi from apparently healthy skin coats of domestic animals. *Indian J. Med. Res.*, 59, 1699-1702.

Gugnani, H.C., Wattal, B.L. and Sandhu R.S. (1975). Dermatophytes and other keratinophilic fungi recovered from small mammals in India. *Mykosen*, 18, 529-536.

Hubalek, Z. (1974). Fungi associated with free living birds in czechoslovakia and yogoslovkia. *Acta Scientarium Naturalium Bmo.*, 8, 1-62.

Hubalek, A. and Balat, F. (1974). The survival of microfungi in the nest of tree sparrow *(Passer montanus L.)* in the nestboxes over the winter season. *Mycopath. Mycol.appl.,* 54, 517-530.

Jain, P.C. (1983). Prevalence of keratinophilic fungi in soils of Madhya Pradesh and Uttar Pradesh, India. *Geobios New Reports,* 2, 10-13.

Jain, P.C. (1996). Antimycotic compounds from higher plants: Assessment of present status and future strategies. In: *Herbal medicines Biodiversity and Conservation Strategies* (*Ed.* Rajak R.C. and M.K. Rai). International Book Publishers and Distributors, Dehradun, India, 31-49.

Jain, P.C. (2000). *Biotechnological potential of keratinophilic fungi in keratin waste management* (*Ed.* P. Shrivastava) APH Publishing Corporation, New Delhi, pp 88-107.

Jain, P.C. and Agrawal, S. C. (1977). Keratinophilic fungi from the soils of Mount Abu (India). *Geobios,* 4, 136-138.

Jain, P.C. and Agrawal, S.C. (1979). Some addition to Indian *Malbranchea* . *Kavaka,* 7: 69-72.

Jain, P.C. S.K. Deshmukh and Agrawal, S.C. (1993): *Chrysosporium gourii*, new species Jain, Deshmukh and Agrawal. *Mycoses,* 36 (3-4), 77-79.

Jain, M., Shukla, P.K. and Srivastava, O.P. (1985). Keratinophilic fungi and dermatophytes in Lucknow soils with their global distribution. *Mykosen*, 2893), 148-153.

Kalpan, W., Lucille, K., George, L.K. and Ajello, L. (1958). Recent development in animal ringworm and their public health implications. *Annals. of New York Academy of Science*, 70, 363-648.

Khudtson, W.W. and Robertstand, G.W. (1970). The isolation of Keratinophilic fungi from soil and wild animals in south Dakota. *Mycopathol. Mycol. Applicata*, 40, 309-323.

Kushwaha, R.K.S. (1980a). A new species of *Gleocladium. Curr. Sci.* 49, 74-75.

Kushwaha, R.K.S. (1980b). *Verticillium* sp. Nov. A. new keratinophilic species from Indian soils. *Curr. Sci.* 49, 968-969.

Kushwaha, R.K.S. (1983). Taxonomy of dermatophytes and related fungi. *Proc. Natl. Symp. Adv. Pl. Sci.* 37-38.

Kushwaha, R.K.S. and Agrawal, S.C. (1976a). A new species of the genus *Acrodontium* de Hoog from India. *Mykosen,* 20, 97-100.

Kushwaha, R.K.S. and Agrawal, S.C. (1976b). Some keratinophilic fungi and related dermatophytes from soil. *Proc. Ind. Natl. Sci. Acad.* 42, 102-110.

Kushwaha, R.K.S. and Shrivastava, J. N. (1989). A new species of *Chrysosporium* from soil. *Curr. Sci.,* 58, 970-971.

Latha, N., A., Hilda and Manjula, V.K. (1992). Occurrence of keratinophilic fungi from playground soils in Arakkonam, Tamil Nadu. *J. Environ. Biol.* 13(2), 107-112.

Marples, M.J. (1967). Non-domestic animals in New Zealand and in Rotalonga as a reservoir of agent of ringworm. *New Zealnd. Medical J.,* 66, 299-302.

Muanza, D.N., Kim, B.W., Euler, K.L., Williams, L. (1994). Antibacterial and antifungal activities of nine medicinal plants from Zaire. *International J. of Pharmacognosy,* 32(4), 337-345.

Nigam, N. and Kushwaha, R.K.S. (1990). Biodeterioration of human hair. *J. Ind. Bot. Soc.,* 69, 469-470.

Nwosu, M. O., Okafor, J.I. (1995). Preliminary studies of the antifungal activities of some medicinal plants against *Basidiobolus* and some other pathogenic fungi. *Mycoses*, 38(5-6), 191-195.

Okafor, J.I. and Gungnani, H.C. (1981). Dermotophytes and other keratinophilic fungi associated with hair of rodents in Nigeria, Mykosen, 24, 616-620.

Orr, G.F. and Kuehn, H.H. (1972). Notes on *Gymnoascaceae* II. Some *Gymnoascaceae* and keratinophilic fungi from Utah. *Mycologia*, 64, 55-72.

Padhye, A.A., Mishra, S.P. and Thirumalachar, M.J. (1966). Occurrence of soil inhabiting fungi from soils in Poona. *Hindustan Antibiot. Bull.* 9, 90-93.

Padhye, A.A., Pawar, V.H., Sukapure, R.S. and Thirumalachar, M.J. (1967). Keratinophilic fungi from marine soils of Bombay, India part I. *Hindustan Antibiot. Bull.*, 10, 138-141.

Puri, H. R. (1961). Isolation of dermatophytes from Indian soils. *Bull. Calcutta Sch. Trop. Med.* 9, 121-122.

Rai, M.K. and Qureshi, S. (1994). Screening of different keratin baits for isolation of keratinophilic fungi, *Mycoses* 37 (7- 8): 295-298.

Randhawa, H.S. and Sandhu, R.S. (1965). A survey of soil inhabiting dermatophytes and related Keratinophilic fungi in India. *Sabouraudia*, 4(2), 71-79.

Randhawa, H.S., Nath, A. and Vishwanathan, R. (1959). Isolation of *Microsporum gypseum* from soil in Delhi. *Sci. Cult.* (India) 25(5), 326-327.

Rippon, J.W. (1982). *Medical mycology*. The pathogenic fungi and Actinomycetes. Philadephia: W.B. Saunders Co. II. Edition P. 154-248.

Rose, A.H. (1980). Microbial Enzymes and Bio-conversions. In: *Economic Microbiology* (*Ed:* A.H. Rose) Vol. 3. Academic press, London, pp 1-147.

Sur, B. and Ghosh, G.R. (1980). Keratinophilic fungi from Orissa India. II. Isolation from feathers of wild birds and domestic fowls. *Sabouraudia*, 18, 275-280.

Verma, T.N., Sinha, B.K., and Das, U.L. (1982). Isolation of keratinophilic fungi from soils in Bihar. *Mykosen,* 25: 449-452.

Van Oorschot, C.A.N. (1980). A revision of *Chrysosporium* and allied genera. Centraal Bureau Voor Schimmel Cultures, Baarn. *Studies in Mycology* No. 20.

Williamson, D. and Iyer, S.R. (1992). Dermatomycoses in India with Special reference to Rajasthan. *Advances in Medical Mycology* Aditya Publishing house, New Delhi, 131-143.

Microbiology and Biotechnology for Sustainable Development (Ed. P.C. Jain),
CBS Publishers & Distributors, New Delhi (2004), pp. 365–368.

B-23

Anti-microbial Activity of Essential Oil Derived from the Flowers of *Lantana camara* Linn

R. Lachoria, M.P. Goutam*, A. Jain and S.C. Agrawal
Department of Applied Microbiology and Biotechnology
Dr. H.S. Gour University, Sagar 470003 (M.P.) India
**Forensic Science Laboratory (FSL) Sagar (M.P.)*

Abstract

"In vitro" antimicrobial activity of essential oil obtained from the flowers of Lantana camara *Linn was tested against 4 bacteria and 7 fungi. In the present study the test essential oil showed its inhibitory action against all test organisms. The oil showed maximum inhibition against the growth of Sacchromyces cerevisiae.*

INTRODUCTION

Essential oils of several plants are frequently used in the preparation of cosmetics, perfumes antiseptics and as an active ingredient in certain medicines. Essential oils are also used for purification of environment since they possess antimicrobial properties. Anti-microbial activity of essential oils has been reported by various workers and has been reviewed time to time (Chaurasia and Jain, 1978; Goutam *et al.*, 1980; Nayak and Rao, 1980; Deshmukh *et al.*, 1986; Chaudhury, 1994; Jain, 1996; Lachoria *et al.*, 1999; Kamboj, 2000).

The shrub *Lantana camara* belongs to the family–Verbenaceae. It is well described by Kirtikar and Basu, 1935, Chopra *et al.*, 1956 and Grewal, 2000. The plant is commonly believed to have acquired poisonous properties since its fruit, leaf and flowers when consumed by animals cause certain disorders in their health. Its air-dried leaves and flowers have been reported to possess 0.2 and 0.07 percent essential oil, respectively(Chopra *et al.*, 1965). The oil contains 80 percent of a Caryophyllene-like sesquiterpene and 1-α-phellandrene with some aldehyde and free alcohol. The fresh leaves of this weed have yielded 0.069 percent of an essential oil containing citral. From the distillation of whole plant, 0.053 percent of aromatic oil containing α-pinene (14%), α-terpinene (10%) p-cymene (6%), sesquiterpenes of caryo-phyllene type (43%) and of cadinene type (21%) have been recovered (Chopra *et al.*, 1965).

In the present study essential oil was obtained from the flowers of *Lantana camara* (family-Verbenaceae) and evaluated for its antifungal and antibacterial properties.

MATERIALS AND METHODS

The materials and methods used for the extraction of oil and to evaluate it's antimicrobial properties are as follows :

1. Extraction of oil

The flowers of this plant were collected from the university campus and Patheria hills of Sagar District (M.P.) India. Flowers were semidried and subjected to hydro distillation to obtain essential oil, it was treated with anhydrous sodium sulfate to remove water molecules and a light yellowish coloured essential oil having a characteristics smell was obtained and was used for the present antimicrobial activity.

2. Evaluation of Antimicrobial property

The anti-bacterial and anti-fungal activity was determined by the "Filter paper disc diffusion method" (Loo *et al.,* 1945) using Malt extract agar medium for the growth of fungi and nutrient agar medium for the growth of bacteria. 20 ml of molten medium was taken in sterilized Petridishes (90 mm in diameter) and allowed to solidify. One ml of spore suspension of each test organisms was spread over the surface of solidified medium. The sterilized filter paper discs (Hi-media sterile discs) having 6 mm diameter were saturated with essential oil. These were placed over the seeded medium with the help of sterilized forceps. These plates were then incubated at 32°C$\pm$1°C for 48 hours and at 28°C$\pm$1°C for the 96 hours in case of bacteria and fungi, respectively. After incubation the diameter of inhibition zones caused by the test essential oil was recorded. For each determinations two set of experiments were run and the results indicate an average of two independent determinations.

RESULTS AND DISCUSSION

After the incubation, the zone of inhibition was measured with the help of divider to the nearest millimeter. All the experiments were conducted in duplicate for each test organisms. The results obtained are given in Table 1. The zones recorded, include the size of filter paper disc (6 mm in diameter).

From the data it is evident that the oil possesses antimicrobial properties. A varying degree of activity was noted in different cases. The oil was found highly effective against *Sacchromyces cerevisiae* (22 mm), *Alternaria* sp. (18 mm) and *Citrobacter* (16 mm). The oils could cause the inhibition zones of 15, 15, 14, 14, 14, 12, 10 and 10 mm against *Fusarium* sp. *Proteus mirabilis, Enterobacter naoniae, Escherichia coli, Aspergillus flavus, Aspergillus fumigatus, Aspergillus niger* and *Penicillium* sp. respectively.

Grewal (2000) has reported activity of essential oil of leaves of *Lantana camara* against *Bacillus subtilis, Escherichia coli, Sarcina lutea* and *Staphylococcus aureus.* He also reported antifungal activity in 1% water extracts of leaves of this plant. Earlier, Satyanarayana *et al.*, (1977) have also noted activity in extracts of leaves of this plant against some bacteria. Their test organisms, include *Bacillus pumilus, B. subtilis, Pseudomonas mangiferae-indicae, Xanthomonas compestris* and *X. malvacearum*. Qureshi *et al.*, (1997) and Lachoria *et al.*, (1999) reported antifungal ingredients in various plants studied by them. They reported antifungal activity in crude extracts of different plant parts.

The essential oil from flowers of test plant gives a pungent odour and hence its use in the treatment of human diseases is not feasible, however, the oil can be successfully used in biological control of plant diseases caused by fungi and bacteria. The results of present investigation are quite encouraging and further work is suggested for its practical application in agriculture and remediation of microbial contaminants in environment.

Table 1: Activity of essential oil of *Lantana camara* against bacteria and fungi

S.No.	Test organisms	Zone of inhibition* (mm)
1.	*Aspergillus niger*	10
2.	*Aspergillus flavus*	14
3.	*Aspergillus fumigatus*	12
4.	*Fusarium* sp.	15
5.	*Penicillum* sp.	10
6.	*Alternaria* sp.	18
7.	*Enterobacter naoniae*	14
8.	*Proteus mirabilis*	15
9.	*Citrobacter* sp.	16
10.	*Escherichia coli*	14
11.	*Sacchromyces cerevisiae*	22

*Including the diameter of filter paper Disc-6 mm.

REFERENCES

Chaudhary, R.R. (1994). Herbal Medicine for Human Health. CBS Publishers and Distributors (P) Ltd., New Delhi, P. 87.

Chaurasia, S.C.and Jain, P.C. (1978). Antibacterial Activity of Essential oils of four Medicinal Plants. *Indian Journal of Hospital Pharmacy,* Volume 166-168.

Chopra, R.N., Badhwar, R.L. and Ghosh, S. (1965). "Poisonous Plants of India" Vol. II, Indian Council of Agricultural Research (ICAR) New Delhi, 698-702.

Chopra, R.N., Nayar, S.L. and Chopra, I.C. (1956). Glossary of Indian Medicinal Plants. Published by CSIR, New Delhi, India, 149-150.

Deshmukh, S.K., Jain, P.C. and Agrawal, S.C. (1986). A note on Mycotoxicity of Some Essential oils. *Fitoterapia,* 57 (4): 295-297.

Goutam, M.P. Jain, P.C. and Singh, K.V. (1980). Activity of Some Essential oils Against Dermatophytes. *Indian drugs,* 17: 269-270.

Grewal, R.C. (2000). "Medicinal Plants" Campus Book International, New Delhi.

Jain, P.C. (1996). Antimycotic components from Higher Plants: Assessment of Present status and future strategies. In *Herbal Medicines, Biodiversity and Conservation Strategies.* (*Ed.* R.C. Rajak and M.K. Rai) International Book Distributors, Dehra Dun, p. 31-49.

Kamboj, V.P. (2000). Herbal Medicine. *Current Science*, 78(1) : 35-39.

Kirtikar, K.K. and Basu, B.D. (1935). Indian medicinal plants, Published by Lalit Mohan Basu, 49, Leader Road, Allhabad, India.

Lachoria, R.; Jain, P.C. and Agrawal, S.C. (1999). Activity of some plant extract against Dermatophytes, *Hind. Antibiot. Bull.,* 14 : 17-21.

Loo, Y.H.; Skell, P.S.; Thornberry, H.H.; John Ehrlich, McGurie, J.M.; Savage, G.M. and Sylvester, J.C. (1945). Assay of streptomycin by the paper-disc plate method. *J. Bact.* 50 : 701-709.

Nayak, M.L. and Rao, J.J. (1980). Antimicrobial studies of plant products : A review. *Indian Drugs,* 17 : 259-265.

Qureshi, S.; Rai, M.K. and Agrawal, S.C. (1997).In vitro Evaluation of Inhibitory Nature of Extracts of 18- Plant Species of Chhindwara Against 3- Keratinophilic Fungi. *Hind. Antibiot. Bull.*, 39 : 56-60.

Satyanarayana, T., Rao, D.P.C. and Sundar Singh, B. (1977). Anti-bacterial Activity of six Medicinal Plant Extracts. *Indian Drugs.* 14 : 200-210.

Microbiology and Biotechnology for Sustainable Development (*Ed.* P.C. Jain),
CBS Publishers & Distributors, New Delhi (2004), pp. 369–372.

B-24

Tinea corporis and Allied Diseases (Dermatophytosis) in Rural and Urban Population at Agra

J.N. Shrivastava, Nidhi Govil, V.P. Bhatnagar, A.K. Bhatnagar,
G.P. Satsangi and Manish Mathur
Microbiology Lab, Department of Botany, Faculty of Science,
Dayalbagh Educational Institute, Dayalbagh, Agra – 282005.

Abstract

A clinical investigation was made to study the correlation between the Tinea causing dermatophytes and keratinophilic fungi in urban and rural population at Agra and patients seeking medical advice from Sarojni Naidu Medical College, Agra to evaluate the occurrence of soil inhabiting keratinophilic fungi at their capability to cause Tinea. It include twelve dermatophytes viz. Epidermophyton floccosum 26.1%, Trichophyton rubrum 26.1%, Microsporum nanum 11%, T.schoenleinii 8%, T.concentricum 8%, T.mentagrophytes 7.1%, T.violaceum 3.7%, M.audouinii 5.5%, T.verrucosum 3.2%, M.canis 3.2%, M.gypseum 2.1%, T.tonsurans 1.6%. Among isolated dermatophytes four were common to urban and rural population at Agra (M.nanum 1.3%, T.rubrum 8.5%, Epidermophyton floccosum 2.7% and T.mentagrophytes 7.7%).

Key words: Dermatophytes, Urban, Rural, Population, tinea.

INTRODUCTION

A fungal infection of animals was reported for the first time from the skin on the face of a monkey by Pinoy(1912). Later on several cases of *Tinea* and other diseases caused by *Trichophyton simii* and other diseases in man and animals caused by dermatophytes and keratinophilic fungi were reported by various workers (Okashi *et al.*, 1966; Gugnani *et al.* 1967a & b; Kiokke and Durairaj, 1967; Gupta *et al.*, 1968; Tewari, 1969; Mohpatra and Mahajan, 1970; Mulay and Garg, 1970; Singh *et al.*, 1992). Most of these cases reported of the fungal dissemination through the soil rich in keratin content. The keratin rich substrates, especially human hair, animal hooves, and feathers etc. are of frequent occurrence in rural areas due to domestication of animals like cow, horse, goat etc. The fungi colonizing the keratin rich substrate are generally called keratinophilic fungi and most of these are potentially pathogenic. In the present study an epidermological diffusion of *Tinea* and allied diseases (dermatophytes and keratinophilic fungi) in rural and urban area was evaluated. The data obtained were also compared with the clinical investigation made at Sarojni Naidu Medical College, Agra and their capacity to cause *Tinea corporis* and *T.capatis*.

MATERIALS AND METHODS

Soil samples were collected from rural and urban areas during a period of 2 years (1999-2000) at Agra. Fungi and related dermatophytes were isolated by hair baiting technique. The fungal growth appeared on keratin bait were picked up with the help of needle and were transferred to the sterilized dishes containing Sabouraud's dextrose agar (S.D.A.) medium and incubated at 25±2°c. The fungal colonies appeared on medium were purified by repeated culturing.

RESULTS AND DISCUSSION

The comparison between the dermatophytes isolated from urban and rural parts of Agra and data collected from S.N. Medical College, Agra (Table 1) reveals that 580 patients reported to S.N. Medical College were suffering from various *Tinea* diseases caused by twelve dermatophytic fungi. Out of 12 species, *Trichophyton rubrum* (26.1%) and *Epidermophyton* (26.1%) had maximum prevalence as mycosis causing fungi while a few patients were infected by *Microsporum canis* (3.2%), *Trichophyton verrucosum* (3.2%) and *T.tonsurans* (1.6%). Four dermatophytic fungi *T.rubrum* (8.6%), *Epidermophyton* (2.7%), *T. mentagrophytes* (7.7%) and *M. nanum* (1.3%) were isolated from soil samples collected from urban and rural surrounding areas of S.N. Medical College, Agra.

Table 1: Comparative analysis of pathogenic fungi isolated from Agra and Data collected from S.N. Medical College, Agra.

Species	% Prevalence of Pathogenic fungi	
	S.N. Medical College, Agra	Urban and Rural parts of Agra
Trichophyton mentagrophytes	7.1	7.7
T. violaceum	5.5	-
T. verrucosum	3.2	-
T. tonsurans	1.6	-
T. schoenleinii	8.0	-
T. concentricum	8.0	-
T. rubrum	26.1	8.5
M. audouinii	5.5	-
M. canis	3.2	-
M. gypseum	2.1	-
M. nanum	11.0	1.3
Epidermophyton floccosum	26.1	2.7

The percentage prevalence of dermatophytic fungi was observed more in urban area while prevalence of *Epidermophyton* (12.0%) and *T. rubrum* (7.6%) was observed in rural areas. Some species of *Trichophyton* (*T.tonsurans* and *T.violaceum*) and *Microsporum* (*M.gypseum* and *M.nanum*) were absent in patients reported to S.N. Medical College, Agra belong to rural area have more pathogenic fungi (*Epidermophyton, M.nanum*) in comparison to urban area.(Table 2). The percentage prevalence of dermatophytes and keratinophilic fungi from soil samples of rural and urban areas is given in Table 3. *Chrysosporium carmichaeli* was dominant in urban areas and had 22.2% prevalence as compared to other fungi. However, *Myceliophthora vellerea* and *Microsporum nanum* were absent in the urban area. *M. vellera* showed maximum percentage prevalence (12.5%) and *M. nanum* showed minimum percentage prevalence (1.3%) in rural areas. *Chrysosporium lucknowense* and *Epidermophyton floccosum* were found in urban and rural areas with minimum percentage prevalence.

Table 2: Prevalence of pathogenic fungi isolated from patients belonging to urban and rural areas.

Species	% Prevalence in patients	
	Urban	Rural
Trichophyton mentagrophytes	5.6	1.5
T. violaceum	5.5	-
T. verrucosum	2.1	1.1
T. tonsurans	1.6	-
T. schoenleinii	5.0	3.0
T. concentricum	4.0	4.0
T. rubrum	18.5	7.6
M. audouinii	3.8	1.7
M. canis	1.8	1.4
M. gypseum	2.1	-
M. nanum	11.0	-
Epidermophyton floccosum	14.1	12.0

Table 3: Dermatophytic and keratinophilic fungi isolated from soil samples collected from urban and rural areas at Agra.

Species	% Prevalence of isolated fungi (%)	
	Urban	Rural
Chrysosporium carmichaeli	22.2	9.1
C. tropicum	8.3	4.1
C. lobatum	3.3	1.3
C. lucknowense	2.7	-
Epidermophyton floccosum	-	2.7
Microsporum nanum	-	1.3
Myceliopthora vellerea	-	12.5
Trichophyton rubrum	2.6	6.0
T. mentagrophytes	2.7	5.0

In the present study the comparison between the soil borne dermatophytes and prevalence of skin mycoses and *Tinea* in Agra was correlated with the data collected from S.N. Medical College, Agra. There is prevalence of skin mycoses or *Tinea corporis* and *Tinea capatis* causing dermatophytes, isolated from the 580 patients during a span of two years in this area.

The more prevalence of *Tinea* causing fungi *T.mentagrophytes* 7.1%, *M.nanum* 11%, *T.rubrum* 26.1% and the *Epidermophyton* 26.1% found at S.N. Medical College, Agra whereas *T. mentagrophytes* 2.7%, *M. nanum* 1.3%, *T. rubrum* 26.1% and *Epidermophyton* 2.7% were in rural areas of Agra. Apart from this *T. violaceum, M. audouinii, T. verrucosum, M. concentricum* were also reported in the samples from S.N. Medical College to be responsible for skin diseases in Agra. However prevalence of *Tinea* disease by the fungi in human being is quite low as compared to their presence in the soil. This may be due to their transmittable nature from one organism to other, the present study established the prominence of skin pathogens of human in soil but it is very difficult to say that whether the fungi responsible for skin diseases in Agra is of soil origin or air borne. On the other hand prevalence of *Tinea* causing pathogens has been reported maximum in urban areas, as compared to rural areas, which is more prevalent. All the keratin rich products especially human hair and hooves of animals after slaughtering and dressing are dumped away from the city in rural area, but the existence of keratinophilic fungi is more in human inhabited area, seems to be unusual.

ACKNOWLEDGEMENT

We are thankful to Prof. P.S. Satsangi, Director, DEI for providing necessary facilities.

REFERENCES

Gugnani, H.C., Shrivastava, J.B. and Gupta, N.P. (1967a). Occurrence of *Arthroderma simii* in soil and on hair of small mammals. *Sabouraudia*, 6: 77-80.

Gugnani, H.C., Mulay, D.N. and Murty, D.K. (1967b). Fungus flora of dermatophytosis and *Trichophyton simii* infection in North India. *Indian Journal of Dermatology and Venereology*, 33: 73-82.

Gupta, P.K., Singh, R.P., and Singh, J.P. (1968). Dermatophytes from man, dogs and Pigs with special reference to *Trichophyton simii* and *Microsporum nanum. Indian journal of Animal health*, 7: 247-253.

Kiokke, A.H. and Durairaj, Padma. (1967). The casual agents of superficial mycoses isolated in rural areas of south India . *Sabouraudia*, 5:153-158.

Mohapatra, L.N. and Mahajan, V.M. (1970). *Trichophyton simii* infection in man and animals *Mycopathologia et. Mycologia .Applicata*, 41: 357-362.

Mulay, D.N. and Garg A.K. (1970). A study on the *Trichophyton simii* infection in man at Delhi. *Indian. Journal. of Dermatology and venereology*, 36: 175-181.

Okashi, S., Takashio, M. and Masegawa, A. (1966). Ring worm caused by *Trichophyton simii* in a captive chimpanzee. *Japanese Journal of medical mycology*, 7: 204-207.

Pinoy, E. (1912). Epidermophyton du singe. *Bulletin de la Societe de Pathologie Exotique (Paris)*, 5: 60-63.

Rippon, J.W. Eng., Anna and Malkensio, F.D. (1968). *Trichophyton simii* infection in United States. *Archives of Dermatology.*

Singh, S.M., Agrawal, A., Naidu, J, Hoog. G.S. de, Figueres. (1992). Cutaneous phaeohyphomycosis caused by *Phialophora richardsiae* and the effect of tropical clotrimazole in its treatments. *Antonie. Van. Leev*. 61: 51-55.

Tewari, R.P. (1969). *Trichophyton simii* infections in chickens, dogs and man in India. *Mycopathologia et. Mycologia Applicata,* 39: 293-298.